LEUKAEMIA
DIAGNOSIS

LEUKAEMIA DIAGNOSIS

Barbara J. Bain

MB BS, FRACP, FRCPath
Reader in Diagnostic Haematology
St Mary's Hospital Campus
Imperial College Faculty of Medicine
and Consultant Haematologist
St Mary's Hospital
London
UK

Third Edition

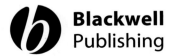
Blackwell
Publishing

© 2003 by Blackwell Publishing Ltd
a Blackwell Publishing company
Blackwell Science, Inc., 350 Main Street, Malden, Massachusetts 02148-5020, USA
Blackwell Publishing Ltd, 9600 Garsington Road, Oxford OX4 2DQ, UK
Blackwell Science Asia Pty Ltd, 550 Swanston Street, Carlton, Victoria 3053, Australia
Blackwell Wissenschafts Verlag, Kurfürstendamm 57, 10707 Berlin, Germany

First published 1990
(Published by Gower Medical Publishing)
Reprinted 1993 (by Wolfe Publishing)
Second edition 1999
Third edition 2003
3   2006

Library of Congress Cataloging-in-Publication Data
Bain, Barbara J.
    Leukaemia diagnosis/Barbara J. Bain.—3rd ed.
        p.   ;   cm.
Includes bibliographical references and index.
    ISBN 1-4051-0661-1   (hardback : alk. paper)
1. Leukemia—Diagnosis.
[DNLM: 1. Leukemia—classification.   2. Leukemia—diagnosis.   WH 15
B162L   2003]
I. Title.
RC643 .B35   2003
616.99′419075—dc21

2002155879

ISBN 13: 978-1-4051-0661-0
ISBN 10: 1-4051-0661-1

A catalogue record for this title is available from the British Library

Set in 9/11$\frac{1}{2}$ pt Meridien by Graphicraft Limited, Hong Kong

Printed and bound in India by Replika Press Pvt. Ltd

Commissioning Editor: Maria Khan
Managing Editor: Elizabeth Callaghan
Production Editor: Rebecca Huxley
Production Controller: Kate Charman

For further information on Blackwell Publishing, visit our website:
http://www.blackwellpublishing.com

CONTENTS

PREFACE

Leukaemias are a very heterogeneous group of diseases, which differ from each other in aetiology, pathogenesis, prognosis and responsiveness to treatment. Accurate diagnosis and classification are necessary for the identification of specific biological entities and underpin scientific advances in this field. The detailed characterization of haematological neoplasms is also essential for the optimal management of individual patients. Many systems for the classification of leukaemia have been proposed. Between 1976 and 1999, a collaborative group of French, American and British haematologists (the FAB group) proposed a number of classifications, which became widely accepted throughout the world. In the case of the acute leukaemias and the related myelodysplastic syndromes, the FAB classifications also provided the morphological basis for more complex classifications such as the morphologic–immunologic–cytogenetic (MIC) classification and the MIC-M classification, which also incorporates molecular genetic analysis. A quarter of a century after the first FAB proposals, a WHO expert group proposed a further system for the classification of leukaemia and lymphoma incorporating aetiology, cytology and the results of cytogenetic analysis. In this book I have sought to illustrate and explain how laboratory techniques are used for the diagnosis and classification of leukaemia.

I have sought to discuss leukaemia diagnosis and classification in a way that will be helpful to trainee haematologists and to laboratory scientists in haematology and related disciplines. However, I have also tried to provide a useful reference source and teaching aid for those who already have expertise in this field. In addition, I hope that cytogeneticists and molecular geneticists will find that this book enhances their understanding of the relationship of their discipline to the diagnosis, classification and monitoring of leukaemia and related disorders.

Acknowledgements. I should like to express my gratitude to various members of the FAB group for their useful advice. In particular I should I like to thank Professor David Galton and Professor Daniel Catovsky, who have given me a great deal of help, but at the same time have left me free to express my own opinions. Professor Galton read the entire manuscript of the first edition and, by debating many difficult points with me, gave me the benefit of his many years of experience. Professor Catovsky also discussed problem areas and kindly permitted me to photograph blood and bone marrow films from many of his patients. My thanks are also due to many others who helped by lending material for photography, including members of the United Kingdom Cancer Cytogenetics Study Group.

Barbara J. Bain 2002

ABBREVIATIONS

AA — all metaphases abnormal (description of a karyotype)

aCML — atypical chronic myeloid leukaemia (a category in WHO classifications)

AL — acute leukaemia

ALIP — abnormal localization of immature precursors

ALL — acute lymphoblastic leukaemia

AML — acute myeloid leukaemia

AN — a mixture of normal and abnormal metaphases (description of a karyotype)

ANAE — α-naphthyl acetate esterase (a cytochemical stain)

ANBE — α-naphthyl butyrate esterase (a cytochemical stain)

ATLL — adult T-cell leukaemia/lymphoma

ATRA — all-*trans*-retinoic acid

BCSH — British Committee for Standards in Haematology

BFU-E — burst-forming unit—erythroid

BM — bone marrow

CAE — chloroacetate esterase (a cytochemical stain)

c — cytoplasmic or, in cytogenetic terminology, constitutional

CD — cluster of differentiation

CFU-E — colony-forming unit—erythroid

CFU-G — colony-forming unit—granulocyte

CFU-GM — colony-forming unit—granulocyte, macrophage

CFU-Mega — colony-forming unit—megakaryocyte

CGL — chronic granulocytic leukaemia

cIg — cytoplasmic immunoglobulin

CLL — chronic lymphocytic leukaemia

CLL/PL — chronic lymphocytic leukaemia, mixed cell type (with prolymphocytoid cells)

CML — chronic myeloid leukaemia

CMML — chronic myelomonocytic leukaemia (a category in the FAB and WHO classifications)

EGIL — European Group for the Immunological Characterization of Leukemias

ERFC — E-rosette-forming cells

FAB — French–American–British classification

FISH — fluorescent *in situ* hybridization

G-CSF — granulocyte colony-stimulating factor

H & E — haematoxylin and eosin (a stain)

Hb — haemoglobin concentration

HCL — hairy cell leukaemia

HLA-DR — histocompatibility antigens

Ig — immunoglobulin

JCML — juvenile chronic myeloid leukaemia

JMML — juvenile myelomonocytic leukaemia (a category in WHO classifications)

LGLL — large granular lymphocyte leukaemia

M0-M7 — categories of acute myeloid leukaemia in the FAB classification

MAC — morphology–antibody–chromosomes (technique)

McAb — monoclonal antibody

MDS — myelodysplastic syndrome/s

MDS-U — myelodysplastic syndrome, unclassified (a category in WHO classifications)

MGG — May–Grünwald–Giemsa (a stain)

MIC — morphologic–immunologic–cytogenetic (classification)

MIC–M — morphological–immunological–cytogenetic–molecular genetic (classification)

MPO	myeloperoxidase		blasts, 2 (a category in the WHO classification)
mRNA	messenger RNA		
NAP	neutrophil alkaline phosphatase	RAEB-T	refractory anaemia with excess of blasts in transformation (a category in the FAB classification)
NASA	naphthol AS acetate esterase (a cytochemical stain)		
NASDA	naphthol AS-D acetate esterase (a cytochemical stain)	RARS	refractory anaemia with ring sideroblasts (a category in the FAB and WHO classifications)
NCI	National Cancer Institute		
NK	natural killer	RCMD	refractory cytopenia with multilineage dysplasia (a category in the WHO classification)
NN	all metaphases normal (description of a karyotype)		
NSE	non-specific esterase (a cytochemical stain)	RCMD-RS	refractory cytopenia with multilineage dysplasia and ring sideroblasts (a category in the WHO classification)
PAS	periodic acid–Schiff (a cytochemical stain)	RQ-PCR	real time quantitative polymerase chain reaction
PB	peripheral blood		
PcAb	polyclonal antibody	RT-PCR	reverse transcriptase PCR
PCR	polymerase chain reaction	SB	Southern blot
PLL	prolymphocytic leukaemia	SBB	Sudan black B (a cytochemical stain)
PPO	platelet peroxidase	SLVL	splenic lymphoma with villous lymphocytes
RA	refractory anaemia (a category in the FAB and WHO classifications)		
		Sm	surface membrane (of a cell)
RAEB	refractory anaemia with excess of blasts (a category in the FAB classification)	SmIg	surface membrane immunoglobulin
		TCR	T-cell receptor
RAEB-1	refractory anaemia with excess of blasts, 1 (a category in the WHO classification)	TdT	terminal deoxynucleotidyl transferase
		TF	transcription factor
		TRAP	tartrate-resistant acid phosphatase
RAEB-2	refractory anaemia with excess of	WHO	World Health Organization

CHAPTER 1

ACUTE LEUKAEMIA
Cytology, Cytochemistry and the FAB Classification

The nature of leukaemia

Leukaemia is a disease resulting from the neoplastic proliferation of haemopoietic or lymphoid cells. It results from a mutation in a single stem cell, the progeny of which form a clone of leukaemic cells. Often there is a series of genetic alterations rather than a single event. Genetic events contributing to malignant transformation include inappropriate expression of oncogenes and loss of function of tumour suppressor genes. The cell in which the leukaemic transformation occurs may be a lymphoid precursor, a myeloid precursor or a pluripotent stem cell capable of differentiating into both myeloid and lymphoid cells. Myeloid leukaemias can arise in a lineage-restricted cell or in a multipotent stem cell capable of differentiating into cells of erythroid, granulocytic, monocytic and megakaryocytic lineages.

Genetic alterations leading to leukaemic transformation often result from major alterations in the chromosomes of a cell, which can be detected by microscopic examination of cells in mitosis. Other changes are at a submicroscopic level but can be recognized by analysis of DNA or RNA.

Leukaemias are broadly divided into: (i) acute leukaemias, which, if untreated, lead to death in weeks or months; and (ii) chronic leukaemias, which, if untreated, lead to death in months or years. They are further divided into lymphoid, myeloid and biphenotypic leukaemias, the latter showing both lymphoid and myeloid differentiation. Acute leukaemias are characterized by a defect in maturation, leading to an imbalance between proliferation and maturation; since cells of the leukaemic clone continue to proliferate without maturing to end cells

and dying there is continued expansion of the leukaemic clone and immature cells predominate. Chronic leukaemias are characterized by an expanded pool of proliferating cells that retain their capacity to differentiate to end cells.

The clinical manifestations of the leukaemias are due, directly or indirectly, to the proliferation of leukaemic cells and their infiltration into normal tissues. Increased cell proliferation has metabolic consequences and infiltrating cells also disturb tissue function. Anaemia, neutropenia and thrombocytopenia are important consequences of infiltration of the bone marrow, which in turn can lead to infection and haemorrhage.

Lymphoid leukaemias need to be distinguished from lymphomas, which are also neoplastic proliferations of cells of lymphoid origin. Although there is some overlap between the two categories, leukaemias generally have their predominant manifestations in the blood and the bone marrow whilst lymphomas have their predominant manifestations in lymph nodes and other lymphoid organs.

The classification of acute leukaemia

The purpose of any pathological classification is to bring together cases that have fundamental similarities and that are likely to share features of causation, pathogenesis and natural history. Acute leukaemia comprises a heterogeneous group of conditions that differ in aetiology, pathogenesis and prognosis. The heterogeneity is reduced if cases of acute leukaemia are divided into acute myeloid leukaemia (AML) (in North America often designated 'acute non-lymphoblastic leukaemia'), acute lymphoblastic leukaemia (ALL) and acute biphenotypic leukaemia; even then, however, considerable heterogeneity remains within each of the groups. The recognition of homogeneous groups of biologically similar cases is important as it permits an improved understanding of the leukaemic process and increases the likelihood of causative factors being recognized. Since such subgroups may differ from each other in the cell lineage affected and in their natural history and their prognosis following treatment, their recognition permits the development of a more selective therapeutic approach with a resultant overall improvement in the prognosis of acute leukaemia.

Although the best criteria for categorizing a case of acute leukaemia as myeloid or lymphoid may be disputed, the importance of such categorization is beyond doubt. Not only does the natural history differ but the best current modes of treatment are still sufficiently different for an incorrect categorization to adversely affect prognosis. Assigning patients to

subtypes of acute myeloid or acute lymphoblastic leukaemia is becoming increasingly important as the benefits of more selective treatment are identified. Similarly, the suspected poor prognosis of biphenotypic acute leukaemia suggests that the identification of such cases may lead to a different therapeutic approach and an improved outcome. Cases of acute leukaemia can be classified on the basis of morphology, cytochemistry, immunophenotype, cytogenetic abnormality, molecular genetic abnormality, or by combinations of these characteristics. Morphology and cytochemistry will be discussed in this chapter and other diagnostic techniques in Chapter 2. The cytochemical stains most often employed are summarized in Table 1.1 [1, 2].

Patients may be assigned to the same or different subgroups depending on the characteristics studied and the criteria selected for separating subgroups. All classifications necessarily have an element of arbitrariness, particularly since they need to incorporate cut-off points for continuous variables such as the

Table 1.1 Cytochemical stains of use in the diagnosis and classification of acute leukaemia [1, 2].

Cytochemical stain	Specificity
Myeloperoxidase	Stains primary and secondary granules of cells of neutrophil lineage, eosinophil granules (granules appear solid), granules of monocytes, Auer rods; granules of normal mature basophils do not stain
Sudan black B	Stains primary and secondary granules of cells of neutrophil lineage, eosinophil granules (granules appear to have a solid core), granules of monocytes, Auer rods; basophil granules are usually negative but sometimes show metachromatic staining (red/purple)
Naphthol AS-D chloroacetate esterase ('specific' esterase)	Stains neutrophil and mast cell granules; Auer rods are usually negative except in AML associated with t(15;17) and t(8;21)
α-naphthyl acetate esterase ('non-specific' esterase)	Monocytes and macrophages, megakaryocytes and platelets, most T lymphocytes and some T lymphoblasts (focal)
α-naphthyl butyrate esterase ('non-specific' esterase)	Monocytes and macrophages, variable staining of T lymphocytes
Periodic acid–Schiff*	Neutrophil lineage (granular, increasing with maturation), leukaemic promyelocytes (diffuse cytoplasmic), eosinophil cytoplasm but not granules, basophil cytoplasm (blocks), monocytes (diffuse plus granules), megakaryocytes and platelets (diffuse plus granules), some T and B lymphocytes, many leukaemic blast cells (blocks, B more than T)
Acid phosphatase*	Neutrophils, most T lymphocytes, T lymphoblasts (focal), variable staining of eosinophils, monocytes and platelets, strong staining of macrophages, plasma cells and megakaryocytes and some leukaemic megakaryoblasts
Toluidine blue	Basophil and mast cell granules
Perls' stain	Haemosiderin in erythroblasts, macrophages and, occasionally, plasma cells

*These cytochemical stains are largely redundant if immunophenotyping is available.

percentage of cells falling into a defined morphological category, positivity for a certain cytochemical reaction, or the presence of a certain immunological marker. An ideal classification of acute leukaemia must be biologically relevant. If it is to be useful to the clinical haematologist, as well as to the research scientist, it should also be readily reproducible and easily and widely applicable. Rapid categorization should be possible so that therapeutic decisions can be based on the classification. The classification should be widely acceptable and should change as little as possible over time so that valid comparisons can be made between different groups of patients. Ideal classifications of acute leukaemia do not yet exist, although many have been proposed.

The development of the French–American–British (FAB) classification of acute leukaemia by a collaborating group of French, American and British haematologists [3–7] was a major advance in leukaemia classification, permitting a uniform classification of these diseases over two decades. It appears likely that the WHO classification, published in its definitive form in 2001 [8], will gradually take the place of the FAB classification. However, since application of the WHO classification requires knowledge of the results of cytogenetic analysis it appears equally likely that haematologists will make an initial diagnosis in FAB terms, pending the availability of results of cytogenetic or molecular genetic analysis. It is important that FAB designations (which have a precise, carefully defined meaning) are not applied to WHO categories for which the diagnostic criteria differ. For maximum clarity, all publications relating to acute leukaemia and the myelodysplastic syndromes (MDS) should state which classification is being used and should adhere strictly to the criteria of the relevant classification.

The FAB group both established diagnostic criteria for acute leukaemia and proposed a system of classification. There is usually no difficulty in recognizing that a patient with ALL is suffering from acute leukaemia, although arbitrary criteria are necessary to distinguish ALL from the closely related lymphoblastic lymphomas. In the case of AML, more difficulty can arise because of the necessity to distinguish between acute leukaemia and MDS. The latter term indicates a group of related conditions, characterized by an acquired intrinsic defect in the maturation of myeloid cells, which has been designated myelodysplasia or dysmyelopoiesis. MDS is a clonal,

neoplastic disorder, which is closely related to, and in some patients precedes, acute leukaemia. In other patients MDS persists unchanged for many years or leads to death from the complications of bone marrow failure without the development of acute leukaemia; it is therefore justifiable to regard the myelodysplastic syndromes as diseases in their own right rather than merely as preludes to acute leukaemia. As the prognosis of MDS is generally better than that of acute leukaemia, and because therapeutic implications differ, it is necessary to make a distinction between acute leukaemia (with or without coexisting myelodysplasia or a preceding MDS) and cases of MDS in which acute leukaemia has not supervened. The FAB group proposed criteria for making the distinction between acute leukaemia and MDS, and for further categorizing these two groups of disorders. The distinction between AML and MDS will be discussed in this chapter and the further categorization of MDS in Chapter 3.

The FAB classification

The FAB classification of acute leukaemia was first published in 1976 and was subsequently expanded, modified and clarified [3–7]. It deals with both diagnosis and classification.

Diagnosing acute leukaemia

The diagnosis of acute leukaemia usually starts from a clinical suspicion. It is uncommon for this diagnosis to be incidental, resulting from the performance of a blood count for a quite different reason. Clinical features leading to suspicion of acute leukaemia include pallor, fever consequent on infection, pharyngitis, petechiae and other haemorrhagic manifestations, bone pain, hepatomegaly, splenomegaly, lymphadenopathy, gum hypertrophy and skin infiltration. A suspicion of acute leukaemia generally leads to a blood count being performed and, if this shows a relevant abnormality, to a bone marrow aspiration. The diagnosis then rests on an assessment of the peripheral blood and bone marrow.

The FAB classification requires that peripheral blood and bone marrow films be examined and that differential counts be performed on both. In the case of the bone marrow, a 500-cell differential count is required. Acute leukaemia is diagnosed if:

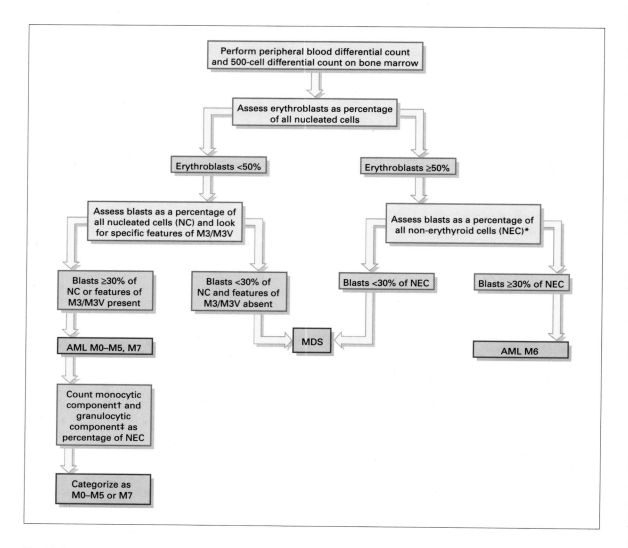

Fig. 1.1 A procedure for diagnosing acute myeloid leukaemia (AML) and for distinguishing it from the myelodysplastic syndromes [6]. *Excludes also lymphocytes, plasma cells, mast cells and macrophages. †Monoblasts to monocytes. ‡Myeloblasts to polymorphonuclear leucocytes.

1 at least 30%* of the total nucleated cells in the bone marrow are blast cells; or
2 if the bone marrow shows erythroid predominance (erythroblasts ≥50% of total nucleated cells) and

*It should be noted that the criterion of at least 30% blast cells has been altered, in the WHO classification, to at least 20% blast cells (see page 127).

at least 30% of non-erythroid cells are blast cells (lymphocytes, plasma cells and macrophages also being excluded from the differential count of non-erythroid cells); or
3 if the characteristic morphological features of acute promyelocytic leukaemia (see page 16) are present (Fig. 1.1).

Cases of ALL will be diagnosed on the first criterion since erythroid hyperplasia does not occur in this condition, but the diagnosis of all cases of AML requires application also of the second and third criteria. The bone marrow in acute leukaemia is usually hypercellular, or at least normocellular, but this is not necessarily so since some cases meet

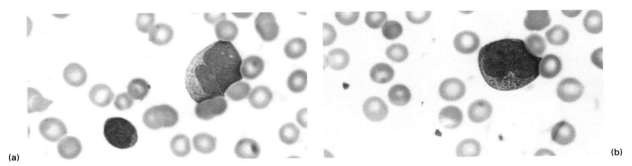

(a)   (b)

Fig. 1.2 The peripheral blood (PB) film of a patient with AML showing: (a) a type II blast with scanty azurophilic granules; (b) a promyelocyte with more numerous granules and a Golgi zone in the indentation of the nucleus. May–Grünwald–Giemsa (MGG) × 870.

the above criteria when the bone marrow is hypocellular.

Defining a blast cell

The enumeration of blasts in the bone marrow is crucial in the diagnosis of acute leukaemia and the definition of a blast cell is therefore important. Whether immature myeloid cells containing small numbers of granules are classified as blasts is a matter of convention. The FAB group chose to classify such cells as myeloblasts rather than promyelocytes. They recognized two types of myeloblast [9]. Type I blasts

lack granules and have uncondensed chromatin, a high nucleocytoplasmic ratio and usually prominent nucleoli. Type II blasts resemble type I blasts except for the presence of a few azurophilic granules and a somewhat lower nucleocytoplasmic ratio. Cells are categorized as promyelocytes rather than type II blasts when they develop an eccentric nucleus, a Golgi zone, chromatin condensation (but with the retention of a nucleolus), numerous granules and a lower nucleocytoplasmic ratio. The cytoplasm, except in the pale Golgi zone, remains basophilic. Cells that have few or no granules, but that show the other characteristics of promyelocytes, are regarded as hypogranular or agranular promyelocytes rather than as blasts. Examples of cells classified as type II myeloblasts and promyelocytes, respectively, are shown in Figs 1.2 and 1.3. The great majority of lymphoblasts lack granules and are therefore type I blasts; they resemble myeloblasts but are often

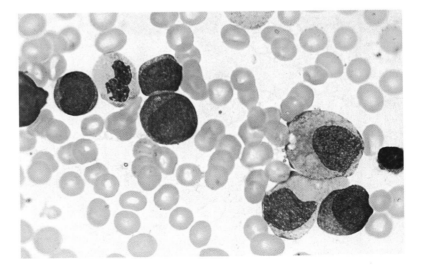

Fig. 1.3 Bone marrow (BM) of a patient with AML (M2/t(8;21)) showing a cell that lacks granules but nevertheless would be classified as a promyelocyte rather than a blast because of its low nucleocytoplasmic ratio; defective granulation of a myelocyte and a neutrophil is also apparent. Type I and type II blasts are also present. MGG × 870.

smaller with scanty cytoplasm and may show some chromatin condensation (see Table 1.11, p. 43).

Distinguishing between AML and ALL

The diagnosis of acute leukaemia requires that bone marrow blast cells (type I plus type II) constitute at least 30% either of total nucleated cells or of non-erythroid cells. The further classification of acute leukaemia as AML or ALL is of critical importance. When the FAB classification was first proposed, tests to confirm the nature of lymphoblasts were not widely available. The group therefore defined as AML cases in which at least 3% of the blasts gave positive reactions for myeloperoxidase (MPO) or with Sudan black B (SBB). Cases that appeared to be non-myeloid were classed as 'lymphoblastic'. The existence of cases of AML in which fewer than 3% of blasts gave cytochemical reactions appropriate for myeloblasts was not established at this stage, and no such category was provided in the initial FAB classification. In the 1980s and 1990s the wider availability and application of immunological markers for B- and T-lineage lymphoblasts, supplemented by ultrastructural cytochemistry and the application of molecular biological techniques to demonstrate rearrangements of immunoglobulin and T-cell receptor genes, demonstrated that the majority of cases previously classified as 'lymphoblastic' were genuinely lymphoblastic but that a minority were myeloblastic with the blast cells showing only minimal evidence of myeloid differentiation.† These latter cases were designated M0 AML [7]. It should be noted that SBB is more sensitive than MPO in the detection of myeloid differentiation and more cases will be categorized as M1 rather than M0 if it is used [10].

Correct assignment of patients to the categories of AML and ALL is very important for prognosis and choice of therapy. Appropriate tests to make this distinction must therefore be employed. Despite the advances in immunophenotyping, cytochemical reactions remain useful in the diagnosis of AML

---

†In discussing the FAB classification I have used the terms 'differentiation' and 'maturation' in the sense in which they were used by the FAB group, that is with differentiation referring to an alteration in gene expression that commits a multipotent stem cell to one pathway or lineage rather than another, and maturation indicating the subsequent changes within this cell and its progeny as they mature towards end cells of the lineage.

[11]. The FAB group recommended the use of MPO, SBB and non-specific esterase (NSE) stains. If cytochemical reactions for myeloid cells are negative, a presumptive diagnosis of ALL must be confirmed by immunophenotyping. When immunophenotyping is available the acid phosphatase reaction and the periodic acid–Schiff (PAS) reaction (the latter identifying a variety of carbohydrates including glycogen) are no longer indicated for the diagnosis of ALL. When cytochemical reactions indicative of myeloid differentiation and immunophenotyping for lymphoid antigens are both negative, immunophenotyping to demonstrate myeloid antigens and thus identify cases of M0 AML is necessary. It should be noted that when individuals with an inherited MPO deficiency develop AML, leukaemic cells will give negative reactions for both MPO and SBB.

The incidence of acute leukaemia

AML has a low incidence in childhood, less than 1 case per 100 000/year. Among adults the incidence rises increasingly rapidly with age, from approximately 1/100 000/year in the fourth decade to approximately 10/100 000/year in those over 70 years. AML is commoner in males than in females. ALL is most common in childhood, although cases occur at all ages. In children up to the age of 15 years the overall incidence is of the order of 2.5–3.5/ 100 000/year; the disease is more common in males than in females. ALL has also been observed to be more common in white people than in black people, but this appears to be related to environmental factors rather than being a genetic difference since the difference disappears with an alteration in socio-economic circumstances.

The classification of AML

Once criteria for the diagnosis of AML have been met and cases have been correctly assigned to the broad categories of myeloid or lymphoid, further classification can be carried out. The FAB group suggested that this be based on a peripheral blood differential count and a 500-cell bone marrow differential count, supplemented when necessary by cytochemistry, studies of lysozyme concentration in serum or urine, and immunophenotyping; with the greater availability of immunophenotyping, measurement of lysozyme concentration is no longer in current use. Broadly speaking, AML is categorized as acute

Table 1.2 Criteria for the diagnosis of acute myeloid leukaemia of M0 category (acute myeloid leukaemia with minimal evidence of myeloid differentiation).

Blasts ≥30% of bone marrow nucleated cells
Blasts ≥30% of bone marrow non-erythroid cells*
<3% of blasts positive for Sudan black B or for myeloperoxidase by light microscopy
Blasts demonstrated to be myeloblasts by immunological markers or by ultrastructural cytochemistry

*Exclude also lymphocytes, plasma cells, macrophages and mast cells from the count.

myeloblastic leukaemia without (M1) and with (M2) maturation, acute hypergranular promyelocytic leukaemia and its variant (M3 and M3V), acute myelomonocytic leukaemia (M4), acute monoblastic (M5a) and monocytic (M5b) leukaemia, acute erythroleukaemia (M6) and acute megakaryoblastic leukaemia (M7). M0 is AML without maturation and with minimal evidence of myeloid differentiation. In addition to the above categories there are several very rare types of AML, which are not included in the FAB classification. These include mast cell leukaemia and Langerhans' cell leukaemia. In addition, the diagnosis of hypoplastic AML requires consideration. Transient abnormal myelopoiesis of Down's syndrome may also be regarded as a variant of AML.

AML with minimal evidence of myeloid differentiation—M0 AML

The FAB criteria for the diagnosis of M0 AML are shown in Table 1.2 and morphological and immunocytochemical features are illustrated in Figs 1.4 and 1.5. The blasts in M0 AML usually resemble M1 myeloblasts or L2 lymphoblasts (see page 45) but in a minority of cases they resemble the monoblasts of M5 AML. Associated dysplastic features in erythroid and megakaryocyte lineages may provide indirect evidence that a leukaemia is myeloid, not lymphoid. Dysplastic features are present in up to a quarter of cases. Definite evidence of myeloid differentiation may be provided by:

1 demonstration of ultrastructural features of cells of granulocytic lineage, e.g. characteristic basophil granules (Table 1.3) [12–17];
2 demonstration of MPO activity by ultrastructural cytochemistry (Table 1.4) [13, 18, 19] (Fig. 1.6);
3 demonstration of MPO protein by immunocytochemistry with an anti-MPO monoclonal antibody;
4 demonstration of other antigens characteristic of myeloid cells by the use of monoclonal antibodies such as CD13, CD14, CD15, CD33, CD64, CD65 and

CD117 (but without expression of platelet-specific antigens, which would lead to the case being categorized as AML M7).

Although not included in the criteria suggested by the FAB group, the demonstration of messenger RNA (mRNA) for MPO could also be taken as evidence of myeloid differentiation [20], but its expression may not be restricted to myeloid cells [21].

Immunophenotyping is now widely used for identifying cases of M0 AML and as a consequence ultrastructural examination and ultrastructural cytochemistry are rarely used. However, these techniques remain useful for the identification of immature cells of basophil, mast cell and eosinophil lineage. Immunophenotyping shows that the most specific lymphoid markers—cytoplasmic CD3, cytoplasmic CD79a and cytoplasmic CD22—are not expressed in M0 AML but there may be expression of less specific lymphoid-associated antigens such as CD2, CD4, CD7, CD10 and CD19, in addition to CD34, HLA-DR and terminal deoxynucleotidyl transferase (TdT).

M0 AML is associated with adverse cytogenetic abnormalities and poor prognosis [22, 23]. The molecular genetic abnormalities recognized include a high incidence of mutations of the *AML1* gene, most of which are biallelic [24].

Cytochemical reactions in M0 AML

By definition fewer than 3% of blasts are positive for MPO, SBB and CAE since a greater degree of positivity would lead to the case being classified as M1 AML. Similarly, blast cells do not show NSE activity, since positivity would lead to the case being classified as M5 AML. Maturing myeloid cells may show peroxidase deficiency or aberrant positivity for both chloroacetate and non-specific esterase [25].

AML without maturation—M1 AML

The criteria for diagnosis of M1 AML are shown in

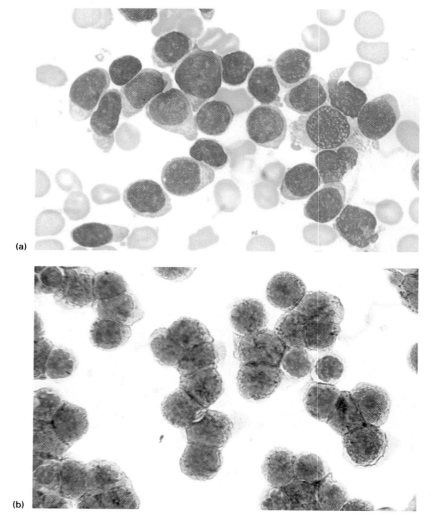

(a)

(b)

Fig. 1.4 PB and BM preparations from a patient with M0 AML: (a) BM film stained by MGG showing agranular blasts; (b) immunoperoxidase reaction of PB cells with a CD13 monoclonal antibody (McAb) showing many strongly positive blasts; the blasts were also positive for CD34, HLA-DR and terminal deoxynucleotidyl transferase (TdT). × 870.

Table 1.5 and the cytological features are illustrated in Figs 1.7–1.10. M1 blasts are usually medium to large in size with a variable nucleocytoplasmic ratio, a round or oval nucleus, one or more nucleoli, which range from inconspicuous to prominent, and cytoplasm that sometimes contains Auer rods, a few granules or some vacuoles. Auer rods are crystalline cytoplasmic structures derived from primary granules either just after their formation in the cisternae of the Golgi apparatus or by coalescence of granules within autophagic vacuoles. Auer rods may thus be seen as cytoplasmic inclusions or, less often, within a cytoplasmic vacuole. In children, the presence of Auer rods has been found to be associated with a better prognosis [26]. In M1 AML the blasts are predominantly type I blasts. In some cases the blasts are indistinguishable from L2 or even L1 lymphoblasts (see page 43).

M1 is arbitrarily separated from M2 AML by the requirement that no more than 10% of non-erythroid cells in the bone marrow belong to the maturing granulocytic component (promyelocytes to neutrophils).

The M1 category accounts for 15–20% of AML.

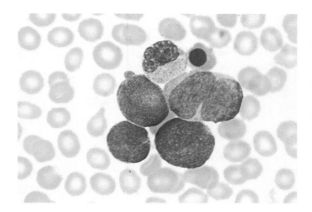

Fig. 1.5 BM film of a patient with M0 AML showing agranular pleomorphic blasts with a high nucleocytoplasmic ratio; the presence of a neutrophil with a nucleus of abnormal shape suggests the correct diagnosis. MGG × 870.

Cytochemical reactions in M1 AML

By definition M1 AML has a minimum of 3% of blasts that are positive for MPO or SBB. Hayhoe and Quaglino [2] found that the SBB reaction is a more sensitive marker of early granulocyte precursors than MPO. M1 blasts are usually positive for CAE, although this marker is usually less sensitive than either MPO or SBB in the detection of neutrophilic differentiation. Myeloblasts give a weak or negative reaction for a number of esterases that are more characteristic of the monocyte lineage, and that are collectively referred to as non-specific esterases. In the case of α-naphthyl acetate esterase (ANAE) and α-naphthyl butyrate esterase (ANBE) the reaction is usually negative, whereas in the cases of naphthol AS-D acetate esterase (NASDA) there is usually a weak fluoride-resistant reaction. Myeloblasts show

Table 1.3 Ultrastructural characteristics distinguishing blast cells and other immature leukaemic cells from each other [12, 13].

Myeloblasts of neutrophil lineage
Small, medium or large granules; sometimes Auer rods, which may be homogeneous or be composed of longitudinal tubules or dense material with a periodic substructure [14]

Promyelocytes of promyelocytic leukaemia
In hypergranular promyelocytic leukaemia the cytoplasm is packed with granules ranging from 120 to 1000 nm in diameter [15, 16]; in the variant form of hypergranular promyelocytic leukaemia the granules are much smaller, ranging from 100 to 400 nm, with some cells being packed with granules and other being agranular. Auer rods in promyelocytic leukaemia differ from those in M1 and M2 AML; they are composed of hexagonal structures and have a different periodicity from other Auer rods [16]; microfibrils and stellate configurations of rough endoplasmic reticulum are also characteristic of M3 AML, particularly M3 variant [17]

Myeloblasts of eosinophil lineage
Granules tend to be larger than those of neutrophil series; homogeneous in early cells, in later cells having a crystalline core set in a matrix; sometimes there is asynchrony with granules lacking a central core, despite a mature nucleus; Auer rods similar to those of the neutrophil lineage may be present [14]

Myeloblasts of basophil or mast cell lineage*
Basophil granules may be any of three types: (i) large electron-dense granules composed of coarse particles; (ii) pale granules composed of fine particles; (iii) θ (theta) granules, which are small granules containing pale flocculent material and bisected by a membrane [13]. Mast cell precursors sometimes have granules showing the scrolled or whorled pattern that is characteristic of normal mast cells

Monoblasts and promonocytes
Monoblasts are larger than myeloblasts and cytoplasm may be vacuolated. Granules are smaller and less numerous

Megakaryoblasts
More mature megakaryoblasts show α granules, bull's eye granules and platelet demarcation membranes

Early erythroid precursors
Immature cells can be identified as erythroid when they contain aggregates of ferritin molecules or iron-laden mitochondria or when there is rhopheocytosis (invagination of the surface membrane in association with extracellular ferritin molecules)

*Sometimes in myeloid leukaemias and myeloproliferative disorders there are cells containing a mixture of granules of basophil and mast cell type.

Table 1.4 Ultrastructural cytochemistry in the identification of blast cells and other immature cells of different myeloid lineages.

Myeloblasts of neutrophil lineage
Myeloperoxidase (MPO) activity in endoplasmic reticulum, perinuclear space, Golgi zone, granules and Auer rods (if present); detected by standard technique for MPO and by platelet peroxidase (PPO) techniques (reviewed in [13])

Myeloblasts of eosinophil lineage
MPO-positive granules and Auer rods (if present) detected by MPO and PPO techniques

Myeloblasts of basophil or mast cell lineage
Granules may be peroxidase positive or negative; endoplasmic reticulum, perinuclear space and Golgi zone are rarely positive; more cases are positive by PPO technique than MPO technique

Promyelocytes of acute promyelocytic leukaemia
MPO-positivity is seen in granules, Auer rods, perinuclear space and some rough endoplasmic reticulum profiles [17]; strong lysozyme activity of granules and Auer rods is seen in M3 AML whereas in M3 variant AML activity varies from weak to moderately strong [17]

Monoblasts and promonocytes
The first granule to appear in a monoblast is a small, peripheral acid phosphatase-positive granule [18]. MPO activity appears initially in the perinuclear envelope, Golgi apparatus and endoplasmic reticulum. Subsequently, mainly at the promonocyte stage, there are small MPO-positive granules. A PPO technique is more sensitive in the detection of peroxidase-positive granules than an MPO technique. Non-specific esterase activity can also be demonstrated cytochemically

Megakaryoblasts
PPO activity in endoplasmic reticulum and perinuclear space only [13, 19]

Proerythroblasts
PPO-like activity may be present in the Golgi zone

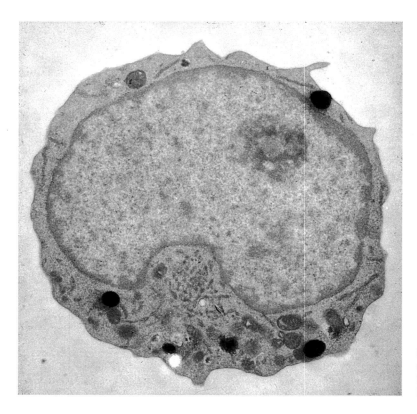

Fig. 1.6 Ultrastructural cytochemistry showing peroxidase-positive granules in a myeloblast (with thanks to Professor D Catovsky, London).

Table 1.5 Criteria for the diagnosis of acute myeloid leukaemia of M1 category (acute myeloid leukaemia without maturation).

Blasts ≥30% of bone marrow cells
Blasts ≥90% of bone marrow non-erythroid cells*
≥3% of blasts positive for peroxidase or Sudan black B
Bone marrow maturing monocytic component (promonocytes to monocytes) ≤10% of non-erythroid cells
Bone marrow maturing granulocytic component (promyelocytes to polymorphonuclear leucocytes) ≤10% of non-erythroid cells

*Exclude also lymphocytes, plasma cells, macrophages and mast cells from the count.

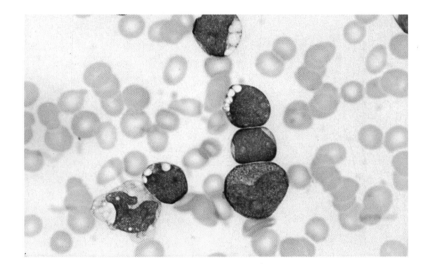

Fig. 1.7 PB film of a patient with M1 AML showing type I and type II blasts, some of which are heavily vacuolated, and a promyelocyte. MGG × 870.

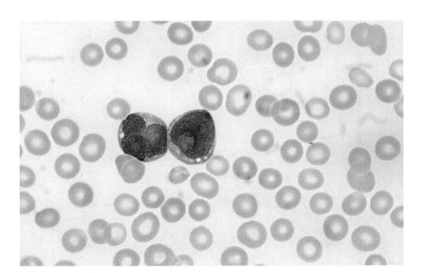

Fig. 1.8 PB film of a patient with M1 AML showing type I blasts with cytoplasmic vacuolation and nuclear lobulation. MGG × 870.

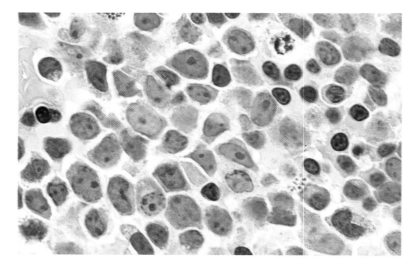

Fig. 1.9 Histological section of a trephine biopsy of a patient with M1 AML. The majority of cells present are blasts with a high nucleocytoplasmic ratio and prominent nucleoli; there are also some erythroblasts. Plastic embedded, haematoxylin and eosin (H & E) × 870.

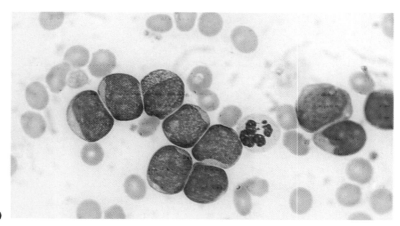

(a)

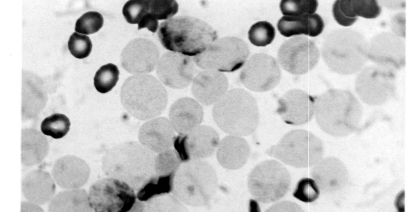

(b)

Fig. 1.10 Cytochemical reactions in a patient with M1 AML: (a) MGG-stained PB film showing largely type I blasts which in this patient are morphologically similar to lymphoblasts. One leukaemic cell is heavily granulated and would therefore be classified as a promyelocyte; this cell and the presence of a hypogranular neutrophil suggest that the correct diagnosis is M1 AML. MGG × 870. (b) myeloperoxidase (MPO) stain of BM showing two leukaemic cells with peroxidase-positive granules and two with Auer rods. × 870.

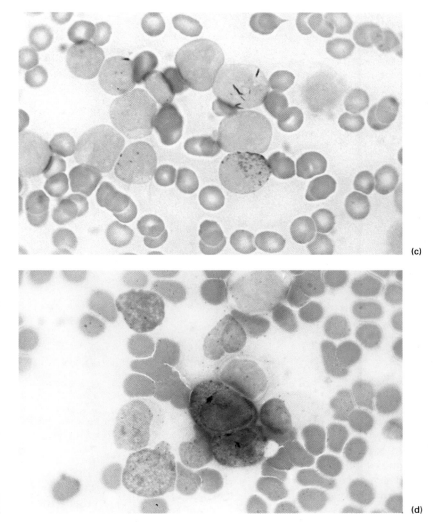

(c)

(d)

Fig. 1.10 (*Continued*) (c) Sudan black B (SBB) stain of BM showing some blasts with Auer rods and some with granules. × 870. (d) Chloroacetate esterase (CAE) stain of BM showing a positive neutrophil and a positive blast; other blasts present are negative. × 870.

diffuse acid phosphatase activity, which varies from weak to strong. The PAS reaction is usually negative, but may show a weak diffuse reaction with superimposed fine granular positivity.

Auer rods give positive reactions for MPO and SBB and occasionally weak PAS reactions. The reaction with CAE is usually weak or negative [2] except in M2 AML associated with t(8;21) (see page 78) in which Auer rods are often positive with CAE [1]. Although Auer rods are often detectable on a Romanowsky stain, they are more readily detectable on an MPO or SBB stain and larger numbers are apparent. Sometimes they are detectable only with

cytochemical stains. Typical cytochemical stains in a case of M1 AML are shown in Fig. 1.10.

AML with maturation—M2 AML

The criteria for the diagnosis of M2 AML are shown in Table 1.6. In this context cells included in the maturing granulocytic category are promyelocytes, myelocytes, metamyelocytes and granulocytes, and also cells that differ cytologically from normal promyelocytes but that are too heavily granulated to be classified as blasts. Typical cytological and cytochemical features in M2 AML are shown in Figs 1.11–1.13.

Blasts ≥30% of bone marrow cells

Blasts 30–89% of bone marrow non-erythroid cells

Bone marrow maturing granulocytic component (promyelocytes to polymorphonuclear leucocytes) >10% of non-erythroid cells

Bone marrow monocytic component (monoblasts to monocytes) <20% of non-erythroid cells and other criteria for M4 not met

Table 1.6 Criteria for the diagnosis of acute myeloid leukaemia of M2 category (acute myeloid leukaemia with maturation).

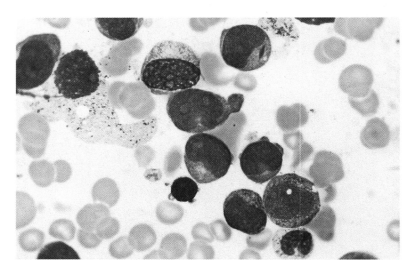

Fig. 1.11 BM film of a patient with M2 AML showing blasts (one of which contains an Auer rod), promyelocytes and a neutrophil. Note the very variable granulation. MGG × 870.

In contrast to M1 AML, blasts are often predominantly type II. Auer rods may be present. In children, Auer rods have been associated with a better prognosis [26], probably because of an association between Auer rods and t(8;21) (see page 78). Dysplastic features, such as hypo- or hypergranularity or abnormalities of nuclear shape are common in the differentiating granulocytic component of M2 AML. Maturation of myeloblasts to promyelocytes occurs in both M2 and M3 AML, and promyelocytes are prominent in some cases of M2 AML. Such cases are distinguished from M3 AML by the lack of the specific features of the latter condition (see below). M2 AML is distinguished from M4 AML by the monocytic component in the bone marrow being less than 20% of non-erythroid cells and by the lack of other evidence of significant monocytic differentiation. In most cases of M2 AML, maturation is along the neutrophil pathway but eosinophilic or basophilic maturation occurs in a minority. Such cases may be designated M2Eo or M2Baso. Other morphologically distinctive categories within M2, associated with specific cytogenetic abnormalities, are recognized (see Chapter 2).

The M2 subtype accounts for about 30% of cases of AML.

Cytochemical reactions in M2 AML

The cytochemical reactions in M2 AML are the same as those in M1 AML, but generally reactions are stronger and a higher percentage of cells are positive for MPO and SBB. CAE is more often positive in M2 than in M1 AML and reactions are stronger. Auer rods show the same staining characteristics as in M1 AML but are more numerous. When leukaemic myeloblasts undergo maturation, as in M2 AML, there may be a population of neutrophils, presumably derived from leukaemic blasts, which lack SBB and MPO activity. This may be demonstrated cytochemically or by means of an automated differential counter based on the peroxidase reaction, which shows a low mean peroxidase score and an abnormally placed neutrophil cluster. The neutrophil cluster

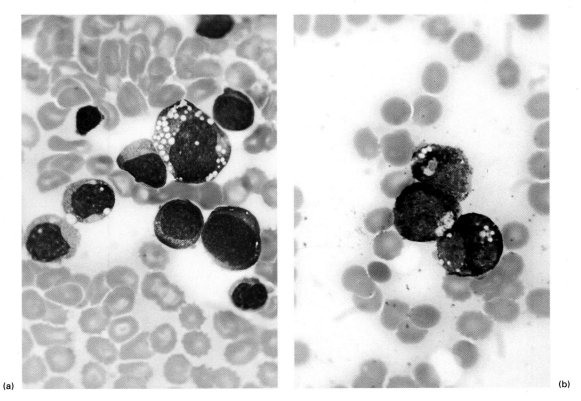

(a)

(b)

Fig. 1.12 BM film of a patient with M2 AML stained by (a) MGG and (b) SBB. In this patient both blasts and maturing cells were heavily vacuolated. × 870.

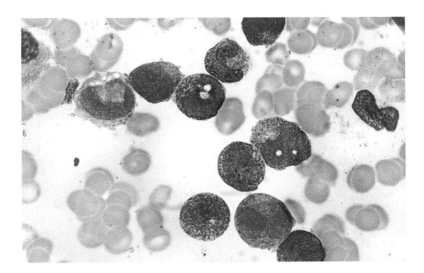

Fig. 1.13 BM film of a patient with M2 AML showing unusually heavy granulation of neutrophils and precursors (courtesy of Dr D. Swirsky, Leeds). MGG × 870.

with such automated instruments is often dispersed in AML in contrast to the normal compact cluster in ALL. The neutrophil alkaline phosphatase (NAP) score is often low in M2 AML.

Acute hypergranular promyelocytic leukaemia—M3 AML

In acute hypergranular promyelocytic leukaemia the predominant cell is a highly abnormal promyelocyte. In the majority of cases, blasts are fewer than 30% of bone marrow nucleated cells. The distinctive cytological features are sufficient to permit a diagnosis and cases are classified as M3 AML despite the low blast percentage. M3 AML is associated with a specific cytogenetic abnormality and with abnormal coagulation (see page 85). Because of the prominent haemorrhagic manifestations this diagnosis can sometimes be suspected from clinical features. Typical cytological

and histological features are shown in Figs 1.14–1.16. The predominant cell is a promyelocyte, the cytoplasm of which is densely packed with coarse red or purple granules, which almost obscure the nucleus. There is often nucleocytoplasmic asynchrony with the nucleus having a diffuse chromatin pattern and one or more nucleoli. When the nuclear shape can be discerned it is found, in the majority of cases, to be reniform or folded or bilobed with only a narrow bridge between the two lobes. The nuclear form is often more apparent on histological sections (Fig. 1.16). Auer rods are common. In one series they were noted in fewer than 50% of cases [27] but others have observed them to be almost always present, at least in a minority of cells [28]. In some cases there are giant granules or multiple Auer rods, which are often present in sheaves or 'faggots'. Most cases have a minority of cells that are agranular, have sparse granules or have fine red or rust-coloured dust-like

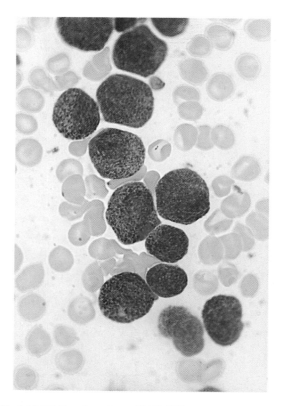

Fig. 1.14 BM film of a patient with M3 AML showing hypergranular promyelocytes, one of which has a giant granule. MGG × 870.

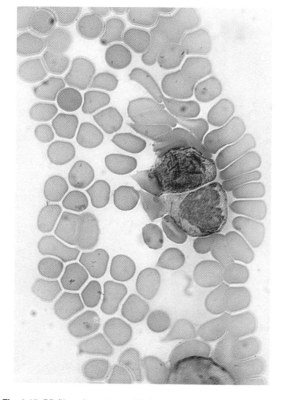

Fig. 1.15 PB film of a patient with M3 AML. One of the abnormal promyelocytes contains loose bundles of Auer rods. MGG × 870.

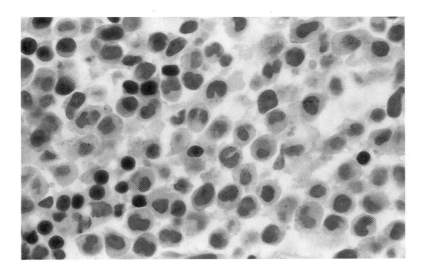

Fig. 1.16 Histological section of a trephine biopsy in a patient with M3 AML. H & E × 870.

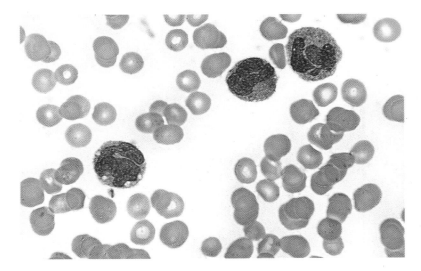

Fig. 1.17 PB film of a patient with M3 AML being treated with all-*trans*-retinoic acid (ATRA) and granulocyte colony-stimulating factor (G-CSF); leukaemic promyelocytes are undergoing maturation into highly abnormal cells. MGG × 870.

granules rather than coarse brightly staining granules. Cells that lack granules but have lakes of hyaline pink material in the cytoplasm may also be seen. There may be basophilic differentiation in M3 AML, in addition to the dominant neutrophilic differentiation. Dysplastic changes in the erythroid and megakaryocyte lineages are usually absent.

Examining an adequate bone marrow aspirate is particularly important in M3 AML, as the white cell count is often low and, even when there is a leucocytosis, typical hypergranular promyelocytes may not be present in the blood. The specimen may clot during attempted aspiration as a consequence of the associated hypercoagulable state, but usually sufficient cells are obtained for diagnosis.

M3 AML has been found to be very sensitive to the differentiating capacity of all-*trans*-retinoic acid (ATRA). Following such therapy an increasing proportion of cells beyond the promyelocyte stage are apparent. Maturing cells are cytologically abnormal (Fig. 1.17). Metamyelocytes and neutrophils may contain Auer rods. The neutrophil count rises and in some patients also the basophil count [29]. M3 AML is also responsive to treatment with arsenic trioxide, As_2O_3. With both ATRA and arsenic trioxide [30] hyperleucocytosis may occur during therapy.

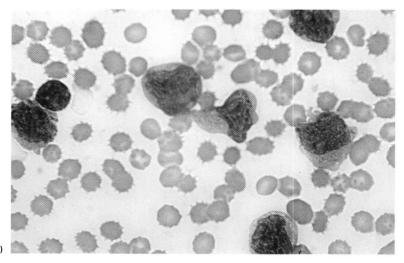

(a)

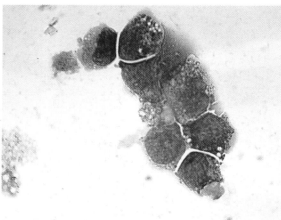

(b)

Fig. 1.18 (a) PB film and (b) film of cultured leukaemic cells from a patient with M3 variant AML showing the acquisition of granules on culture (courtesy of Dr D Grimwade, London). MGG × 870.

The variant form of promyelocytic leukaemia—M3V AML

Some years after the initial description of hypergranular promyelocytic leukaemia it was noted that there were other cases of acute leukaemia that showed the same cytogenetic abnormality and coagulation abnormality but were cytologically different. Such cases were recognized as a variant form of promyelocytic leukaemia, designated microgranular or hypogranular promyelocytic leukaemia [31, 32]. Such cases were subsequently incorporated into the FAB classification as M3 variant (M3V) AML. In addition to cytogenetic and molecular evidence indicating the close relationship of M3 and M3V AML it has been

noted that the cells of M3V may show a marked increase in granularity on culture [32] (Fig. 1.18) and, conversely, cases of M3 AML may have less granular cells on relapse [16]. There is no clear demarcation between cases of classical M3 AML and the variant form—cases with intermediate features are seen. This is not surprising since these are morphological variants of a single biological entity.

Most cases of M3V AML are characterized by a cell with a reniform, bilobed, multilobed or convoluted nucleus and either sparse fine granules or apparently agranular cytoplasm (Figs 1.19 & 1.20). A variable proportion of cells may have multiple Auer rods, fine dust-like granules, or large oval, elliptiform or somewhat angular cytoplasmic inclusions with the same

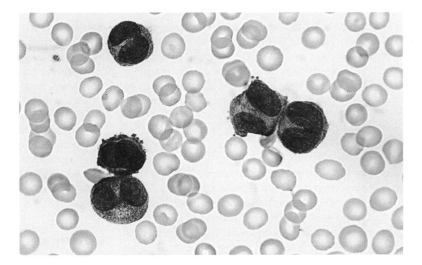

Fig. 1.19 PB film of a patient with M3V AML showing cells with bilobed and reniform nuclei and sparse, fine granules. One binucleate cell is present and one cell with basophilic cytoplasm and cytoplasmic projections. MGG × 870.

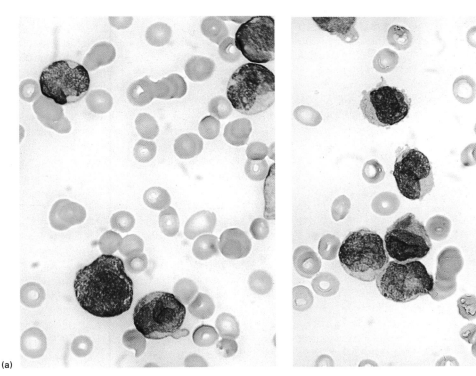

(a)

(b)

Fig. 1.20 PB film of a patient with M3V AML showing (a) predominantly agranular cells with twisted nuclei but with one typical hypergranular cell being present; (b) agranular cells with twisted nuclei; one cell contains a large azurophilic inclusion. MGG × 870.

staining characteristics as primary granules. Typical hypergranular promyelocytes constitute a small minority of the leukaemic cells in the peripheral blood but they are usually more numerous in the bone marrow. The white cell count is usually higher in M3V than in M3 AML.

In a minority of cases of M3V AML the characteristic cell is a small, abnormal promyelocyte with the same lobulated nucleus as described above but with hyperbasophilic cytoplasm; cytoplasmic projections are sometimes present so that cells may resemble megakaryoblasts [16]. Such cells are seen in the majority of cases of M3V AML, but usually as a minor population (see Fig. 1.19).

M3V may be confused with acute monocytic leukaemia (M5b) if blood and bone marrow cells are not examined carefully and if the diagnosis is not considered. The use of an automated blood cell counter based on cytochemistry (MPO or SBB) is useful for the rapid distinction between M3V and M5 AML (see Fig. 1.69). When M3V appears likely from the cytological and cytochemical features the diagnosis can be confirmed by cytogenetic, molecular genetic or immunophenotypic analysis.

When treated with chemotherapy, the prognosis of M3 variant is somewhat worse than that of M3 AML [33]. This is likely to be related to the higher white cell count (WBC), since the WBC is of prognostic importance in M3/M3V AML [23]. As a higher white cell count remains an adverse prognostic feature when M3/M3V AML is treated with ATRA plus chemotherapy [33] it is likely that M3V also has a worse prognosis with combined modality treatment.

M3 and M3V AML together constitute 5–10% of cases of AML.

Cytochemical reactions in M3 and M3V AML

Hypergranular promyelocytes are usually strongly positive for MPO, SBB and CAE. The PAS reaction usually shows a cytoplasmic 'blush'—a fine diffuse or dust-like positivity; the reaction is stronger than in M1 or M2 AML. PAS-positive erythroblasts are not generally seen. The acid phosphatase reaction is strongly positive. M3V AML usually shows similar cytochemical reactions [16] (Fig. 1.21) but sometimes the reactions are weaker [34]. A potentially confusing cytochemical reaction in both M3 and M3V AML is the presence in some cases of NSE activity [15, 16, 27], a reactivity otherwise characteristic of monocytic rather than granulocytic differentiation. ANAE, ANBE and NASDA may be positive and, as for the monocytic lineage, the reaction is fluoride sensitive. The reaction is weaker than in monocytes, and isoenzymes characteristic of the monocytic lineage are not present [34]. Some cells show double staining for NSE and CAE. Cases

that are positive for ANAE tend to have a weaker reaction for CAE, and occasionally the MPO reaction is unexpectedly weak [27]. The minority of cases that are positive for NSE do not appear to differ from other cases with regard to morphology, haematological or cytogenetic findings or prognosis [27].

Cases with basophilic differentiation show metachromatic staining with toluidine blue.

Auer rods in M3 AML are SBB, MPO and CAE positive, whereas in other categories of AML they are usually negative with CAE; they may be weakly PAS positive. On SBB, MPO and CAE staining, the core of the rod may be left unstained and occasionally the core is ANAE positive on a mixed esterase stain [2].

Acute myelomonocytic leukaemia—M4 AML

The criteria for the diagnosis of AML of M4 subtype, that is, AML with both granulocytic and monocytic differentiation, are shown in Table 1.7 and typical cytological and histological features in Figs 1.22–1.24. The criterion for recognition of a significant granulocytic component is a morphological one; the granulocytic component, which in this context includes myeloblasts as well as maturing cells, must be at least 20% of non-erythroid cells. The recognition of a significant monocytic component requires two criteria to be satisfied, which may be both morphological or one morphological and the other cytochemical, as shown in Table 1.7. In assessing the monocytic component, monoblasts, promonocytes and monocytes are included in the count.

Promonocytes are often heavily granulated and can be difficult to distinguish from promyelocytes. Cytochemistry is useful in making this distinction. The FAB criteria for the recognition of monocytic differentiation are the presence of fluoride-sensitive naphthol AS acetate esterase (NASA) or NASDA activity [3], or the presence of ANAE activity [6]. ANBE activity would also identify monocytic differentiation. Alternatively, lysozyme activity of leukaemic cells can be demonstrated cytochemically or lysozyme concentration can be measured in serum or urine, an elevation to more than three times the normal value being regarded as significant [6]. Careful examination of the peripheral blood is important if all cases of M4 AML are to be recognized since the bone marrow is sometimes morphologically indistinguishable from M2 AML. In M4 AML the granulocytic differentiation is usually along the neutrophil pathway, but in some

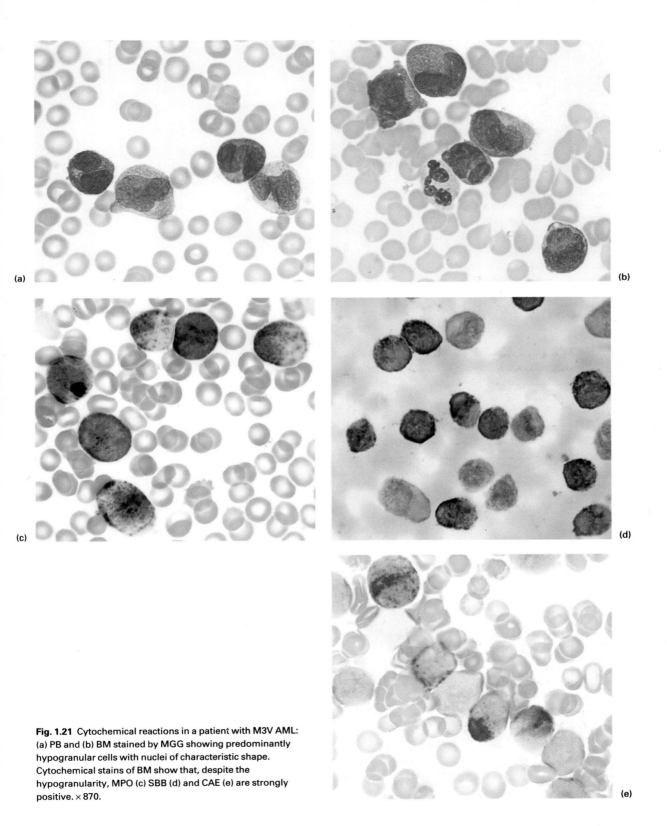

Fig. 1.21 Cytochemical reactions in a patient with M3V AML: (a) PB and (b) BM stained by MGG showing predominantly hypogranular cells with nuclei of characteristic shape. Cytochemical stains of BM show that, despite the hypogranularity, MPO (c) SBB (d) and CAE (e) are strongly positive. × 870.

Table 1.7 Criteria for the diagnosis of acute myeloid leukaemia of M4 category (acute myelomonocytic leukaemia).

Blasts ≥30% of bone marrow cells
Blasts ≥30% of bone marrow non-erythroid cells
Bone marrow granulocytic component (myeloblasts to polymorphonuclear leucocytes) ≥20% of non-erythroid cells
Significant monocytic component as shown by one of the following:
• Bone marrow monocytic component (monoblasts to monocytes) ≥20% of non-erythroid cells and peripheral blood monocytic component ≥5 × 10^9/l, *or*
• Bone marrow monocytic component (monoblasts to monocytes) ≥20% of non-erythroid cells and confirmed by cytochemistry or increased serum or urinary lysozyme concentration, *or*
• Bone marrow resembling M2 but peripheral blood monocyte component ≥5 × 10^9/l and confirmed by cytochemistry or increased serum or urinary lysozyme concentration

---

cases it is eosinophilic (M4Eo) (Fig. 1.23), basophilic (M4Baso) or both (Fig. 1.24).

The M4 subtype accounts for 15–20% of cases of AML.

Cytochemical reactions in M4 AML

In M4 AML some leukaemic cells show cytochemical reactions typical of neutrophilic, eosinophilic or

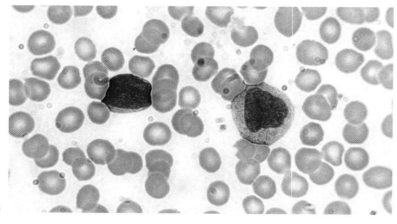

(a)

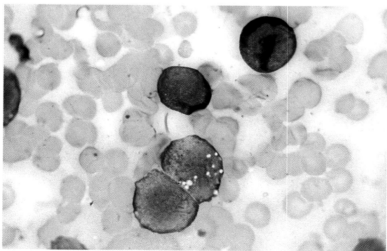

(b)

Fig. 1.22 (a) PB of a patient with M4 AML showing a myeloblast which is of medium size with a high nucleocytoplasmic ratio and a monoblast which is larger with more plentiful cytoplasm and a folded nucleus with a lacy chromatin pattern. MGG × 870. (b) BM of the same patient stained with SBB showing two monoblasts with a weak granular reaction and two cells of the granulocytic series with a much stronger reaction. × 870.

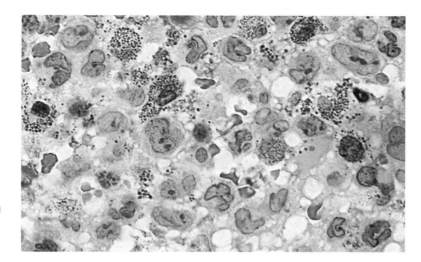

Fig. 1.23 Histological section of a trephine biopsy of a patient with M4Eo AML. Cells are either monoblasts, recognized as large cells with lobulated nuclei containing prominent nucleoli, or eosinophils. Plastic embedded, H & E × 870.

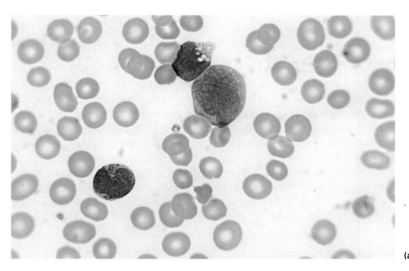

(a)

Fig. 1.24 PB film of a patient with M4 AML—M4Eo/inv(16)—who had both eosinophil and basophil differentiation. (a) a blast cell and two primitive cells containing basophil granules; one of the latter is vacuolated. MGG × 870. (b) Toluidine blue stain showing metachromatic staining of a basophil precursor. × 870. (c) Double esterase stain showing positivity of the granulocyte series with CAE (red) and positivity of the monocyte series with α-naphthyl acetate (non-specific) esterase (brownish-black). × 870.

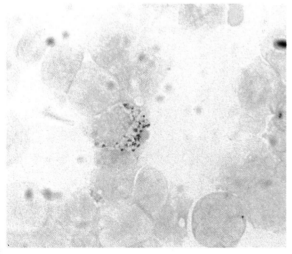

(b)

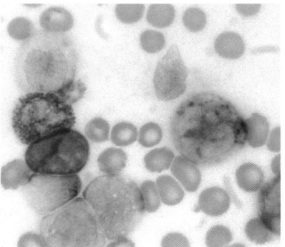

(c)

Table 1.8 Criteria for the diagnosis
of acute myeloid leukaemia of M5
category (acute monoblastic/monocytic
leukaemia).

Blasts ≥30% of bone marrow cells
Blasts ≥30% of bone marrow non-erythroid cells
Bone marrow monocytic component ≥80% of non-erythroid cells

Acute monoblastic leukaemia (M5a)
Monoblasts ≥80% of bone marrow monocytic component

Acute monocytic leukaemia (M5b)
Monoblasts <80% bone marrow monocytic component

basophilic lineages while other cells show reactions typical of the monocytic lineage (see above). A double esterase stain for CAE (neutrophil lineage) and ANAE (monocyte lineage) [35] is a convenient method for demonstrating the pattern of differentiation and maturation in M4 AML (Fig. 1.24c).

Acute monocytic/monoblastic leukaemia—M5 AML

The criteria for the diagnosis of acute monocytic/monoblastic leukaemia, M5 AML, are shown in Table 1.8 and typical cytological and histological features in Figs 1.25–1.28. This diagnosis may be suspected from clinical features when there is infiltration of the skin and the gums. Disseminated intravascular coagulation and increased fibrinolysis are more common in M5 AML than in other categories of AML, with the exception of M3 [36]. M5 AML is further subdivided into M5a AML (acute monoblastic leukaemia) and M5b AML (acute monocytic leukaemia) on the basis of whether monoblasts comprise at least 80% of the total bone marrow monocytic component. Monoblasts are large cells with plentiful cytoplasm, which is sometimes vacuolated and is usually moderately, occasionally strongly, basophilic; scattered fine azurophilic granules may be present. Auer rods are quite uncommon. The nucleus varies from round (in the most primitive monoblasts) to convoluted with a delicate chromatin pattern and one or several nucleoli, which are often large and prominent. Promonocytes have prominent azurophilic granules and cytoplasm that is more basophilic than that of monoblasts. Monocytes have a lower nucleocytoplasmic ratio, a lobulated nucleus and weakly basophilic, often vacuolated, cytoplasm with an irregular outline. In monocytic leukaemias there is often disorderly maturation producing nucleocytoplasmic asynchrony and other dysplastic features. This can make it difficult to assign cells reliably to monoblast, promonocyte and

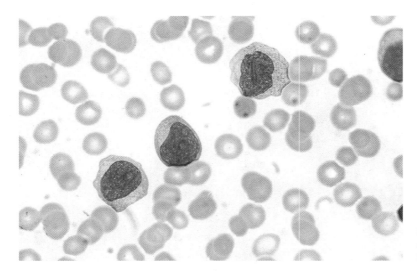

Fig. 1.25 PB film of a patient with M5a AML showing three monoblasts. MGG × 870.

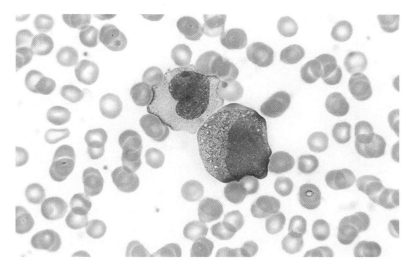

Fig. 1.26 PB of a patient with M5b AML showing a monocyte and a promonocyte; the latter is moderately heavily granulated. MGG × 870.

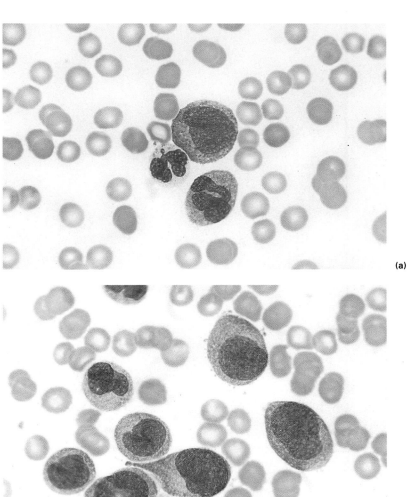

(a)

Fig. 1.27 PB and BM of a patient with M5b AML in whom the PB cells were more mature than the BM cells.
(a) PB showing a promonocyte and a monocyte with a nucleus of abnormal shape; the third cell is probably an abnormal neutrophil. MGG × 870.
(b) BM showing predominantly monoblasts and promonocytes. MGG × 870.

(b)

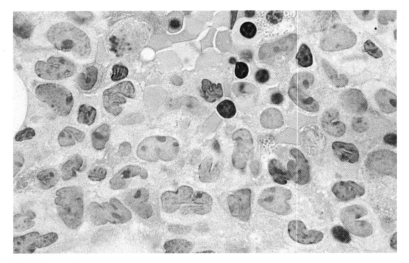

Fig. 1.28 Histological section of trephine biopsy of a patient with M5b AML and myelodysplasia. Monoblasts and monocytes can be identified; the former are the larger cells with a round or lobulated nucleus, a dispersed chromatin pattern and prominent nucleoli whereas the latter are smaller with lobulated nuclei and more chromatin clumping. The cells with smaller dark nuclei are erythroblasts one of which has a nucleus of abnormal shape. H & E × 870.

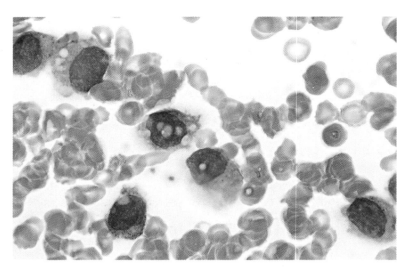

Fig. 1.29 BM film of a patient with leukaemic cells showing histiocytic or macrophage differentiation ('M5c'). MGG × 870.

monocyte categories. Leukaemic cells in the peripheral blood may be more mature than those in the bone marrow (Fig. 1.27). Monocytic differentiation can be confirmed by cytochemistry and by measurement of urinary and serum lysozyme concentrations; immunophenotyping can also be helpful.

In a rare form of acute monocytic leukaemia, cells have cytological features resembling those of macrophages or histiocytes (Fig. 1.29). This may be regarded as the leukaemic phase of malignant histiocytosis. The designation M5c has been suggested [37].

The M5 subtype accounts for about 15% of cases of AML.

Cytochemical reactions in M5 AML

In M5a AML, MPO and SBB reactions are often negative, although a few fine, positive granules may be present. CAE is negative or very weak. Hayhoe and Quaglino [2] found SBB to be more sensitive than MPO in detecting monocytic differentiation; they noted that, with SBB, granules in monoblasts were usually scattered and fine whereas in myeloblasts the reaction was either localized or filled all the cytoplasm. Monoblasts were characteristically negative for MPO. Monoblasts are usually strongly positive for NSE, i.e. ANAE (Fig. 1.30a), ANBE, NASA (Fig. 1.30b,c) and

NASDA. All these esterase activities are inhibited by fluoride but only in the case of NASA and NASDA is it necessary to carry out the reaction with and without fluoride to convey specificity; in the case of ANAE and ANBE the reaction is negative or weak in cells of the granulocytic lineage. Aberrant esterase reactions are sometimes seen; occasional cases have negative reactions for NSE and other cases, when the reaction for NSE is very strong, give a positive reaction also for CAE. Monoblasts show diffuse acid phosphatase activity, which, along with NSE activity, appears in advance of SBB and MPO reactivity. Lysozyme activity, which appears at about the same time as MPO activity, can be demonstrated cytochemically (Fig.

1.30d). The PAS reaction of monoblasts is either negative or diffusely positive with a superimposed fine or coarse granular positivity or, occasionally, superimposed PAS-positive blocks (Fig. 1.30e). In M5 AML, the NAP score is usually normal or high in contrast to the low score that may be seen in cases of AML in which granulocytic maturation is occurring.

It should be noted that in some cases of M5a AML there are negative reactions for SBB, MPO and NSE. Such cases will be recognized as monoblastic only if the cytological features are assessed in relation to the immunophenotype. If the FAB classification is used such cases are classified as M0 AML but an alternative approach would be to classify cases as M5a when the

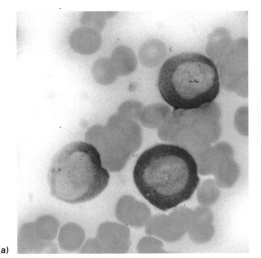

(a)

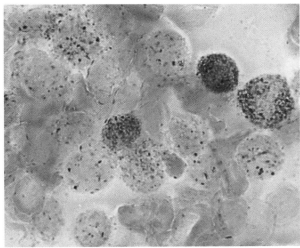

(b)

Fig. 1.30 (a) BM of a patient with M5a AML stained for α-naphthyl acetate (non-specific) esterase activity. × 870. (b, c) BM of a patient with M5b AML stained for naphthol AS acetate esterase (NASA) activity (b) without and (c) with fluoride; inhibition of activity by fluoride is apparent. × 870.

(c)

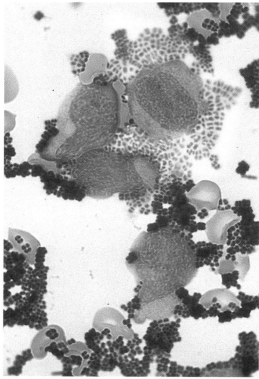

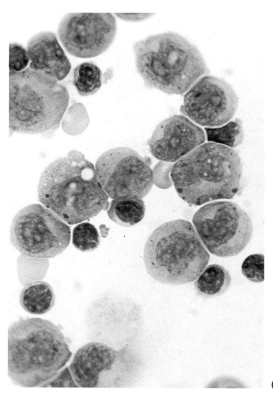

(d)

(e)

Fig. 1.30 (*Continued*) (d) Lysozyme preparation from a patient with M5b AML. Leukaemic cells have been mixed with a suspension of *Micrococcus lysodeikticus* bacteria; some of the leukaemic cells have secreted lysozyme, which has lysed adjacent bacteria so that they appear paler in comparison with intact bacteria (same patient as b and c). MGG × 870. (e) PAS stain of a PB cytospin preparation from a patient with M5a AML showing block positivity superimposed on fine granular and diffuse positivity. × 870.

cytological and immunophenotypic features favour the monocytic lineage.

AML with predominant erythroid differentiation—M6 AML

The FAB criteria for diagnosis of M6 AML are shown in Table 1.9 and cytological and histological features in Figs 1.31–1.37. Many cases of M6 AML represent leukaemic transformation of MDS. Trilineage dysplasia is characteristic. A significant proportion of cases are therapy related and trilineage myelodysplasia and adverse cytogenetic findings are common [38, 39]. Moderate to marked erythroid dysplasia is common, with erythroid precursors showing features such as nucleocytoplasmic asynchrony, nuclear lobulation, karyorrhexis, binuclearity and cytoplasmic vacuolation. There may be coalescence of prominent cytoplasmic vacuoles, this appearance correlating with the cytochemical demonstration of PAS positivity. Giant and multinucleated erythroid cells are sometimes prominent. In some cases, erythropoiesis is predominantly megaloblastic and in others it is macronormoblastic. Phagocytosis, particularly erythrophagocytosis, by abnormal erythroid precursors is sometimes seen.

Table 1.9 Criteria for the diagnosis of acute myeloid leukaemia of M6 category (acute erythroleukaemia).

Erythroblasts ≥50% of bone marrow nucleated cells
Blasts ≥30% of bone marrow non-erythroid cells

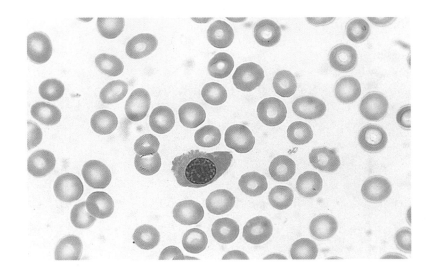

Fig. 1.31 PB film in a patient with M6 AML showing anaemia, severe thrombocytopenia and an abnormal circulating erythroblast. MGG × 870.

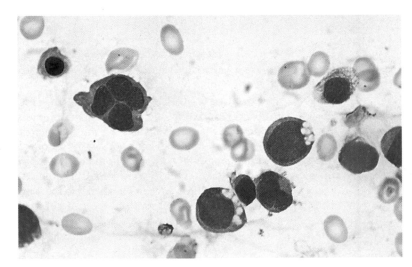

Fig. 1.32 BM film from a patient with M6 AML (erythroleukaemia) showing a multinucleated erythroblast and two heavily vacuolated myeloblasts. MGG × 870.

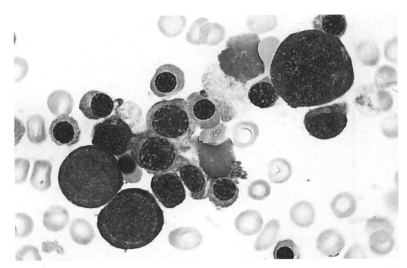

Fig. 1.33 BM film from a patient with M6 AML showing marked erythroid hyperplasia but only mild dyserythropoiesis; one binucleated erythroblast is present. MGG × 870.

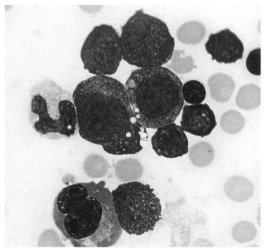

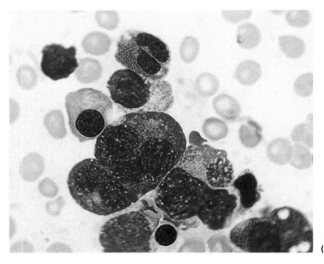

(a)

(b)

Fig. 1.34 BM film from a patient with M6 AML showing: (a) a binucleated erythroblast and two vacuolated erythroblasts; (b) a giant multinucleated erythroblast. MGG × 870.

In some cases proerythroblasts and basophilic erythroblasts are markedly increased as a percentage of total erythroblasts. Circulating erythroblasts which may show dysplastic features are present in some cases. The non-erythroid component of M6 may resemble any other FAB category with the exception of M3/M3V AML. Myeloblasts may show Auer rods.

FAB criteria for M6 AML require that at least 50% of bone marrow nucleated cells are recognizable erythroblasts and that at least 30% of non-erythroid cells are blasts. There are also cases of AML in which the leukaemic cells appear by light microscopy to be undifferentiated blasts but can be shown by immunophenotyping or ultrastructural analysis to be primitive erythroid cells. When such cases lack a significant non-erythroid component including more than 30% of non-erythroid blasts, they do not fit the FAB criteria for M6 AML. Nevertheless, it seems reasonable that such cases (which are rare except when AML occurs in Down's syndrome [40]) should be assigned to the M6 category. Use of the term M6 variant is appropriate [39, 41].

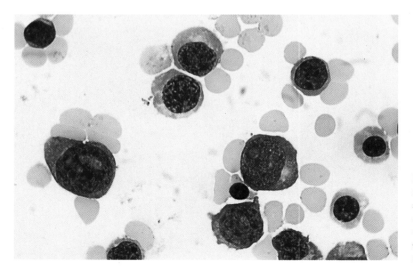

Fig. 1.35 A cytospin preparation of BM cells of a patient with M6 AML showing late erythroblasts and three undifferentiated blasts. A positive reaction of the blast cells with a McAb to glycophorin A showed that these were primitive erythroid cells. MGG × 870.

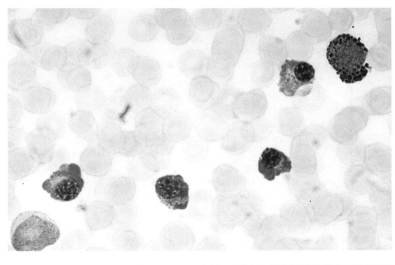

(a)

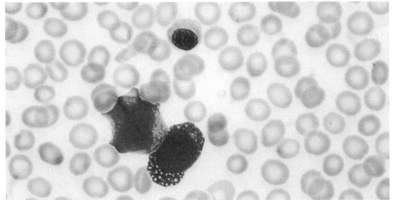

(b)

Fig. 1.36 (a, b) BM aspirate in M6 AML showing diffuse PAS positivity in late erythroblasts and block positivity in an early erythroblast; the corresponding MGG stain shows vacuolation of an early erythroblast, the vacuoles being attributable to the solubility of glycogen. (a) Periodic acid–Schiff (PAS) stain × 870; (b) MGG × 870.

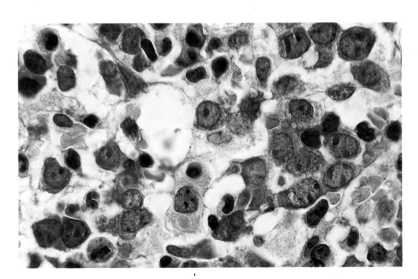

Fig. 1.37 BM trephine biopsy in M6 AML showing primitive erythroid cells, which can be distinguished from granulocyte precursors by their linear nucleoli, some of which abut on the nuclear membrane, and by their more basophilic cytoplasm (readily apparent on a Giemsa stain). H & E × 870.

Overall the M6 category accounts for about 3–4% of cases of AML. The frequency is higher in the elderly [42]. Prognosis appears to be worse than for AML in general [23, 43]. The survival of patients with M6 variant AML was a great deal worse than the survival of patients with FAB M6 AML in one series of patients [38] but in another both had an equally bad prognosis [39].

Cytochemical reactions in M6 AML

In M6 AML, myeloblasts and any Auer rods show the same cytochemical reactions as in other categories of AML. The NAP score may be reduced or increased and a population of neutrophils lacking SBB and MPO activity may be present.

On a PAS stain the erythroblasts show diffuse or finely granular positivity with or without coarse granular or block positivity (Fig. 1.36). Hayhoe and Quaglino [2] have described a characteristic block or granular positivity in early erythroblasts and diffuse positivity in late erythroblasts and some erythrocytes. PAS positivity is not pathognomonic of M6 AML, being seen also in iron deficiency anaemia, severe haemolytic anaemia and thalassaemia major and in occasional cases of megaloblastic anaemia. PAS positivity is seen also in MDS and in other categories of AML (overall in about one in five cases) and suggests that the erythroblasts, even when they are fewer than 50% of nucleated cells, are part of the leukaemic or myelodysplastic clone. Erythroblasts in M6 AML may have focal acid phosphatase activity, which is localized to the Golgi zone [13]; they are usually positive for ANAE and ANBE [2]. These reactions differentiate M6 erythroblasts from the erythroblasts of congenital dyserythropoietic anaemia, in which acid phosphatase and NSE reactions are negative; however, positive reactions can also be seen in megaloblastic anaemia consequent on pernicious anaemia [2]. A Perls' stain for iron may show coarse siderotic granules; in a minority of cases numerous ring sideroblasts are present.

Acute megakaryoblastic leukaemia—M7 AML

Acute megakaryoblastic leukaemia was not included in the original FAB classification of AML but, following the demonstration that in some cases apparently undifferentiated blasts were actually megakaryoblasts, this category was added [5] (Table 1.10). M7

Table 1.10 Criteria for the diagnosis of acute myeloid leukaemia of M7 category (acute megakaryoblastic leukaemia).

Blasts ≥30% of bone marrow nucleated cells
Blasts demonstrated to be megakaryoblasts by immunological markers, ultrastructural examination or ultrastructural cytochemistry

AML shows a markedly increased incidence in children with Down's syndrome. In infants and children, M7 AML may be associated with t(1;22)(p13;q13) (see page 109) and, in adults, a significant proportion of cases are associated with abnormalities of chromosome 3. Leukaemic megakaryoblasts are often highly pleomorphic. Prominent and multiple nucleoli and cytoplasmic basophilia have been noted [13]. Binuclearity and clumping of blast cells have been noted to be frequent features [44]. In some cases the diagnosis can be suspected from the cytological features when the blasts show cytoplasmic protrusions or blebs, or when blasts coexist with apparently bare nuclei, with large bizarre platelets or with more mature cells showing megakaryocytic differentiation. In other cases the blasts cannot be distinguished from myeloblasts or resemble lymphoblasts, being small with a high nucleocytoplasmic ratio and with some chromatin condensation. The WBC is often reduced rather than elevated [45]. A minority of patients with M7 AML have thrombocytosis rather than thrombocytopenia. The nature of megakaryoblasts may be suggested by the pattern of cytochemical reactions (see below) but a reliable identification requires immunophenotyping ultrastructural examination (Fig. 1.38) or ultrastructural cytochemistry (Fig. 1.39). The clinical picture designated acute myelofibrosis, i.e. pancytopenia with bone marrow fibrosis, is usually a consequence of acute megakaryoblastic leukaemia. Cytological and histological features of M7 AML are shown in Figs 1.40–1.42. Some cases show some maturation to dysplastic megakaryocytes, as is shown in Fig. 1.42. With the exception of cases among children with Down's syndrome, the prognosis in both children and adults appears to be poor [23, 44, 45].

Cytochemical reactions in M7 AML

Megakaryoblasts are negative for MPO, SBB and CAE. The more mature cells of this lineage are PAS positive and have partially fluoride-sensitive NSE activity, demonstrated with ANAE. ANBE activity is demon-

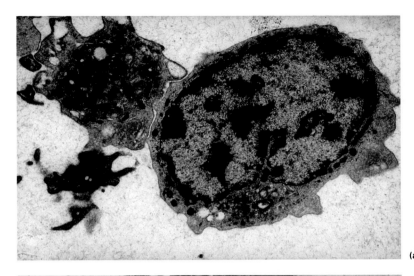

(a)

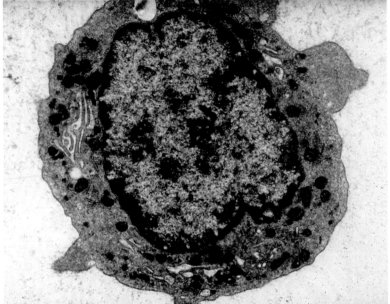

(b)

Fig. 1.38 Ultrastructural examination of peripheral blood cells from a patient with megakaryoblastic transformation of chronic granulocytic leukaemia showing: (a) a blast cell and a giant platelet; the megakaryoblast has characteristic granules including several bull's eye granules; (b) a megakaryoblast with platelet demarcation membranes (courtesy of Professor D Catovsky).

strable in only a minority of cases [44]. On PAS staining there are positive granules on a diffusely positive background. In some cases, those showing more cytoplasmic maturation, there are positive granules or block positivity, localized to the periphery of the cell or packed into the cytoplasmic blebs. A PAS stain can highlight the presence of micromegakaryocytes and megakaryoblasts with cytoplasmic maturation (Fig. 1.43). Esterase activity is usually multifocal punctate [44] but is sometimes localized to the Golgi

zone [17, 44]. There is a similar localization of acid phosphatase activity, which is tartrate sensitive [13]. In very immature megakaryoblasts PAS and NSE reactions are negative.

Acute eosinophilic leukaemia

Cases of eosinophilic leukaemia with a minimum of 30% bone marrow blast cells should be categorized as AML. They can be assigned to FAB categories with

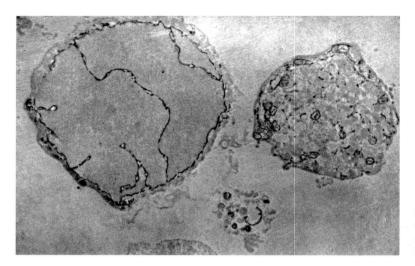

Fig. 1.39 Ultrastructural cytochemistry of blast cell showing a positive platelet peroxidase reaction (courtesy of Professor D Catovsky).

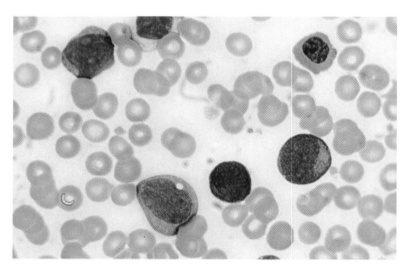

Fig. 1.40 PB film from a patient with Down's syndrome with M7 AML (acute megakaryoblastic leukaemia); blasts are pleomorphic with no specific distinguishing features. The nature of the leukaemia was demonstrated by a positive reaction with a McAb to platelet glycoprotein IIb/IIIa (CD61). MGG × 870.

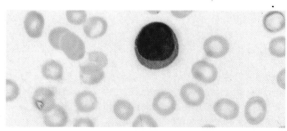

(a)

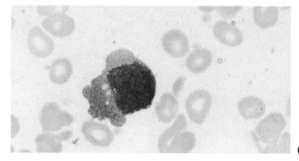

(b)

Fig. 1.41 PB and BM films from a patient with M7 AML presenting as acute myelofibrosis; the nature of the leukaemia was demonstrated by a positive reaction for platelet peroxidase. (a) PB showing mild anisocytosis and a blast cell with no distinguishing features; (b) BM showing megakaryoblast. MGG × 870.

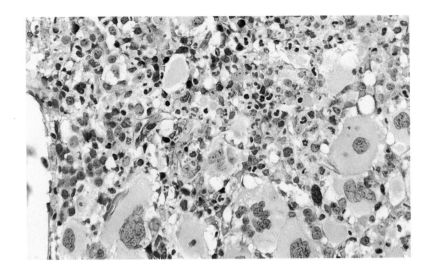

Fig. 1.42 Trephine biopsy sections from a patient with M7 AML showing increased blasts and large dysplastic megakaryocytes. H & E × 348.

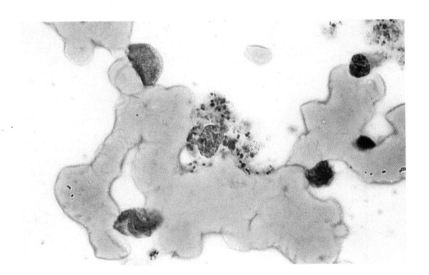

Fig. 1.43 BM aspirate in M7 showing a micromegakaryocyte with cytoplasmic blebs, which are PAS positive. PAS stain × 870.

the addition of the abbreviation 'Eo' to indicate the eosinophilic differentiation, e.g. M2Eo and M4Eo. Such cases may have cardiac and other tissue damage as a consequence of release of eosinophil granule contents. Generally there is both neutrophilic and eosinophilic differentiation. Occasional cases show only eosinophilic differentiation. A minimum of 5% of bone marrow eosinophils has been suggested as a criterion for the recognition of significant eosinophilic differentiation [46]. In cases with maturation, eosinophils are readily recognizable by the characteristic staining of their granules. However, recognition

of eosinophil precursors in M1Eo AML may require cytochemistry or the ultrastructural demonstration of characteristic granule structure (see Table 1.3), since primitive eosinophil granules differ little in their staining characteristics from the granules of neutrophil lineage myeloblasts (Fig. 1.44). Mature eosinophils often show vacuolation, degranulation and nuclear hyper- or hypolobulation. However, these cytological abnormalities are not specific for eosinophilic leukaemia, being seen also in reactive eosinophilia. The bone marrow in acute eosinophilic leukaemia sometimes shows the presence of Charcot–Leyden crystals,

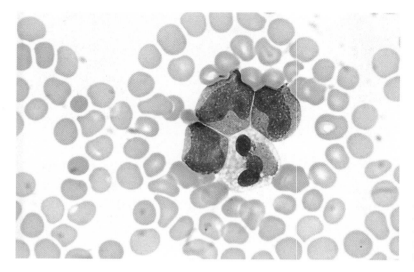

Fig. 1.44 PB in acute eosinophilic leukaemia with abnormal eosinophil precursors showing a mixture of eosinophilic and azurophilic granules; maturing eosinophils were degranulated and some had nuclei of bizarre shapes (courtesy of Dr A Smith, Southampton). MGG × 870.

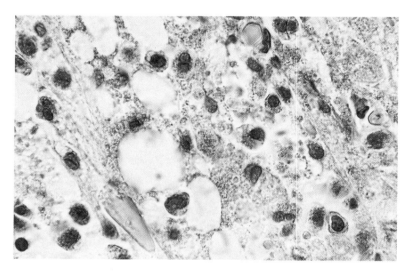

Fig. 1.45 Trephine biopsy in acute eosinophilic leukaemia showing numerous eosinophils and part of a Charcot–Leyden crystal (same case as Fig. 1.44, courtesy of Dr A Smith and Dr Bridget Wilkins, Newcastle-on-Tyne). H & E × 870

either free or within macrophages (Fig. 1.45). Occasionally similar crystals are seen within leukaemic cells (Fig. 1.46).

Cytochemistry in eosinophilic leukaemia

Blast cells of eosinophil lineage are positive with MPO and SBB. With the SBB stain, the granule core may be left unstained. Peroxidase activity differs from that of the neutrophil lineage in being resistant to cyanide [35]. Cells of the eosinophil lineage are usually CAE negative but neoplastic eosinophils are sometimes positive (see page 92). A combined cytochemical stain for CAE and cyanide-resistant peroxidase activity is a convenient means of distinguishing cells of neutrophil and eosinophil lineage [35].

Acute basophilic leukaemia

Cases of basophilic leukaemia with a minimum of 30% bone marrow blasts should be classified as AML. They can be assigned to FAB categories with the abbreviation 'Baso' to indicate the basophilic differentiation. Some cases show maturation and can be

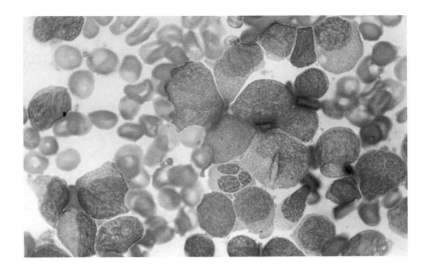

Fig. 1.46 BM aspirate from a patient with acute eosinophilic leukaemia showing a Charcot–Leyden crystal within a leukaemic cell. MGG × 870.

categorized as M2Baso or M4Baso. Others show very little maturation and fall into the M1Baso category. Cases that do not meet the minimal criteria for M1 AML but show evidence of basophil differentiation can be categorized as M0Baso. Cases of M2Baso and M4Baso AML usually have mixed neutrophilic and basophilic differentiation, whereas cases with very primitive basophil precursors (M1 and M0Baso AML) may show only basophilic differentiation. Patients with acute basophilic leukaemia do not usually show features of histamine excess [47] but some patients have had urticaria or gastrointestinal disturbance [48] and anaphylactoid reactions can occur following chemotherapy [49].

In cases with maturation, basophils are usually easily recognized by their cytological and cytochemical characteristics (Fig. 1.47). In other cases with little or no maturation, ultrastructural examination (see Table 1.3) is necessary. Sometimes there are granules with whorls or scrolls (characteristic of mast cells) in addition to typical basophil granules [49]. Blasts of basophil lineage may contain Auer rods [50].

Acute basophilic leukaemia is recognized in the WHO classification [51] (see page 127).

Cytochemistry in basophilic leukaemia

In acute basophilic leukaemia without maturation [52], SBB is commonly negative and MPO is negative by light microscopy. Often CAE is also negative,

although it is weakly positive in later cells of basophil lineage. In cases showing maturation there is positivity with SBB, MPO and CAE, and metachromatic staining with toluidine blue, alcian blue and astra blue. Sometimes, staining with SBB is also metachromatic, granules being grey, black, pinkish or red while granules of the eosinophil and neutrophil lineages are greenish-black. ε-amino caproate activity [53] is specific for the basophil lineage. At an ultrastructural level, ruthenium red can be used to identify basophil granules [52].

Mast cell leukaemia

Mast cell leukaemia can occur either *de novo* or as the terminal phase of urticaria pigmentosa or systemic mastocytosis. However, it should be noted that systemic mastocytosis terminates in other types of AML more often than in mast cell leukaemia. The peripheral blood shows mast cells (Fig. 1.48), which are often immature or morphologically abnormal with hypogranularity or nuclear lobulation. The bone marrow is hypercellular and infiltrated by mast cells (Fig. 1.49). Ultrastructural examination can confirm the diagnosis but it should be noted that in some cases cells show both basophil and mast cell characteristics [54]. As for acute basophilic leukaemia, anaphylactoid reactions may follow chemotherapy [55]. In some patients there is differentiation to both myeloblasts and mast blasts (Fig. 1.50) [56].

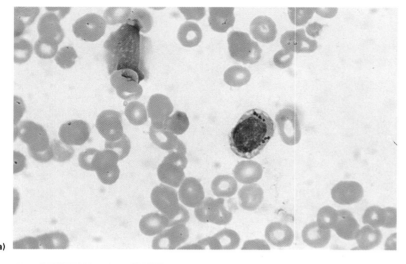

(a)

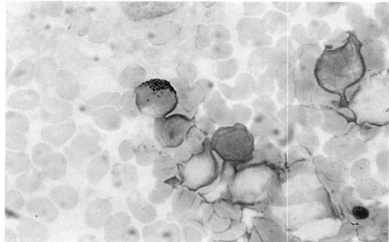

(b)

Fig. 1.47 BM in acute basophilic leukaemia. (a) Vacuolated blast with large granules. MGG × 870. (b) Metachromatic staining, toluidine blue stain × 870.

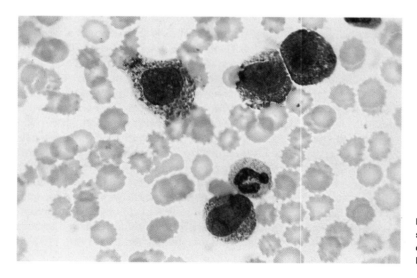

Fig. 1.48 PB in mast cell leukaemia showing a neutrophil and four mast cells (courtesy of Dr I Bunce and Miss Desley Scott, Brisbane). MGG × 870.

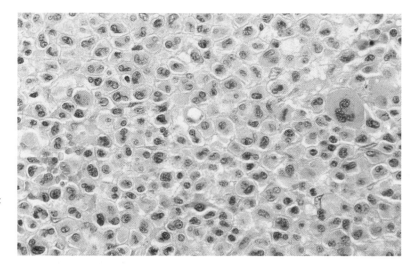

Fig. 1.49 Trephine biopsy from a patient with acute mast cell leukaemia showing irregular nuclei and voluminous cytoplasm (courtesy of Professor G Mufti, London). MGG × 348.

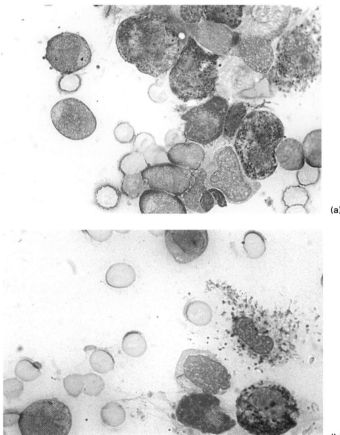

(a)

(b)

Fig. 1.50 BM film from a patient with acute leukaemia showing mast cell and neutrophilic differentiation; (a) blast cells and immature abnormal mast cells; (b) abnormal mast cells and a blast cell containing an Auer rod (courtesy of Dr Neelam Varma, Chandigar). MGG × 870.

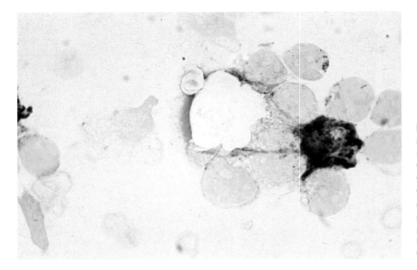

Fig. 1.51 BM film from a patient with acute mast cell leukaemia showing a mature mast cell packed with granules that are strongly positive for mast cell tryptase and several blast cells with tryptase-positive granules; these latter cells are therefore identified as blast cells of mast cell lineage (same patient as Fig. 1.50) (courtesy of Dr Neelam Varma, Chandigar and Dr Bridget Wilkins).

Cytochemistry in mast cell leukaemia

Mast cells stain metachromatically with a Giemsa stain and with toluidine blue, alcian blue and astra blue. They are CAE positive. When cells are relatively agranular, immunocytochemistry for mast cell tryptase is more sensitive than cytochemical staining (Fig. 1.51) [56].

Langerhans' cell and dendritic cell leukaemias

Rare cases of AML show features of Langerhans' cells [57] (Fig. 1.52). Such cases may occur *de novo* but it is likely that cases resembling M5 AML supervening in Langerhans' cell histiocytosis [58] also represent a leukaemia of Langerhans' cells. The diagnosis is made by assessment of cytology and immunophenotype (CD1a is expressed) with the demonstration of Birbeck granules by ultrastructural examination providing a definitive diagnosis. A case of AML showing features of dendritic cell differentiation *in vitro* has also been reported; it resembled M2 AML cytologically and cytochemically [59].

Hypoplastic or hypocellular AML

The majority of cases of AML have a hypercellular bone marrow. However, in a minority of cases the

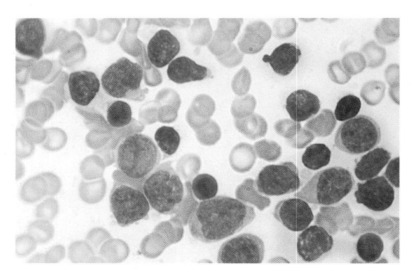

Fig. 1.52 Langerhans' cell leukaemia (courtesy of Dr BIS Srivastava, Buffalo, New York). MGG × 870.

bone marrow is hypocellular. Hypoplastic AML has been variously defined as AML with bone marrow cellularity being less than 50% [60], less than 40% [61], less than 30% [62] or, in the WHO classification, less than 20% [63]. Hypoplastic AML can occur *de novo* or supervene in one of the myelodysplastic syndromes. Often examination of the peripheral blood and bone marrow does not permit a distinction from myelodysplasia since there is often pancytopenia with few circulating blast cells and a hypocellular bone marrow aspirate. Diagnosis is then dependent on identifying more than 30% (or 20%) of blast cells on examination of bone marrow trephine biopsy sections. Hypocellular AML can be assigned to FAB categories, often falling into M0, M1 or M2 categories. Because of the high percentage of lymphoid cells in hypocellular AML it has been suggested that the FAB criteria for the diagnosis of AML should be modified in respect to this subtype so that blasts are counted as a percentage of all nucleated cells with the exception of lymphocytes [64]. Hypocellular AML often has a smouldering clinical course. However, intensive chemotherapy often achieves a complete remission, which may be associated with restoration of normal bone marrow cellularity [64].

Transient abnormal myelopoiesis in Down's syndrome

Neonates with Down's syndrome have been observed to have a condition that closely resembles acute leukaemia but that resolves spontaneously to be later followed, in some but not all cases, by acute leukaemia, which does not resolve. This phenomenon has sometimes been regarded as a leukaemoid reaction. However, in a number of cases there has been an additional clonal cytogenetic abnormality in the proliferating cells and in others clonality has been shown by molecular genetic analysis [65, 66]. It therefore seems likely that transient abnormal myelopoiesis is actually a spontaneously remitting leukaemia. These cases have hepatosplenomegaly, anaemia and sometimes thrombocytopenia with large numbers of blasts in the blood and marrow (Figs 1.53 & 1.54). Hydrops fetalis can occur [67]. Some affected fetuses die *in utero* and some babies die as a result of bone marrow and liver dysfunction. The abnormal cells are often megakaryoblasts but sometimes have features of primitive erythroid cells or of basophiloblasts [68]. The acute leukaemia that follows in some cases, usually after an interval of years, is not necessarily of the same morphological type and may show the same or a different cytogenetic abnormality. These transient leukaemias may be described morphologically according to the FAB classification, but they should not be grouped with other cases of acute leukaemia in neonates since the prognosis differs and in view of the high probability of spontaneous remission it is generally considered that only supportive treatment is indicated.

In the WHO classification, transient abnormal myelopoiesis of Down's syndrome is recognized as a variant of acute megakaryoblastic leukaemia [51].

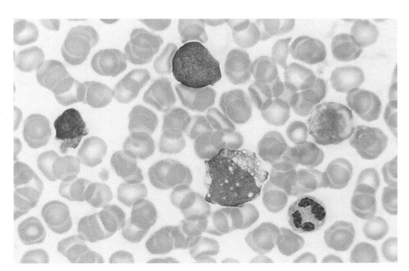

Fig. 1.53 PB of a neonate with transient abnormal myelopoiesis of Down's syndrome showing a neutrophil, a giant platelet, an unidentifiable abnormal cell, a blast cell and a micromegakaryocyte. The blast cells were demonstrated to be megakaryoblasts by immunophenotyping. MGG × 870.

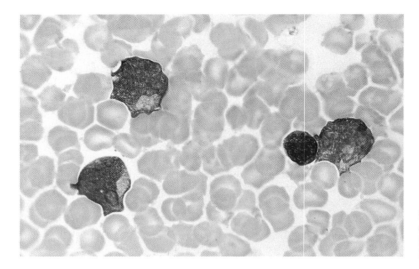

Fig. 1.54 BM film of the same patient as shown in Fig. 1.53 showing a lymphocyte and three pleomorphic blasts. MGG × 870.

The immunophenotype in transient abnormal myelopoiesis differs from that in AML occurring in older infants with AML (see page 65).

Clinical correlates of FAB categories of AML

The FAB category of M3 AML is a distinct disease entity (see page 85). Otherwise there are only minor clinical differences between FAB categories. M4 and M5 AML are associated with more hepatosplenomegaly, skin infiltration and gum infiltration. M0 AML [69] and M6 AML are associated with complex cytogenetic abnormalities and with a worse prognosis than other categories. In general the morphological–immunological–cytogenetic–molecular genetic (MIC–M) categories of AML, as described in Chapter 2, are of more clinical significance than the FAB categories.

The classification of ALL

ALL was initially largely a diagnosis of exclusion. Although some cases had characteristic cytological features, others were categorized as 'lymphoid' only because they did not show any definite cytological or cytochemical evidence of myeloid differentiation. With the availability of a wide range of monoclonal antibodies directed at antigens expressed on lymphoid cells, the diagnosis of ALL should now be based on positive criteria. The role of immunophenotyping

in the diagnosis and classification of ALL will be discussed in detail in Chapter 2. It is sufficient at this stage to say that ALL is classified broadly as B lineage and T lineage. B-lineage ALL includes a small minority of cases with the immunophenotypic features of mature B cells (regarded as non-Hodgkin's lymphoma rather than as acute lymphoblastic leukaemia in the WHO classification) and a large majority of cases with the immunophenotype of B-cell precursors. The latter group includes a major subset designated common ALL.

The FAB group have assigned ALL to three cytological categories: L1, L2 and L3. The classification is summarized in Table 1.11. Apart from a strong correlation between L3 cytological features and a mature B phenotype there is little relationship between the cytological features and the immunophenotype. The recognition of ALL L3 is generally straightforward but the categorization of a case as L1 or L2 can be difficult. However, it is of little clinical significance whether the cytological features are those of L1 or L2 ALL.

It should be noted that although myeloblasts do not show any appreciable chromatin condensation, lymphoblasts may do so. This is often noticeable in some of the smaller blasts in common ALL of L1 type. It has also been noted that a minority of cases of T-lineage ALL, particularly those with a relatively mature immunophenotype, have leukaemic cells that are difficult to recognize as blasts because of

Table 1.11 Morphological features of ALL subtypes.

FAB category	L1 ALL	L2 ALL	L3 ALL
Cell size	Mainly small	Large, heterogeneous	Large, homogeneous
Nuclear chromatin	Fairly homogeneous, may be condensed in some cells	Heterogeneous	Finely stippled, homogeneous
Nuclear shape	Mainly regular	Irregular; clefting and indentation common	Regular; oval or round
Nucleolus	Not visible or small and inconspicuous	Usually visible, often large	Usually prominent
Amount of cytoplasm	Scanty	Variable, often abundant	Moderately abundant
Cytoplasmic basophilia	Slight to moderate	Variable	Strong
Cytoplasmic vacuolation	Variable	Variable	Often prominent

chromatin condensation and inconspicuous nucleoli [70]; immunophenotyping is of importance in these cases.

ALL of L1 subtype

In L1 ALL [3] small cells, up to twice the diameter of a red cell, predominate. They have a high nucleo-cytoplasmic ratio. The nucleus is regular in shape with only occasional clefting or indentation, the chromatin pattern is fairly homogeneous (although smaller cells may show a greater degree of chromatin condensation) and the nucleoli, if visible at all, are small and inconspicuous. The scanty cytoplasm is slightly to moderately basophilic, rarely intensely basophilic, and in some cases shows a variable degree of vacuolation. In a minority of cases there are small numbers of azurophilic granules. Typical examples of L1 ALL are shown in Figs 1.55 and 1.56 and ultrastructural features in Fig. 1.57. The L1 category

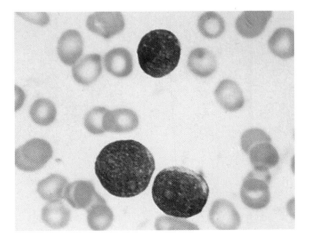

Fig. 1.55 PB film of a patient with L1 acute lymphoblastic leukaemia (ALL). MGG × 870.

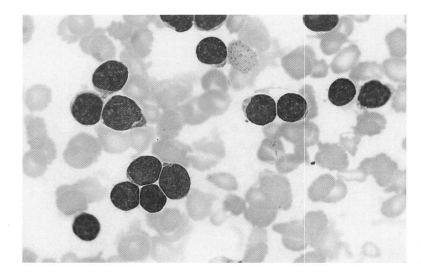

Fig. 1.56 BM film from a patient with L1 ALL. MGG × 870.

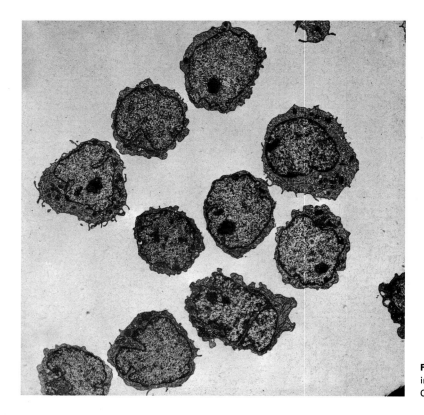

Fig. 1.57 Ultrastructure of lymphoblasts in L1 ALL (courtesy of Professor D Catovsky).

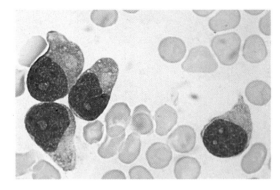

Fig. 1.58 BM film from a patient with L2 ALL showing large pleomorphic blasts; the cells were CD10 (common ALL antigen) positive. MGG × 870.

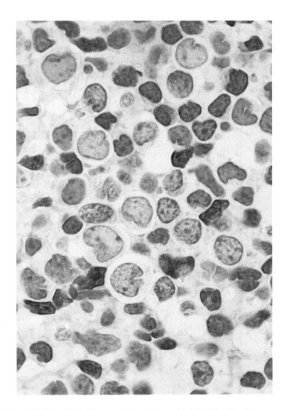

Fig. 1.60 Trephine biopsy of a patient with L2 ALL. Plastic embedded, H & E × 870.

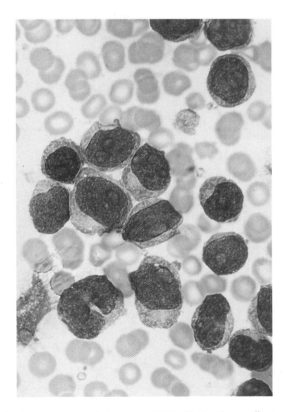

Fig. 1.59 BM film from a patient with L2 ALL showing medium to large pleomorphic blasts which were CD10 negative but positive for CD19, HLA-DR and TdT. MGG × 870.

includes the majority of cases of ALL; in childhood 70–80% of cases fall into this category. L1 ALL may be of B or T lineage.

ALL of L2 subtype

In L2 ALL [3] the blasts are larger and more heterogeneous. The nucleocytoplasmic ratio is variable from cell to cell but the cytoplasm, which shows a variable degree of basophilia, may be moderately abundant. The nuclei are irregular in shape with clefting, folding and indentation being common, and with heterogeneity also of the chromatin pattern. Nucleoli are usually present and may be large. A variable degree of cytoplasmic vacuolation may be present, and in a minority of cases there are small numbers of azurophilic, but peroxidase-negative, granules. Typical examples of L2 ALL are shown in Figs 1.58–1.60. About a quarter of cases of ALL fall into the L2 category. L2 ALL may be of B or T lineage.

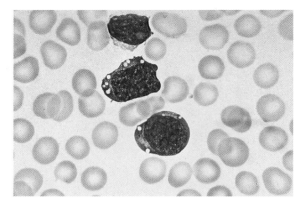

Fig. 1.61 PB film of a patient with L3 ALL with the immunological phenotype being mature B cell. MGG × 870.

ALL of L3 subtype

In L3 ALL [3] the blast cells are large but homogeneous. The nucleocytoplasmic ratio is lower than in L1 ALL. The nucleus is regular in shape, varying from round to somewhat oval. The chromatin pattern is uniformly stippled or homogeneous, with one or more prominent, sometimes vesicular, nucleoli. In contrast to L1 and L2 ALL, in which mitotic figures are uncommon, the mitotic index is high and many apoptotic cells are seen. The cytoplasm is strongly basophilic with variable but prominent-vacuolation. Typical examples of L3 ALL are shown in Figs 1.61–1.64. L3 ALL constitutes only 1–2% of cases of ALL.

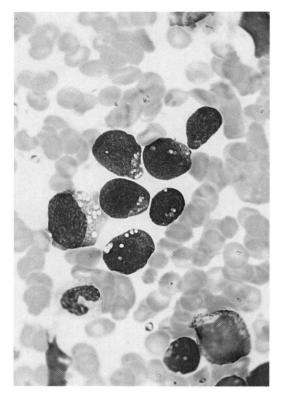

Fig. 1.62 BM film of a patient with L3 ALL with the immunological phenotype being mature B cell. MGG × 870.

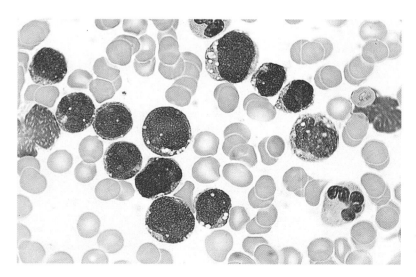

Fig 1.63 PB film of a case of L3 ALL which was unusual in being of T lineage and having a t(7;9) translocation. MGG × 870.

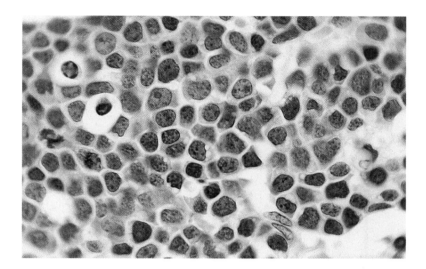

Fig. 1.64 Trephine biopsy from a patient with L3 ALL, B-cell phenotype; vacuolation of some of the blasts can be observed and there are two blasts undergoing apoptosis. Paraffin embedded, H & E × 870.

ALL of L3 subtype is often the leukaemic equivalent of Burkitt's lymphoma, since an aspirate performed on a lymph node or other tissue affected by this lymphoma shows cells that are cytologically the same as those of L3 ALL. 'Acute leukaemia with Burkitt's lymphoma cells' was first described in 1972 [71], although the occurrence of bone marrow infiltration and a terminal leukaemic phase of endemic African Burkitt's lymphoma had been recognized earlier than this.

The great majority of cases of L3 ALL have a mature B-cell immunophenotype, i.e. they express surface membrane immunoglobulin (SmIg). Less often cases have a common ALL phenotype, a pre-B immunophenotype (cytoplasmic immunoglobulin positive) [72] or even a T-cell [73] (Fig. 1.63) or a hybrid B–T phenotype [74]. Cases have also been reported of acute leukaemia with L3 morphology with a lack of B or T markers but with the characteristics of very early erythroid cells [75, 76]; as these latter cases had cytogenetic findings usually associated with L3 ALL or Burkitt's lymphoma (see page 124) the involvement of a primitive cell with the potential for both B lymphoid and erythroid differentiation is suggested. Rarely L3 morphology can be found in association with biphenotypic acute leukaemia [77], acute myelomonocytic leukaemia or undifferentiated carcinoma [78].

When a patient shows L3 cytological features, further investigation is essential. This should be initially immunophenotyping and, in B-lineage cases, cytogenetic or molecular genetic analysis. Cases with a mature B phenotype may have specific Burkitt's lymphoma-related translocations; they do poorly with standard ALL management but have a much more favourable prognosis with specific protocols. However, patients with L3 morphology and a mature B phenotype may also have t(14;18)(q32;q21) (see page 125); their prognosis is poor and optimal management has not yet been defined. Cases with L3 cytological features and a B-cell precursor immunophenotype may be found to have t(1;19)(q23;p13) (see page 119); they do not have an adverse prognosis and should be treated as ALL, not with protocols relevant to Burkitt's lymphoma.

Cytochemistry of ALL

There is little relationship between cytochemical reactions and the FAB categories, but somewhat more between cytochemical reactions and immunophenotypic categories.

Lymphoblasts show negative reactions for MPO and CAE. With SBB, very fine, positive cytoplasmic granules may be present but these are usually obscured by the counterstain so that for practical purposes SBB is negative [2]; these very fine granules probably represent mitochondria. Rare cases of apparent ALL have shown coarse granular positivity with SBB [2, 79]. In ALL the great majority of

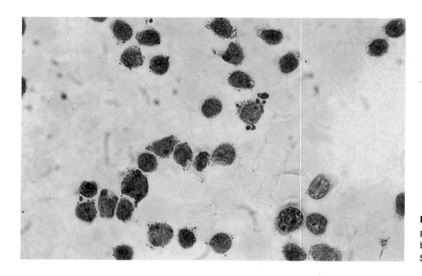

Fig. 1.65 PAS stain of the BM of a patient with common ALL showing block positivity (courtesy of Dr A Eden, Southend-on-Sea). MGG × 870.

neutrophils are MPO positive and show strong positivity with SBB whereas in AML there may be an expanded population of SBB- and MPO-negative neutrophils.

In B-lineage ALL, the PAS stain often shows characteristic block positivity (Fig. 1.65); this is seen also, although perhaps less often, in T-lineage ALL. The blocks and coarse granules of positively staining material are present in PAS-negative cytoplasm, whereas in the case of the block positivity that is seen

much less often in cases of AML (mainly in monoblasts and erythroblasts) the PAS-positive blocks are in cells with a background diffuse or finely granular positivity (see Fig. 1.30e). L3 ALL is usually PAS negative [80].

There is some correlation between PAS positivity and blast vacuolation. In one study of 733 children [81], 28% had more than 10% of vacuolated blasts. This finding correlated strongly with PAS positivity, a relatively low white cell count and the presence of

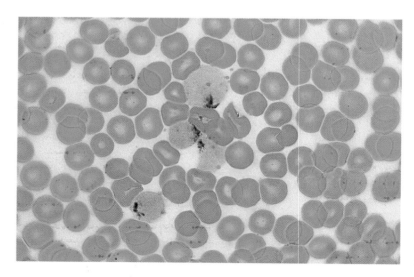

Fig. 1.66 Acid phosphatase stain of the PB of a patient with T-lineage ALL showing focal positivity. MGG × 870.

the common ALL antigen (CD10). When cases had both vacuoles and PAS positivity the chance of CD10 being positive was 98%. Although PAS staining can be useful in the diagnosis of ALL it is important to recognize that PAS block positivity alone is not a sufficient basis for this diagnosis.

The presence of strong localized positivity for acid phosphatase is common in T-lineage ALL (Fig. 1.66) but rare in B-lineage ALL. This pattern should not, however, be regarded as pathognomonic for T-lineage ALL as a similar pattern of staining is not uncommon in M6 AML and may also be seen in M7 AML [13]. In a minority of cases of ALL, the presence of azurophilic granules on the Romanowsky stain can be related to the presence of lysosomal granules, which also show punctate acid phosphatase activity [82]. This phenomenon correlates with B-lineage ALL (mainly common ALL) and with L2 morphology. T lymphoblasts may also have localized coarse granular positivity for NSE (NASDA, ANAE and ANBE), whereas B-lineage blasts either give negative reactions or have scattered fine granules. Neither pattern resembles the strong generalized positivity that is characteristic of cells of monocyte lineage.

In L3 ALL, the vacuoles stain with Oil red O, demonstrating that they contain lipid [80]. However, Oil red O-positive vacuoles are sometimes seen in L1 and L2 ALL, and were also noted in the case of metastatic carcinoma that simulated L3 ALL [78].

Because of their lack of specificity, cytochemical stains should be regarded as redundant in the diagnosis of ALL unless immunophenotyping is unavailable [83] and, when used, there must be a constant awareness of their lack of specificity.

Clinical correlates of FAB categories of ALL

Many cases of L3 ALL represent a distinct entity that requires specific management. However, the categorization of a case as L1 or L2 ALL is of little importance. The FAB L1 category includes more childhood cases with a relatively good prognosis. The incidence of ALL L1 falls with increasing age whereas the incidence of ALL L2 does not vary much with age. ALL L2 has generally been found to have a worse prognosis, although the difference is not major. In some series the prognostic difference disappears if age is allowed for whereas, in others, FAB category is an independ-

ent prognostic factor [84]. The immunophenotype and, to an even greater extent, the cytogenetic and molecular genetic characteristics are of much greater relevance to prognosis and treatment choice than is the FAB category.

Natural killer cell leukaemia

A rare type of leukaemia that is not included in the FAB classification is aggressive natural killer cell leukaemia [85]. The blasts have azurophilic granules and may show natural killer cell function. They do not express CD3 but express CD16 or CD56. Whether it is more appropriate to classify this type of leukaemia with the acute leukaemias or with large granular lymphocyte leukaemia is not yet clear. This entity is discussed further in Chapter 5 (see page 235).

There are other cases expressing CD56 together with a limited range of myeloid markers [86]. These cases express CD7 and CD45 and express CD13, CD33 or both [87]. Some also have MPO detected immunophenotypically, although not cytochemically [87]. In the FAB classification, such cases would be categorized as M0 AML. It has been suggested that they represent leukaemia derived from a myeloid/NK cell precursor [86].

The co-expression of CD56 and myeloid markers is further discussed on page 66.

Problems with the FAB classification of acute leukaemia

Since its inception, there have been criticisms of the FAB classification. These centred on (i) the necessarily arbitrary criteria for FAB categories (ii) the lack of reproducibility between observers (iii) the appropriateness of the criteria for distinguishing between AML and MDS, particularly the requirement for 30% of bone marrow blast cells (iv) the occurrence of unclassifiable cases (v) the failure to include all relevant information in the classification, e.g. there is no consideration of the presence of bi- or tri-lineage dysplasia (Figs 1.67 & 1.68) or of cytogenetic and molecular genetic abnormalities, and immunophenotyping had only a limited role so that biphenotypic leukaemia is not recognized. These criticisms have been largely, although not entirely, addressed by later classifications incorporating new methods of investigation

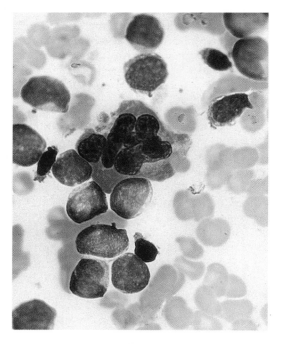

Fig. 1.67 BM of a patient with M1 AML showing a giant erythroid cell. MGG × 870.

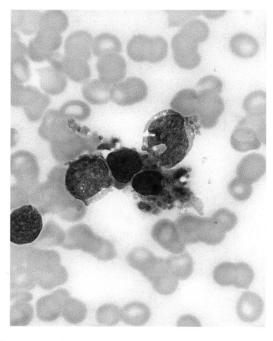

Fig. 1.68 BM of a patient with M4 AML showing two micromegakaryocytes. MGG × 870.

(see Chapter 2) and do not detract from the major significance of the FAB classifications. The FAB classifications brought clarity to a previously confused area. The degree of standardization that was achieved within and between countries greatly improved communication between haematologists and provided a framework for the major advances that subsequently occurred in the genetics and molecular genetics of haematological neoplasms. No other proposed classification was so widely accepted or stood the test of time.

Results of automated full blood counts in acute leukaemia

Modern automated instruments that perform full blood counts detect the majority of cases of AML and ALL, identifying blast cells by means of their light scattering, cytochemical and other characteristics. Current automated Bayer instruments, the H.1 series and Advia, include peroxidase cytochemistry and

produce scatterplots, which are of some use in the further classification of AML (Fig. 1.69) [88]. Cases of ALL and M0 and M7 AML show an abnormal cluster of large, peroxidase-negative cells (Fig. 1.69b). In M1 AML it is apparent that blasts have peroxidase activity (Fig. 1.69c) and in M2 AML the peroxidase activity is stronger (Fig. 1.69d), giving a higher mean peroxidase score. In M3 and M3V AML there is very strong peroxidase activity, giving a characteristic scatterplot, which can provide rapid confirmation of a provisional diagnosis of M3V AML (Fig. 1.69e). M4 (Fig. 1.69f, g) and M5 AML show blasts cells with variable peroxidase activity.

ABX and related instruments employ Sudan black B instead of peroxidase cytochemistry and give similar information to Bayer instruments. Other automated instruments, e.g. those produced by Beckman-Coulter, Sysmex and Abbott, also produce abnormal scatterplots in acute leukaemia. These show some difference between AML and ALL but do not differentiate well between FAB subclasses [89].

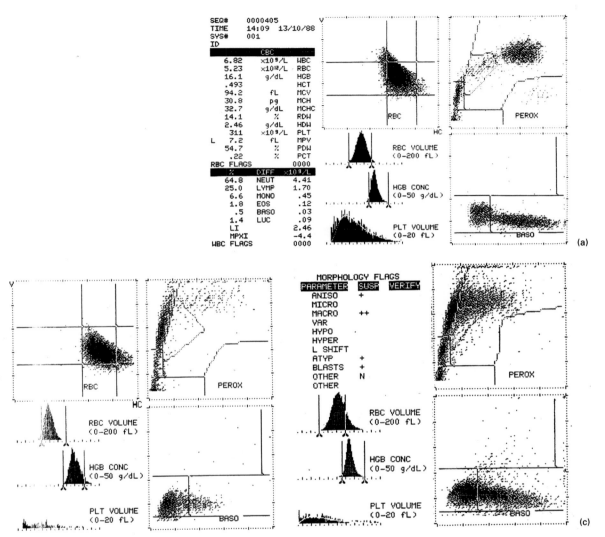

Fig. 1.69 Printouts from Bayer-Technicon H.1 series instruments on blood samples from a healthy volunteer and from patients with AML. (a) Histograms, red cell cytogram and scatterplots on a normal blood sample using a Bayer-Technicon H2 automated blood cell analyser: in the peroxidase cytogram separate clusters are identified, which represent neutrophils, eosinophils, monocytes, lymphocytes and 'large unstained (i.e. peroxidase-negative) cells' (LUC); in the basophil-lobularity channel there is a rounded head, which represents mononuclear cells (monocytes and lymphocytes) and an extended tail, which represents neutrophils and eosinophils. Basophils fall above the horizontal threshold. (b) Histograms, red cell cytogram and scatterplots on a blood sample from a patient with M0 AML performed on a Bayer-Technicon H2 automated analyser: the blasts are peroxidase negative and therefore fall into the LUC area; the only indication that this is an acute myeloid not an acute lymphoblastic leukaemia is that the neutrophil cluster is more dispersed than normal indicating neutrophil dysplasia; note also the dense mononuclear cluster expanded leftwards in the basophil-lobularity channel, which indicates the presence of blasts; the platelet histogram shows that there is severe thrombocytopenia. Similar scattergrams to this are also seen in M7 AML. (c) Histograms and scatterplots on a blood sample from a patient with M1 AML performed on a Bayer-Technicon H2 automated analyser: some of the blasts fall into the LUC area but others have peroxidase activity and thus fall into the areas normally occupied by monocytes and neutrophils; the platelet histogram shows thrombocytopenia. (*Continued on p. 52*)

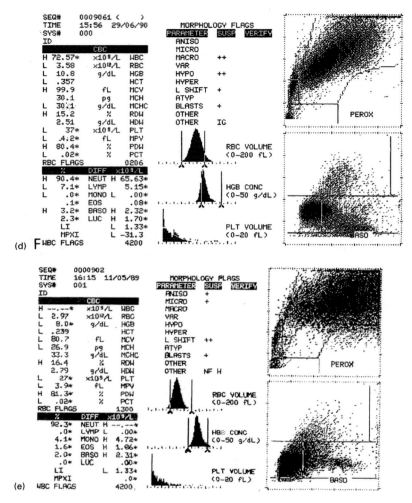

Fig. 1.69 (*Continued*) (d) Histograms and scatterplots on a blood sample from a patient with M2 AML performed on a Bayer-Technicon H2 automated analyser: the blasts show more peroxidase activity than those in the case of M1 AML, falling further to the right in the peroxidase histogram; the basophil-lobularity histogram shows the presence of blasts expanding the mononuclear cluster leftwards and, in addition, causing pseudobasophilia since some of them fall in the area normally occupied by basophils; there is also thrombocytopenia. (e) Histograms and scatterplots on a blood sample from a patient with M3V AML performed on a Bayer-Technicon H2 automated analyser; the abnormal promyelocytes are intensely peroxidase positive and form a triangular cluster based on the right-hand margin; there is pseudobasophilia and thrombocytopenia; the scattergrams in M3 AML show the same features as are shown in this case of M3V AML. (*Continued on p. 53*)

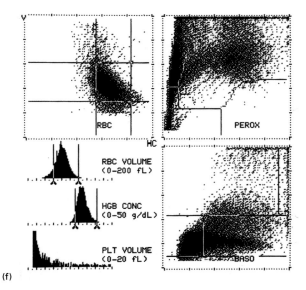

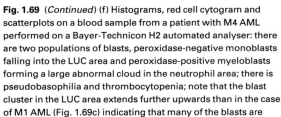

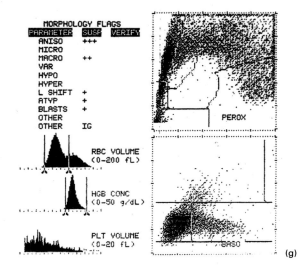

Fig. 1.69 (*Continued*) (f) Histograms, red cell cytogram and scatterplots on a blood sample from a patient with M4 AML performed on a Bayer-Technicon H2 automated analyser: there are two populations of blasts, peroxidase-negative monoblasts falling into the LUC area and peroxidase-positive myeloblasts forming a large abnormal cloud in the neutrophil area; there is pseudobasophilia and thrombocytopenia; note that the blast cluster in the LUC area extends further upwards than in the case of M1 AML (Fig. 1.69c) indicating that many of the blasts are very large. (g) Histograms and scatterplots on a blood sample from a patient with M4Eo AML performed on a Bayer-Technicon H2 automated analyser: the peroxidase scatterplot is similar to that seen in M4 AML but extension into the eosinophil area is apparent; there is pseudobasophilia and thrombocytopenia; the double population shown in the red cell histogram is a result of blood transfusion, the patient having macrocytic red cells and the transfused cells being normocytic.

References

1 Swirsky D and Bain BJ (2001) Erythrocyte and leucocyte cytochemistry—leukaemia classification. In Lewis SM, Bain BJ and Bates I (Eds), *Dacie and Lewis Practical Haematology*. Ninth edition. Churchill Livingstone, London, pp. 269–295.

2 Hayhoe FGJ and Quaglino D (1988) *Haematological Cytochemistry*. Second edition. Churchill Livingstone, Edinburgh.

3 Bennett JM, Catovsky D, Daniel MT, Flandrin G, Galton DAG, Gralnick HR and Sultan C (1976) Proposals for the classification of the acute leukaemias (FAB cooperative group). *Br J Haematol*, **33**, 451–458.

4 Bennett JM, Catovsky D, Daniel MT, Flandrin G, Galton DAG, Gralnick HR and Sultan C (1980) A variant form of acute hypergranular promyelocytic leukaemia (M3). *Br J Haematol*, **44**, 169–170.

5 Bennett JM, Catovsky D and Daniel M-T (1985) Criteria for the diagnosis of acute leukemia of megakaryocytic lineage (M7): a report of the French–American–British cooperative group. *Ann Intern Med*, **103**, 460–462.

6 Bennett JM, Catovsky D, Daniel MT, Flandrin G, Galton DAG, Gralnick HR and Sultan C (1985) Proposed revised criteria for the classification of acute myeloid leukemia. *Ann Intern Med*, **103**, 626–629.

7 Bennett JM, Catovsky D, Daniel MT, Flandrin G, Galton DAG, Gralnick HR and Sultan C (1991) Proposal for the recognition of minimally differentiated acute myeloid leukaemia (AML M0). *Br J Haematol*, **78**, 325–329.

8 Jaffe ES, Harris NL, Stein H and Vardiman JW (Eds) (2001) *World Health Organization Classification of Tumours: Pathology and Genetics of Tumours of Haematopoietic and Lymphoid Tissues*. IARC Press, Lyon.

9 Bennett JM, Catovsky D, Daniel MT, Flandrin G, Galton DAG, Gralnick HR and Sultan C (1982) Proposals for the classification of the myelodysplastic syndromes. *Br J Haematol*, **51**, 189–199.

10 Cuneo A, Ferrant A and Michaux JL (1995) Cytogenetic profile of minimally differentiated (FAB M0) acute

myeloid leukaemia: correlation and clinicobiologic findings. *Blood*, **85**, 3688–3695.

11 Li C-Y and Yam LT (1994) Cytochemistry and immuno-chemistry in hematologic diagnoses. *Hematol Oncol Clin North Am*, **8**, 665–681.

12 Parkin JL, McKenna RW and Brunning RD (1982) Philadelphia-positive blastic leukaemia: ultrastructural and ultracytochemical evidence of basophil and mast cell differentiation. *Br J Haematol*, **52**, 663–677.

13 Polli N, O'Brien M, Tavares de Castro J, Matutes E, San Miguel JF and Catovsky D (1985) Characterization of blast cells in chronic granulocytic leukaemia in transformation, acute myelofibrosis and undifferentiated leukaemia. *Br J Haematol*, **59**, 277–296.

14 Cawley JC and Hayhoe FGJ (1973) *The Ultrastructure of Haemic Cells*. WB Saunders Company, London.

15 Golomb HM, Rowley JD, Vardiman JW, Testa JR and Butler A (1980) 'Microgranular' acute promyelocytic leukaemia: a distinct clinical, ultrastructural and cytogenetic entity. *Blood*, **55**, 253–259.

16 McKenna RW, Parkin J, Bloomfield CD, Sundberg RD and Brunning RD (1982) Acute promyelocytic leukaemia: a study of 39 cases with identification of a hyperbasophilic microgranular variant. *Br J Haematol*, **50**, 201–214.

17 Shaft D, Shtalrid M, Berebi A. Catovsky D and Resnitzky P (1998) Ultrastructural characteristics and lysozyme content of hypergranular and variant type of acute promyelocytic leukaemia. *Br J Haematol*, **103**, 729–739.

18 O'Brien M, Catovsky D and Costello C (1980) Ultrastructural cytochemistry of leukaemic cells. Characterization of the early small granules of monoblasts. *Br J Haematol*, **45**, 201–208.

19 Breton-Gorius J, Van Haeke D, Pryzwansky KB, Guichard J, Tabilio A, Vainchenker W and Carmel R (1984) Simultaneous detection of membrane markers with monoclonal antibodies and peroxidatic activities in leukaemia: ultrastructural analysis using a new method of fixation preserving the platelet peroxidase. *Br J Haematol*, **58**, 447–458.

20 Crisan D, Kaplan SS, Penchansky L and Krause JR (1993) A new procedure for cell lineage determination in acute leukemias: myeloperoxidase mRNA detection. *Diagn Mol Pathol*, **2**, 65–73.

21 Kaleem Z and White G (2001) Diagnostic criteria for minimally differentiated acute myeloid leukemia (AML-M0): evaluation and a proposal. *Am J Clin Pathol*, **115**, 876–884.

22 Cascavilla N, Melillo L, d'Arena G, Greco MM, Carella AM, Sajeva MR *et al.* (2000) Minimally differentiated acute myeloid leukemia (AML M0): clinicobiological findings in 29 cases. *Leuk Lymphoma*, **37**, 105–113.

23 Löwenberg B (2001) Prognostic factors in acute myeloid leukaemia. *Bailliere's Clin Haematol*, **14**, 65–75.

24 Preudhomme C, Warot-Loze D, Roumier C, Grardel-Duflos N, Garand R, Lai JL *et al.* (2000) High incidence of biallelic point mutations in the Runt domain of the AML/PEGBP2αB gene in M0 acute myeloid leukemia and in myeloid malignancies with acquired trisomy 21. *Blood*, **96**, 2862–2869.

25 Elghetany MT (1999) Double esterase staining of the bone marrow contributes to lineage identification in a case of minimally differentiated acute myeloid leukaemia (AML M0). *Clin Lab Haematol*, **21**, 293–295.

26 Creutzig U, Zimmermann M, Ritter J, Henze G, Graf N, Löffler H and Schellong G (1999) Definition of a standard-risk group in children with AML. *Br J Haematol*, **104**, 630–639.

27 Matsuo T, Jain NC and Bennett JM (1988) Nonspecific esterase of acute promyelocytic leukemia. *Am J Hematol*, **29**, 148–151.

28 Brunning RD and McKenna RW (1994) *Tumors of the Bone Marrow*. Third Series, fascicle 9. Armed Forces Institute of Pathology, Washington.

29 Koike T, Tatewaki W, Aoki A, Yoshimoto H, Yagisawa K, Hashimoto S *et al.* (1992) Brief report: severe symptoms of hyperhistaminaemia after the treatment of acute promyelocytic leukemia with tretinoin (all-*trans*-retinoic acid). *N Engl J Med*, **327**, 385–387.

30 Roberts TF, Sprague K, Schenkein D, Miller KB and Relias V (2000) Hyperleucocytosis during induction therapy with arsenic trioxide for relapsed acute promyelocytic leukemia associated with central nervous system infarction. *Blood*, **96**, 4000–4001.

31 Testa JR, Golomb HM, Rowley JD, Vardiman JW and Sweet DL (1978) Hypergranular promyelocytic leukaemia (APL): cytogenetic and ultrastructural specificity. *Blood*, **52**, 272–280.

32 Berger R, Bernheim A, Daniel M-T, Valensi F and Flandrin G (1981) Karyotype and cell phenotypes in primary acute leukemias. *Blood Cells*, **7**, 287–292.

33 Fenaux P, Chomienne C and Degos L (2001) Treatment of acute promyelocytic leukaemia. *Bailliére's Clin Haematol*, **14**, 153–174.

34 Scott CS, Patel D, Drexler HG, Master PS, Limbert HJ and Roberts BE (1989) Immunophenotypic and enzymatic studies do not support the concept of mixed monocytic–granulocytic differentiation in acute promyelocytic leukaemia (M3): a study of 44 cases. *Br J Haematol*, **71**, 505–509.

35 Yam LT, Li CY and Crosby WH (1971) Cytochemical identification of monocytes and granulocytes. *Am J Clin Pathol*, **55**, 283–290.

36 Weltermann A, Pabinger I, Geissler K, Jäger U, Gisslinger H, Knöbl P *et al.* (1998) Hypofibrinogenemia in non-M3 acute myeloid leukemia. Incidence, clinical and laboratory characteristics and prognosis. *Leukemia*, **12**, 1182–1186.

37 Laurencet FM, Chapuis B, Roux-Lombard P, Dayer JM and Beris P (1994) Malignant histiocytosis in the leukemic stage: a new entity (M5c-AML) in the FAB classification? *Leukemia*, **8**, 502–506.

38 Mazzalle FM, Kowal-Vern A, Shrit A, Wibowo AL, Rector JT, Cotelingam JD, Collier J *et al.* (1998) Acute

erythroleukemia: evaluation of 48 cases with reference to classification, cell proliferation, cytogenetics, and prognosis. *Am J Clin Pathol*, **110**, 590–598.

39 Park S, Picard F, Azgui Z, Viguie F, Merlat A, Guesnu M et al. (2002) Erythroleukemia: a comparison between previous FAB approach and the WHO classification. *Leuk Res*, 26, 423–429.

40 Villeval JL, Cramer F, Lemoine A, Henri A, Bettaieb A, Bernaudin F et al. (1986) Phenotype of early erythroblastic leukaemias. *Blood*, **68**, 1167–1174.

41 Hasserjian RP, Howard J, Wood A, Henry K and Bain B (2001) Acute erythremic myelosis (true erythroleukaemia): a variant of AML FAB-M6. *J Clin Pathol*, **54**, 205–209.

42 Yoshida S, Kuriyama K, Miyazaki Y, Taguchi J, Fukushima T, Honda M et al. (2001) De novo acute myeloid leukemia in the elderly: a consistent fraction of long-term survivors by standard-dose chemotherapy. *Leuk Res*, **25**, 33–38.

43 Davey FR, Abraham N, Brunetto VL, MacCallum JM, Nelson DA, Ball ED et al. (1995) Morphological characteristics of erythroleukemia (acute myeloid leukemia; FAB M6): a CALGB study. *Am J Hematol*, **49**, 29–38.

44 Athale UH, Razzouk BI, Raimondi SC, Tong X, Behm FG, Head DR et al. (2001) Biology and outcome of childhood acute megakaryoblastic leukemia: a single institution's experience. *Blood*, **87**, 3727–3732.

45 Tallman MS, Neuberg D, Bennett JM, Franscois CJ, Paietta E, Wiernik PH et al. (2000) Acute megakaryocytic leukemia: the Eastern Cooperative Oncology Group experience. *Blood*, **96**, 2405–2411.

46 Swirsky DM, Li YS, Matthews JG, Flemans RJ, Rees JKH and Hayhoe FGJ (1984) 8;21 translocation in acute granulocytic leukaemia: cytological, cytochemical and clinical features. *Br J Haematol*, **56**, 199–213.

47 Peterson LC, Parkin JL, Arthur DC and Brunning RD (1991) Acute basophilic leukaemia: a clinical, morphologic, and cytogenetic study of eight cases. *Am J Clin Pathol*, **96**, 160–170.

48 Duchayne E, Demur C, Rubie H, Robert A and Dastugue N (1999) Diagnosis of acute basophilic leukemia. *Leuk Lymphoma*, **32**, 269–278.

49 Bernini JC, Timmons CF and Sandler ES (1995) Acute basophilic leukemia in a child: anaphylactoid reaction and coagulopathy secondary to vincristine-mediated degranulation. *Cancer*, **75**, 110–114.

50 Castoldi G and Cuneo A (1996) Special cytological subtypes of acute myeloid leukaemias and myelodysplastic syndromes. *Bailliére's Clin Haematol*, **9**, 19–33.

51 Brunning RD, Matutes E, Flandrin G, Vardiman J, Bennett J, Head D and Harris NL (2001) Acute myeloid leukaemia, not otherwise categorized. In Jaffe ES, Harris NL, Stein H and Vardiman JW (Eds), *World Health Organization Classification of Tumours: Pathology and Genetics of Tumours of Haematopoietic and Lymphoid Tissues*. IARC Press, Lyon, pp. 91–105.

52 Wick MR, Li C-Y and Pierre RV (1982) Acute nonlymphocytic leukemia with basophilic differentiation. *Blood*, **60**, 38–45.

53 Yam LT, Yam C-F and Li CY (1980) Eosinophilia and systemic mastocytosis. *Am J Clin Pathol*, **73**, 48–54.

54 Schmiegelow K (1990) Philadelphia chromosome-negative acute hemopoietic malignancy: ultrastructural, cytochemical and immunocytochemical evidence of mast cell and basophil differentiation. *Eur J Haematol*, **44**, 74–77.

55 Labar B, Mrsić M, Boban D, Batinic′ D, Markovic′-Glamoak M, Hitrec V et al. R (1994) Acute mastocytic leukaemia—case report. *Br J Haematol*, **87**, Suppl 1, 13.

56 Varma N, Varma S and Wilkins B (2000) Acute myeloblastic leukaemia with differentiation to myeloblasts and mast cell blasts. *Br J Haematol*, **111**, 991.

57 Srivastava BIS, Srivastava A and Srivastava MD (1994) Phenotype, genotype and cytokine production in acute leukaemia involving progenitors of dendritic Langerhans' cells. *Leuk Res*, **18**, 499–512.

58 Fontana J, Koss W, McDaniel D, Jenkins J and Whelton W (1989) Histiocytosis X and acute monocytic leukaemia. *Am J Med*, **82**, 137–142.

59 Santiago-Schwarz F, Coppock DL, Hindenberg AA and Kern J (1994) Identification of malignant counterpart of the monocyte–dendritic cell progenitor in an acute myeloid leukemia. *Blood*, **84**, 3054–3062.

60 Needleman SW, Burns P, Dick FR and Armitage JO (1981) Hypoplastic acute leukaemia. *Cancer*, **48**, 1410–1414.

61 Howe RB, Bloomfield CD and McKenna RW (1982) Hypoplastic acute leukaemia. *Cancer*, **48**, 1410–1414.

62 Cheson BD, Cassileth PA, Head DR, Schiffer CA, Bennett JM, Bloomfield CD et al. (1990) Report of the National Cancer Institute-sponsored workshop on definitions of diagnosis and response in acute myeloid leukemia. *J Clin Oncol*, **8**, 813–819.

63 Brunning RD, Matutes E, Harris NL, Flandrin G, Vardiman J, Bennett J and Head D (2001) Acute myeloid leukaemia: introduction. In Jaffe ES, Harris NL, Stein H and Vardiman JW (Eds), *World Health Organization Classification of Tumours: Pathology and Genetics of Tumours of Haematopoietic and Lymphoid Tissues*. IARC Press, Lyon, pp. 77–80.

64 Nagai K, Kohno T, Chen Y-X, Tsushima H, Mori H, Nakamura H, Jinnai I, Matsuo T, Kuriyama K, Tomonaga M and Bennett JM (1996) Diagnostic criteria for hypocellular acute leukemia: a clinical entity distinct from overt acute leukemia and myelodysplastic syndrome. *Leuk Res*, **20**, 563–574.

65 Bain B (1991) Down's syndrome—transient abnormal myelopoiesis and acute leukaemia, *Leuk Lymphoma*, **3**, 309–317.

66 Bain BJ (1994) Transient leukaemia in newborn infants with Down's syndrome. *Leuk Res*, **18**, 723–724.

67 Bain BJ, Haynes A, Prentice AG, Luckit J, Swirsky D, Williams Y, Bhavnani M, Barton C and Ezekwesili R (1999) British Society for Haematology Slide Session,

Annual Scientific Meeting, Brighton, 1999. *Clin Lab Haematol*, **21**, 417–425.

68 Bessho F, Hayashi Y, Hayashi Y and Ohga K (1988) Ultrastructural studies of peripheral blood of neonates with Down's syndrome and transient abnormal myelopoiesis. *Am J Clin Pathol*, **88**, 627–633.

69 Venditti A, Del Poeta G, Buccisano F, Tamburini A, Cox C, Stasi R *et al.* (1997) Minimally differentiated acute myeloid leukemia (AML-M0): comparison with 25 cases with other French–American–British subtypes. *Blood*, **89**, 621–629.

70 Gassman W, Haferlach T, Ludwig W-D, Löffler H, Thiel E and Hoelzer D (1996) Diagnostic problems in T-ALL—morphological and cytochemical analysis of the German ALL Study Group Diagnostic Review Panel. *Br J Haematol*, **93**, Suppl 2, 56–57.

71 Stevens DA, O'Conor GT, Levine PH and Rosen RB (1972) Acute leukemia with 'Burkitt's lymphoma cells' and Burkitt's lymphoma. Simultaneous onset in American siblings; description of a new entity. *Ann Intern Med*, **76**, 967–973.

72 Ganick DJ and Finlay JL (1980) Acute lymphoblastic leukemia with Burkitt cell morphology and cytoplasmic immunoglobulin. *Blood*, **56**, 311–314.

73 Koziner B, Mertelsmann R, Andreeff M, Arlin Z, Hansen H, de Harven E *et al.* (1980) Heterogeneity of cell lineages in L3 leukemias. *Blood*, **53**, 694–698.

74 Berman M, Minowada J, Loew JM, Ramsey MM, Ebie N and Knospe WH (1985) Burkitt cell acute lymphoblastic leukemia with partial expression of T-cell markers and subclonal chromosome abnormalities in a man with acquired immunodeficiency syndrome. *Cancer Genet Cytogenet*, **16**, 341–347.

75 Ekblom M, Elonen E, Vuopio P, Heinonen K, Knuutila S, Gahmberg CG and Andersson LC (1982) Acute erythroleukaemia with L3 morphology and the 14q+ chromosome. *Scand J Haematol*, **29**, 75–82.

76 Knuutila S, Elonem E, Heinonen K, Borgström GH, Lakkala-Paranko T, Perkkiö M *et al.* (1984) Chromosome abnormalities in 16 Finnish patients with Burkitt's lymphoma or L3 acute lymphoblastic leukemia. *Cancer Genet Cytogenet*, **13**, 139–151.

77 Wright S, Chucrallah A, Chong YY, Kantarjian H, Keating M and Albitar M (1996) Acute lymphoblastic leukaemia with myeloperoxidase activity. *Leuk Lymphoma*, **51**, 147–151.

78 Castella A, Davey FR, Kurec AS and Nelson DA (1982) The presence of Burkitt-like cells in non-Burkitt's neoplasms. *Cancer*, **50**, 1764–1770.

79 Tricot G, Broeckaert-Van Orshoven, Van Hoof A and Verwilghen RL (1982) Sudan Black B positivity in acute lymphoblastic leukaemia. *Br J Haematol*, **51**, 615–621.

80 Flandrin G, Brouet JC, Daniel MT and Preud'homme JL (1975) Acute leukemia with Burkitt's tumor cells: a study of six cases with special reference to lymphocyte surface markers. *Blood*, **45**, 183–188.

81 Lilleyman JS, Hann IM, Stevens RF, Richards SM and Eden OB (1988) Blast vacuoles in childhood lymphoblastic leukaemia. *Br J Haematol*, **70**, 183–186.

82 Darbyshire PJ and Lilleyman JS (1987) Granular acute lymphoblastic leukaemia of childhood: a morphological phenomenon. *J Clin Pathol*, **40**, 251–253.

83 General Haematology Task Force of the British Committee for Standards in Haematology (1996) The role of cytology, cytochemistry, immunophenotyping and cytogenetic analysis in the diagnosis of haematological neoplasms. *Clin Lab Haematol*, **18**, 231–236.

84 Mandelli F, Annino L and Rotoli B for the GIMEMA Cooperative Group Italy (1996) The GIMEMA ALL 0183 trial: analysis of 10-year follow-up. *Br J Haematol*, **92**, 665–672.

85 Prieto J, Rios E, Parrado A, Martin A, de Blas JM and Rodriguez JM (1996) Leukaemia of natural killer cell large granular lymphocyte type with HLA-DR-CD16-CD56[bright+] phenotype. *J Clin Pathol*, **49**, 1011–1013.

86 Suzuki R, Yamamoto K, Seto M, Kagami Y, Ogura M, Yatabe Y *et al.* (1997) CD7+ and CD56+ myeloid/natural killer cell precursor acute leukemia: a distinct hematolymphoid disease. *Blood*, **90**, 2417–2148.

87 Inaba T, Shimazaki C, Sumikuma T, Ochiai N, Okano A, Hatsuse M *et al.* (2001) Clinicopathological features of myeloid/natural killer (NK) cell precursor acute leukemia. *Leuk Res*, **25**, 109–113.

88 d'Onofrio G and Zini G, translated by Bain BJ (1997) *Morphology of the Blood.* Verduci Editore, Rome, and Heinemann, London.

89 Hoyer JD, Fisher CP, Soppa VM, Lantis KL and Hanson CA (1996) Detection and classification of acute leukemia by the Coulter STKS Hematology Analyzer. *Am J Clin Pathol*, **106**, 352–358.

CHAPTER 2

ACUTE LEUKAEMIA

Immunophenotypic, Cytogenetic and Molecular Genetic Analysis in the Classification of Acute Leukaemia—the EGIL, MIC, MIC–M and WHO Classifications

Introduction

Cytology and cytochemistry are fundamental to the diagnosis and classification of the acute leukaemias but important and often essential information is also gained from immunophenotyping, cytogenetic analysis and molecular genetic (DNA or RNA) analysis.

Leukaemic cells of different types express characteristic nuclear, cytoplasmic and cell surface antigens. This is referred to as the immunophenotype of the cell. Characterization of the immunophenotype is referred to as immunophenotyping and is achieved by means of labelled antibodies that recognize specific epitopes of cellular antigens. In general, the most useful antibodies are monoclonal antibodies (McAb) produced by hybridoma technology but, for some antigens, polyclonal antibodies (PcAb) (antisera) are better. The technique employed for immunophenotyping may be immunocytochemistry or, much more often, flow cytometry. Immunophenotyping is essential for the diagnosis of B- or T-lineage acute lymphoblastic leukaemia (ALL). In acute myeloid leukaemia (AML), immunophenotyping is particularly important in the diagnosis of M0 and M7 AML and AML with an early erythroid phenotype. Immunophenotyping is essential for the identification of biphenotypic leukaemia and undifferentiated stem cell leukaemia (see below). The immunophenotype can form the sole basis of a classification of AML [1] as well as ALL but more often it is used in conjunction with a morphological classification.

Cytogenetic analysis is conventionally carried out by microscopic analysis of the chromosomes of cells in metaphase. The chromosomes are stained with Giemsa or other cytochemical (sometimes fluorescent) stains to establish a banding pattern characteristic of each chromosome. Cytogenetic analysis can be supplemented by *in situ* hybridization techniques, particularly fluorescence *in situ* hybridization (FISH).

Molecular genetic analysis may be based on analysis of DNA by techniques such as Southern blot analysis or the polymerase chain reaction (PCR) or on analysis of RNA by reverse transcriptase PCR (RT-PCR). The purpose of molecular genetic analysis may be either the establishment of clonality, by detection of rearrangement of immunoglobulin or T-cell receptor (*TCR*) genes in ALL, or the identification of a molecular rearrangement characteristic of a specific type of AML or ALL. The results of cytogenetic and molecular genetic analysis should be interpreted only in the light of the cytological features since the same chromosomal abnormalities may be found in both acute and chronic leukaemia, in both AML and ALL, or in both AML and the myelodysplastic syndromes (MDS). However, there are some cytogenetic abnormalities that identify a subtype of AML with such high specificity that the subtype may be defined more accurately by the karyotype than by the morphology.

Immunophenotypic and cytogenetic information can be combined with the French–American–British (FAB) classification subtype to describe individual cases of acute leukaemia more fully and to divide patients into distinct groups with differing prognoses. This was the basis of the proposals made by the morphologic–immunologic–cytogenetic (MIC) classification groups [2, 3]. Since the MIC classifications were proposed, there have been major advances in the molecular genetics of leukaemia and there is now a need to add this to the classification, creating a MIC–M classification [4]. For both AML and ALL, the underlying cytogenetic and molecular genetic abnormality is of more importance for prognosis and choice of treatment than the morphological or even the immunophenotypic features. It is therefore likely that classifications based on MIC–M principles will become increasingly important. The WHO classification adopts this principle for a number of the entities for which adequate information is available [5].

Immunophenotyping in acute leukaemia

Immunophenotyping is indicated in all cases of acute leukaemia that are not obviously myeloid, in order to make a positive diagnosis of ALL and recognize all cases of M0 and M7 AML. A possible further indication is the recognition of an immunophenotype that is likely to indicate a specific subtype of acute leukaemia. If the detection of minimal residual disease becomes important in the management of patients with acute leukaemia, as appears very likely, the application of immunophenotyping for the recognition of a leukaemia-associated immunophenotype may also become important. Specific surface membrane antigens of normal and leukaemic cells can be recognized by antibodies. Using appropriate techniques, cytoplasmic and intranuclear antigens can also be recognized. The antibodies used may be

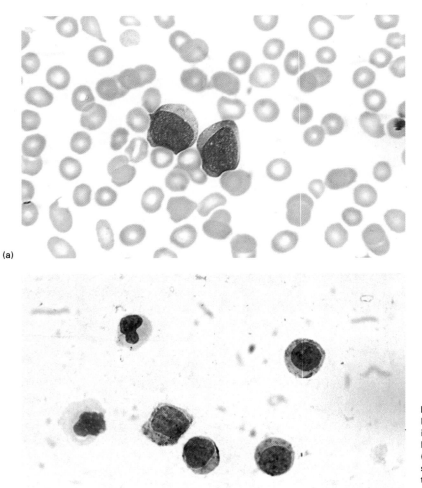

(a)

(b)

Fig. 2.1 M0 acute myeloid leukaemia (AML) investigated by immunophenotyping. (a) Peripheral blood (PB) film. May–Grünwald–Giemsa (MGG) × 870. (b) Cytospin preparation stained by immunoperoxidase technique with a CD13 monoclonal antibody, showing two negative lymphocytes and four positive blasts. Immunoperoxidase × 870.

polyclonal, raised by the immunization of an animal, usually a rabbit, with normal or leukaemic cells. More often antibodies are monoclonal, being secreted by clones of cells obtained by hybridizing an antibody-producing cell with a mouse myeloma cell, thus immortalizing it. McAb resulting from this hybridoma technology are stable and their specificity can be defined. A large number of antibodies have been characterized by a number of workshops (the International Workshops on Human Leukocyte Differentiation Antigens) and those recognizing the same antigen have been allocated to a cluster of differentiation, identified by a CD number. Hybridoma technology has led to the wide availability of antibodies suitable for typing leukaemic cells and has made the standardization of techniques possible.

The identification of antigens within or on the surface of leukaemic cells is known as immunophenotyping. Flow cytometry techniques may identify only surface membrane antigens but, if the cell is fixed or 'permeabilized', cytoplasmic and nuclear antigens can also be recognized. Techniques for recognizing that an antibody has bound to a cell include immunoenzymatic and immunofluorescence techniques. Immunoenzymatic techniques are applicable to fixed cells and therefore permit recognition of both surface and intracellular antigens. Either the primary antibody or a second antibody directed against antigens of the primary antibody is conjugated to an enzyme such as peroxidase or alkaline phosphatase, which produces a brown or red reaction product, visible by light microscopy. Use of both peroxidase and alkaline phosphatase conjugated to different antibodies permits detection of co-expression of two antigens on a single cell. Immunocytochemical techniques have the advantage that the cytological characteristics of the cells can be identified (Fig. 2.1) but because such techniques are very labour-intensive they have largely been replaced by flow cytometry.

In immunofluorescence techniques, the antibody is bound to a fluorochrome, which emits light detectable by fluorescence microscopy or flow cytometry. Flow cytometry immunophenotyping is a technique by which a stream of cells, labelled with an antibody conjugated to a fluorescent dye, flows past a detector so that cells can be counted, sized (by forward light scatter) and characterized (by means of sideways light-scatter, which reflects, particularly, granularity); cytoplasmic vacuolation affects both forward and sideways light scatter. Flow cytometry can also

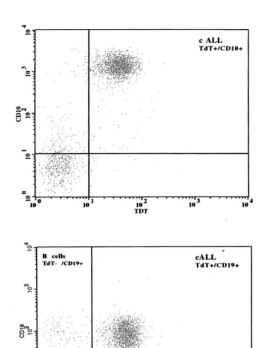

Fig. 2.2 Immunophenotyping of a case of acute leukaemia by flow cytometry with two-colour immunofluorescence: the upper scatterplot shows leukaemic cells which are positive for CD10 and terminal nucleotidyl transferase (TdT), the cells that are negative for both being residual normal cells; the lower plot shows cells that are positive for both CD19 and TdT, which represent leukaemic cells, while there are two clusters of TdT-negative cells, which are positive and negative respectively, for CD19—these represent residual normal B cells and T cells (courtesy of Mr Ricardo Morilla, London).

be used to identify and exclude non-viable cells by differential binding of specific dyes. These methods are applicable to either unaltered cells, in which case only surface antigens are detected, or 'permeabilized' cells, permitting detection of intracellular antigens [6]. Co-expression of antigens on single cells or populations of cells can be detected by using two or more antibodies conjugated to different fluorochromes with specific emission spectrums (Fig. 2.2). Flow cytometry has the advantage that it is rapid and quantification of the percentage of positive cells is more precise

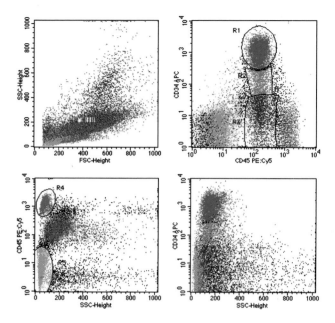

Fig. 2.3 Four-colour flow cytometry immunophenotyping showing characteristics of various types of cell. Standard analysis regions (R1–R3) are set to delinate stages of myeloid blast cell differentiation: R1, the most immature blast cells (CD34+++); R2, maturing blast cells (CD34+); R3, mature blast cells and maturing granulocytes; R4, normal lymphocytes (based on CD45+++ expression and sideways scatter (SSC) characteristics (SSC+); R5, nucleated red cells, which are CD45–, SSC–. These regions can be systematically applied to simultaneously assess a series of antibody combinations relevant to the classification of AML (courtesy of Dr S. Richards, Leeds).

because many more cells are evaluated. On the one sample, it is possible to determine forward and sideways light scatter, examine the co-expression of up to four antigens and quantitate the strength of antigen expression more precisely than is possible by immunocytochemical techniques (Fig. 2.3). Results of flow cytometry may be more accurate if analysis is performed on abnormal cell populations that have initially been selected by a process known as 'gating', e.g. by the use of expression of CD45 (common leucocyte antigen) combined with side-scatter analysis; CD45 expression increases as cells mature and side scatter of light is also greater in the case of more mature cells [7]. Alternatively it is possible to gate on B cells, T cells or probable blast cells (the latter identified by their light-scattering characteristics and CD45 expression).

Several standard panels for the initial phenotyping of acute leukaemia have been proposed [2, 8–14]. The more important McAb and PcAb used in acute leukaemia diagnosis and classification are shown in Table 2.1 [15] and the panels recommended by the European Group for the Immunological Characterization of Leukemias (EGIL) [11], the US-Canadian Consensus Group [13] and the British Committee for Standards in Haematology (BCSH) [14] in Tables 2.2 to 2.4. Approaches to the selection of an antibody panel differ. One approach is to have a relatively

small primary panel, which is chosen according to the provisional diagnosis, and a secondary panel, which is applied selectively, depending on the results with the first panel [14]. This is the only approach that can be followed if there is only limited material available and it has the advantage that it is economical with reagents. However, it does require the application of judgement and, if the provisional diagnosis or the initial interpretation is wrong, an inappropriate panel of antibodies may be applied. An alternative approach is to use a general comprehensive panel. This means that a large amount of information is gathered speedily without the need for decisions to be made with regard to the choice of antibodies. Reagent costs are necessarily higher but there is a greater probability that all necessary data will be collected.

In addition to its role in the recognition of myeloid, lymphoid and biphenotypic acute leukaemia, immunophenotyping often reveals an aberrant phenotype. This can be useful in monitoring minimal residual disease after induction of remission. Minimal residual disease has been found to be of prognostic significance and in the future its assessment is likely to influence patient management [16, 17]. Multiparameter flow cytometry with a large panel of antibodies permits detection of a leukaemia-related immunophenotype in more than 90% of childhood cases of acute leukaemia [16, 17]. Because the

Table 2.1 Monoclonal (or polyclonal) antibodies useful in the diagnosis and classification of acute leukaemia.

Cluster of differentiation or other specificity*	Specificity within haemopoietic lineage
Antibodies identifying antigens expressed mainly in haemopoietic precursors	
CD34	B-lineage lymphoblasts, early T-cell precursors, myeloid progenitors, blast cells in most cases of AML and undifferentiated acute leukaemia
HLA-DR	Major histocompatibility complex, class II antigens; expressed on B lymphocytes and B-lymphocyte progenitors, activated T lymphocytes, blast cells of a small minority of cases of T lineage ALL, monocytes and their precursors, myeloid precursors, blast cells of most cases of AML
Anti-TdT (terminal deoxynucleotidyl transferase)	Blast cells of ALL (stronger in B-lineage than T-lineage blasts), more weakly expressed in blasts in 10–20% of AML
Antibodies identifying antigens expressed in all leucocytes	
CD45	Common leucocyte antigen; use of CD45 permits gating on blast cells which express CD45 and have low sideways light scatter—however note that leukaemic blast cells, particularly B-lineage lymphoblasts may fail to express CD45 or may express it weakly; cells of neutrophil lineage show increased CD45 expression with maturation; monocytes and eosinophils show stronger expression than neutrophils
Antibodies identifying antigens expressed mainly in B cells	
CD10	Common ALL antigen; expressed on a subset of B-cell progenitors, blast cells of about 90% of cases of B-lineage ALL, more weakly expressed in some T-lineage ALL (*c.* 15–20%), some follicular lymphomas and multiple myeloma cells, expressed by neutrophils
CD19	B lymphocytes and B-lymphocyte precursors, blast cells of B-lineage ALL
CD20	B lymphocytes, some B-lymphocyte precursors, blast cells of some B-lineage ALL
CD22	B lineage: as a surface antigen in B lymphocytes, as a cytoplasmic antigen in B-lymphocyte precursors, as a surface antigen in some B-lineage ALL and as a cytoplasmic antigen in *c.* 98%
CD24	B lymphocytes and precursors, blast cells of B-lineage ALL, activated T lymphocytes, granulocytes (neutrophils and eosinophils)
CD79a	Part of the B-cell receptor; expressed by B cells and their precursors and plasma cells
CD79b	Part of the B-cell receptor; expressed by most normal and abnormal B cells (but not chronic lymphocytic leukaemia cells) and late B-cell precursors (from the pre-B cell onwards)
Anti-immunoglobulin and anti-γ, α, μ, δ immunoglobulin heavy chains	Surface membrane expression in B cells (SmIg), cytoplasmic expression in pre-B cells (cμ chain) and in late B lymphocytes and plasma cells (cIg)
Anti-κ, λ (anti-immunoglobulin light chains)	Surface membrane expression in B lymphocytes and cytoplasmic expression in late B lymphocytes and plasma cells
Antibodies identifying antigens expressed mainly in T cells	
CD1 or CD1a	Cortical thymocytes, blast cells of about 20% of T-lineage ALL, subset of B cells, Langerhans' cells
CD2	Cortical and late thymocytes, mature T lymphocytes, most NK cells, blast cells of *c.* 80% of T-lineage ALL, leukaemias of mature T cells
CD3	Part of the TCR complex; membrane antigen in late thymocytes and mature T lymphocytes, expressed by blast cells in *c.* 25% of T-lineage ALL and in leukaemias of mature T cells, cytoplasmic expression is found in the majority of thymocytes and blast cell of most T-lineage ALL
CD4	Cortical thymocytes (co-expressed with CD8), late thymocytes, subset of mature T cells, some leukaemias of mature T cells (see Table 5.4, p. 207), immature myeloid cells, monocytes and eosinophils

Continued p. 62

Table 2.1 (*Continued*)

Cluster of differentiation or other specificity*	Specificity within haemopoietic lineage
CD5	Cortical and late thymocytes, some early thymocytes, T lymphocytes, blast cells of some T-lineage ALL, small subset of B lymphocytes, some leukaemias and lymphomas of mature B cells and mature T cells (see Tables 5.1, 5.2 and 5.4, p. 204)
CD7	Thymocytes, majority of mature T cells, NK cells, blast cells of T-lineage ALL, subset of immature myeloid cells, blast cells of 5–15% of AML, some leukaemias of mature T cells (see Table 5.4)
CD8	Cortical thymocytes (co-expressed with CD4), late thymocytes, subset of mature T cells, some leukaemias of mature T cells (see Table 5.4)
TCR αβ	Subset of T lymphocytes and some T-lineage ALL
TCR γδ	Small subset of T lymphocytes and blast cells of some T-lineage ALL

Antibodies identifying antigens expressed mainly in myeloid cells

CD11b	C3bi receptor; expressed on mature monocytes, cells of neutrophil lineage with expression increasing with maturation—however mature neutrophils show weaker expression than mature monocytes; blast cells of most monocytic and some granulocytic leukaemias, macrophages, NK cells
CD13	Pan-myeloid: membrane expression in blast cells of c. 80% of cases of AML, cytoplasmic expression in a higher proportion
CD14	Monocytes, macrophages, granulocytes to a lesser extent, blast cells of monocytic and some granulocytic leukaemias
CD15	Maturing myeloid cells (granulocytic more than monocytic)
CD16	Neutrophils and NK cells, weakly expressed on monocytes
CD33	Myeloid progenitors and some maturing myeloid cells (myeloblasts, promyelocytes, myelocytes, monocytes-cells of neutrophil lineage express somewhat less CD33 as they mature and monocytes express CD33 more strongly than neutrophils), blast cells of about 80% of cases of AML
CD36	Platelet glycoprotein IV; expressed on erythroblasts and progenitors, monocytes, macrophages, megakaryoblasts, megakaryocytes and platelets (useful for identifying erythroid cells if megakaryocyte and other myeloid markers are negative)
CD41	Platelet glycoprotein IIb/IIIa complex (CD41a) and platelet glycoprotein IIb (CD41b); expressed on megakaryoblasts, megakaryocytes, platelets
CD42a	Platelet glycoprotein IX; expressed on megakaryoblasts, megakaryocytes, platelets
CD42b	Platelet glycoprotein Ibα: expressed on megakaryoblasts, megakaryocytes, platelets
CD61	Platelet glycoprotein IIIa; expressed on megakaryoblasts, megakaryocytes, platelets
CD64	Monocytes, macrophages, activated granulocytes
CD65	Cells of granulocytic and monocytic lineages (weaker expression on monocytes)
CD71	Erythroid cells of all stages of maturation but not lineage specific; expressed by immature or activated cells of other lineages
CD117	Stem cell factor receptor, c-kit: haemopoietic precursors, myeloblasts, primitive erythroid cells, some megakaryoblasts, mast cells, blasts of AML, myeloma cells in some cases of multiple myeloma
Anti-myeloperoxidase (anti-MPO)	Myeloid cells (granulocytic more than monocytic)—cytoplasmic expression
Anti-lactoferrin	A marker of maturation in the neutrophil lineage so can help to distinguish leukaemic cells from residual normal cells—cytoplasmic expression
Anti-glycophorin A or C	Erythroid cells

For a complete list of the specificities of monoclonal antibodies assigned to each CD category see [15].
ALL, acute lymphoblastic leukaemia; AML, acute myeloid leukaemia; c, cytoplasmic; CD, cluster of differentiation; NK, natural killer; Sm, surface membrane; TCR, T-cell receptor.

Table 2.2 Panel of antibodies recommended by the European Group for the Immunological Characterization of Leukemias (EGIL) for the diagnosis and classification of acute leukaemia [11].

First panel	
B lymphoid	CD19, cCD22, CD79a, CD10
T lymphoid	cCD3, CD2, CD7
Myeloid	Anti-MPO, CD13, CD33, CD65, CD117
Non-lineage specific	TdT, CD34, HLA-DR
Second panel	
If B lineage	cμ, κ, λ, CD20, CD24
If T lineage	CD1a, SmCD3, CD4, CD5, CD8, anti-TCR αβ, anti-TCR γδ
If myeloid	Anti-lysozyme, CD14, CD15, CD41, CD61, CD64, anti-glycophorin A

c, cytoplasmio; CD, cluster of differentiation; MPO, myeloperoxidase; Sm, surface membrane; TCR, T-cell receptor; TdT, terminal deoxynucleotidyl transferase.

Table 2.3 Panel of antibodies recommended by the US-Canadian Consensus Group for the diagnosis and classification of acute leukaemia [13].

Core panel	
B lymphoid	CD10, CD19, anti-kappa, anti-lambda
T lymphoid	CD2, CD5, CD7
Myeloid	CD13, CD14, CD33
Non-lineage related	CD34, HLA-DR
Supplementary panel	
B lymphoid	CD20, Sm/cCD22,
T lymphoid	CD1a, Sm/cCD3, CD4, CD8
Myeloid	CD15, CD16, CD41, CD42b, CD61, CD64, CD71, CD117, anti-MPO, anti-glycophorin A
Non-lineage related	CD38, TdT

c, cytoplasmic; CD, cluster of differentiation; MPO, myeloperoxidase; Sm, surface membrane; TdT, terminal deoxynucleotidyl transferase.

Table 2.4 Panel of antibodies recommended by the British Committee for Standards in Haematology for the diagnosis and classification of acute leukaemia [14].

Primary panel	
B lymphoid	CD19, cCD22, cCD79a, CD10
T lymphoid	cCD3, CD2
Myeloid	CD13, CD117, anti-MPO
Not lineage restricted	TdT
Supplementary panel for selective application	
B lymphoid	cμ, SmIg, CD138
T lymphoid	CD7
Myeloid	CD33, CD41, CD42, CD61, anti-glycophorin A
Not lineage restricted	CD45
Non-haemopoietic	Antibodies for the detection of small round cell tumours of childhood and other non-haemopoietic neoplasms
Optional and potentially useful	
Myeloid	anti-lysozyme, CD14, CD36, anti-PML(McAb PL-M3), HLA-DR (for negativity In M3 AML)
B lymphoid	CD15 and 7.1/NG2 (for *MLL*-rearranged ALL)
T lymphoid	anti-TCR αβ, anti-TCR γδ

c, cytoplasmic; CD, cluster of differentiation; MPO, myeloperoxidase; PML, the nuclear protein encoded by the *PML* gene; SmIg, surface membrane immunoglobulin; TdT, terminal deoxynucleotidyl transferase; 7.1/NG2, a monoclonal antibody recognizing chondroitin sulphate.

immunophenotype may change at relapse it is desirable, when possible, to identify two leukaemia-associated phenotypes for monitoring purposes.

Immunophenotyping in AML

Immunological markers that identify AML and distinguish it from ALL include reactivity with antibodies of the CD13, CD33, CD65 and CD117 clusters and reactivity with antibodies that recognize the myeloperoxidase (MPO) protein including its proenzyme form. CD117 has a higher degree of specificity for the myeloid lineage than CD13 or CD33. CD13 is most sensitive when used with a technique that allows cytoplasmic antigen to be detected, since the antigen appears earlier in the cytoplasm than on the cell membrane [18].

The use of a wider panel of McAb shows different patterns of reactivity within the different FAB classes, although the correlation is not very tight (Table 2.5) [7, 12, 19–32]. CD13, CD33, CD65 and anti-MPO antibodies show little difference between the FAB classes while other McAb show some selectivity for immature cells, for more mature cells, for granulocytic differentiation or for monocytic differentiation. CD13 antibodies react with the leukaemic cells of the majority of cases of M1 to M5 AML but with a somewhat lower percentage of cases being positive when there is monocytic differentiation (M4 and M5); CD13 usually also gives positive reactions in M0 AML. CD33 antibodies are somewhat less likely to give positive reactions in M0 AML but reactions are generally positive in M1 to M5. Most CD15 antibodies are generally negative in M0 and M1 AML but are positive in M2,

Table 2.5 Pattern of reactivity with monoclonal (or polyclonal) antibodies commonly observed in French–American–British (FAB) categories of acute myeloid leukaemia (AML). (Derived from [7, 12, 19–32] and other sources.)

	Markers of precursor cells			Myeloid markers					Monocyte markers	
	TdT*	HLA-DR†	CD34‡	CD13	CD33	CD117	CD15	CD11b	CD14
M0	Pos. or neg.	Pos.	Pos.	Mainly pos.	Pos. or neg.	Often pos.	Mainly neg.	Mainly neg.	Mainly neg.
M1	Pos. or neg.	Pos.	Mainly pos.	Mainly pos.	Pos.	Often pos.	Mainly neg.	Pos. or neg.	Mainly neg.
M2	Neg.	Pos.	Mainly neg.	Pos.	Pos.	Pos.	Pos.	Pos. or neg.	Mainly neg.
M3§	Neg.	Neg.	Neg.	Pos.	Pos.	Pos. or neg.	Pos. or neg.	Mainly neg.	Mainly neg.
M4	Mainly neg.	Pos.	Pos. or neg.	Mainly pos.	Pos.	Pos. or neg.	Pos.	Pos.	Often pos.
M5	Mainly neg.	Pos.	Pos. or neg.	Pos. or neg.	Pos.	Pos. or neg.	Pos.	Pos.	Often pos.
M6**	Neg.	Pos. or neg.	Pos. or neg.	Pos. or neg.	Pos. or neg.	Pos.	Mainly neg.	Pos. or neg.	Mainly neg.
M7††	Neg.	Mainly pos.	Mainly pos.	Mainly neg.	Pos. or neg.	Often pos.	Mainly neg.	Neg.	Neg.
AML overall	10–20% pos.	About 70% pos.	30–40% pos.	60–90% pos.	70–90% pos.	60–70% pos.	40–70% pos.	50–60% pos.	15–40% pos.

*Also positive in acute lymphoblastic leukaemia (ALL) with the exception of the minority of cases with mature-B phenotype.
†Also positive in ALL of B lineage and in occasional cases of T-lineage ALL.
‡Also positive in many B-lineage ALL but not mature B-ALL.
§CD9 positive.
**CD36 and anti-glycophorin positive.
††CD9, CD36, CD41, CD42a, CD42b, CD61 positive.

M4 and M5b [20, 21, 29]. Reactions of CD15 antibodies in AML M3 and M5a are less consistent.

CD11b, CD14 and CD64 antibodies show some specificity for leukaemias with monocytic differentiation. CD14 antibodies are better than CD11b antibodies for distinguishing M4 and M5 AML from M1, M2 and M3 AML [19, 21, 33]. CD68 is also usually positive in M4 and M5 AML but is positive in about 40% of other subtypes [25]. Cases of AML that are positive for CD33 and negative for CD13 and CD34 are usually of the M5 subtype [7]. M5a and M5b AMLs show some differences in their pattern of reaction with McAb. The less mature cells of M5a are more likely to give negative reactions with antibodies of CD13, CD15, CD11b and CD14 clusters [21]. In comparison with other FAB categories, cases of M0 AML more often express TdT, HLA-DR, CD34 and CD7.

M3 and M3V AML show a characteristic pattern of reaction with McAb, which may be of diagnostic importance in distinguishing M3V AML from M5 AML (see page 86 and Table 2.4).

Cases of M4 and M5 AML are usually CD13, CD33, CD4 and HLA-DR positive. Reactions with CD14, CD16 and CD24 show a high degree of specificity for the monocyte lineage but are not very sensitive. CD64 shows high sensitivity and, if weak reactions in M3 are disregarded, high specificity.

Diagnosis of M6 AML, particularly when the cells have an immature phenotype, is aided by the use of immunological markers, but good immunophenotypic markers for very early erythroid cells are lacking. The earliest recognizable erythroid cells express a number of antigens that are not lineage specific including HLA-DR, the transferrin receptor (CD71), certain blood group antigens (A, B and H; I and i) and CD36. Although not specific, CD71 reactivity is suggestive of erythroid differentiation since strong reactivity is rarely present in other myeloid leukaemias [31]. CD36 McAb also reacts with megakaryoblasts and monocytes [29, 34] but can be useful when interpreted in conjunction with other markers. More mature erythroid cells express lineage-specific antigens detectable with either McAb or PcAb. The most commonly employed antibody is anti-glycophorin A. Others that have been used include anti-haemoglobin, anti-carbonic anhydrase I [35], anti-spectrin and antibodies to the Gerbich red cell antigen. Carbonic anhydrase I, detectable by a PcAb, is said to be the earliest specific immunophenotypic marker of the erythroid lineage [35].

Immunological markers are important in the diagnosis of AML M7 since they are more specific than cytochemistry and much more widely available than the platelet peroxidase (PPO) reaction, which requires ultrastructural cytochemistry for its detection. The usual order of appearance of markers in the megakaryocyte lineage is probably HLA-DR, PPO and acid phosphatase followed by CD33, CD34 and α-naphthyl acetate esterase activity, followed in turn by platelet glycoprotein IIIa (CD61), glycoprotein IIb and the IIb/IIIa complex (CD41), glycoprotein IX and Ib (CD42a and b) and finally periodic acid–Schiff (PAS) positivity and expression of the von Willebrand antigen. CD41 and CD61 McAb have some advantages over CD42 McAb: they are more sensitive since the antigen appears earlier, and also are more specific since occasional cases of ALL and M5 AML have been found to be positive with CD42 McAb [36]. In the megakaryocyte lineage, only early cells —megakaryoblasts and immature megakaryocytes— show reactivity with the myeloid McAb CD33 and with the stem cell antigen CD34. It should be noted that adhesion of platelets to leukaemic blasts can cause false positivity for platelet antigens in subtypes of AML other than M7. It has therefore been recommended that positive results by flow cytometry be confirmed by immunocytochemistry [7]. Expression of CD2 and CD7 is common in M7 AML, being observed in 23% and 50% of cases respectively in one series [37].

The immunophenotype in transient abnormal myelopoiesis of Down's syndrome is characteristic [38]. Blasts are usually positive for CD7, CD33, CD36, CD56, CD41 and CD61 but are more often negative for CD11b, CD13, CD14 and CD15. The immunophenotype in AML occurring in older infants with Down's syndrome is similar but blast cells are usually also positive for CD11b and CD13.

In acute mast cell leukaemia, cells are positive for CD13, CD33, CD117 and mast cell tryptase (see Fig. 1.51). They also express various antigens not expressed on normal mast cells, specifically CD2, CD25 and CD38 [39].

Myeloid leukaemias often express immunophenotypic markers that are not lineage specific such as TdT, HLA-DR and CD34. TdT is a marker of immature haemopoietic and lymphoid cells. It is positive in the great majority of cases of ALL but in only 15–20% of cases of AML. Expression is stronger in B-lineage ALL than T-lineage ALL and is weaker in AML [40];

among cases of AML, expression is common in FAB categories characterized by a lack of maturation, i.e. in M0 and M1 AML. Expression of TdT correlates with expression of CD7 and CD34 [41]. Expression is most common among cases of M0 and M1 AML and in some series also among cases of M2 and M4 AML [19, 24, 29, 42]. HLA-DR is also expressed on haemopoietic precursor cells but continues to be expressed up to the myeloblast stage in granulocytic maturation and up to the mature monocyte stage in monocyte maturation. It is therefore widely expressed among cases of AML but, as mentioned above, is generally negative in M3 AML. CD133 is expressed in about 40% of patients with AML but it does not distinguish AML from ALL [43]; its expression in AML correlates with other markers of immaturity, being most frequent in M0 AML and not a feature of M3 AML [43].

Cases of AML may express antigens that are usually viewed as more characteristic of lymphoid leukaemias. The B-lymphoid antigen CD24 is expressed in the majority of cases of M4 and M5 AML but is rarely expressed in other categories of AML [44]. CD7, which is expressed in T lymphocytes and in many cases of T-ALL, is also expressed in 10–25% of cases of AML with expression being more frequent in M0, M1 and M5 [42]. The T-lymphoid antigen CD4 is often expressed in M4 and M5 AML and is sometimes expressed in other subtypes. The T-lymphoid antigen CD2 is expressed in a quarter of cases of M3 AML and is occasionally expressed in other subtypes [26, 45]. The natural killer cell marker CD56 is expressed in about 20–40% of cases of AML and the natural killer marker CD16 in about a quarter [28, 46].

Whether expression of various immunophenotypic markers is of prognostic significance in AML is controversial with conflicting results having been reported in different series of patients. What prognostic significance has been demonstrated may largely reflect the fact that the immunophenotype provides a surrogate marker of certain cytogenetic abnormalities. Expression of a strongly myeloid phenotype (positivity for MPO, CD13, CD33, CD65 and CD117) has been found to correlate with favourable cytogenetic abnormalities and a better prognosis [47]. Conversely, CD56 expression has been found to correlate with unfavourable cytogenetic abnormalities and with a lower complete remission rate and worse survival [48]. CD7 positivity in AML has, however, been found to not only correlate with prognostically

worse karyotypic abnormalities but also to be indicative of worse prognosis within the group of patients with most adverse karyotypes [49].

Immunophenotyping is usually performed on suspensions of peripheral blood or bone marrow cells but, when necessary, can be carried out on histological sections, albeit with a more limited range of antibodies. This is most likely to be necessary in AML M7 and in the WHO category of acute panmyelosis when there may be few blast cells in the peripheral blood, and bone marrow fibrosis makes it difficult to obtain an adequate aspirate. Useful antibodies applicable to decalcified trephine biopsy sections are shown in Table 2.6 [50–52]. Immunohistochemistry can identify an acute leukaemia as myeloid and can identify certain FAB categories, e.g. M6 AML and M7 AML. In cases of M5 AML showing the least maturation, leukaemic cells are positive only for lysozyme, showing focal positivity. Cases with more maturation have diffuse lysozyme activity and are also positive with CD68 and Mac387 McAb [53].

Immunophenotyping in ALL

Immunophenotyping confirms the diagnosis of ALL and separates cases into leukaemias of B lineage and of T lineage. Immunophenotyping can also demonstrate an aberrant lymphoid population in children who present with bone marrow aplasia as a prodrome to ALL [7]. Useful McAb for the identification of B-lineage blasts are CD19, CD79a and CD22 (the latter being most sensitive when used with a method for detection of cytoplasmic antigen—cCD22). CD79b is expressed later in development than CD79a and is thus less useful. It should be noted that, in the WHO classification, cases showing expression of surface membrane (Sm) immunoglobulin (Ig) are categorized as non-Hodgkin's lymphoma whereas the FAB and EGIL classifications categorized such cases as ALL. The WHO approach reflects the fact that immunologically the cells are mature B cells not precursor cells. For T-lineage blasts, the most specific antibody is CD3, which is most sensitive when used with a technique for detection of cytoplasmic antigen (cCD3). Anti-TCR $\alpha\beta$ and anti-TCR $\gamma\delta$ probably have similar specificity. CD2, CD4 and CD7 are all less specific. Since CD7 is also expressed in some cases of AML, it is inappropriate to classify a case of acute leukaemia as T-lineage ALL on the basis of reactivity with CD7 alone.

Table 2.6 Monoclonal antibodies and polyclonal antisera (Pc) useful in the diagnosis of acute leukaemia on paraffin-embedded decalcified trephine biopsy specimens* [50–52].

Category	Antibody	Specificity
CD45	2B11, PD726 RP2/18 RP2/22	Leucocyte common antigen: strong reactions in most lymphoid cells (T and B lineage), weak reactions in blasts of myeloid lineage
TdT	NPT26 or Pc	Terminal deoxynucleotidyl transferase: positive in lymphoblasts but negative in mature lymphoid cells, positive in blasts in a minority of cases of acute myeloid leukaemia (AML)
CD34	QBend 10	Haemopoietic and lymphoid precursors, endothelial cells
CD79a	JCB117, Mb1 HP47/A9	Positive in B-lineage lymphoblasts and lymphocytes
CD10	56C6	Common and pre-B ALL and some mature B ALL/Burkitt's lymphoma; also positive in follicular lymphoma
CD20	L26	Positive in B-lineage lymphocytes, some B-lineage lymphoblasts and follicular dendritic cells
CD3	CD3-12 and Pc	Positive in T-lineage lymphoblasts and lymphocytes
Anti-MPO	Pc	Myeloperoxidase: positive in blasts in AML except in M7 AML and some cases of M0 AML
Anti-neutrophil elastase	NP57	Maturing cells of granulocyte lineage
CD14	Leu M3, NCL-CD14-223	Positive in blasts in some cases of AML, mainly M4 and M5
CD15	Leu M1, BY87	Positive in blasts in some cases of AML, Reed–Sternberg cells and mononuclear Hodgkin's cells
CD68	KP1, PGM1	Positive in blasts in many cases of AML (also monocytes, macrophages, mast cells and cells of some cases of hairy cell leukaemia and chronic lymphocytic leukaemia); note that KP1 has broad specificity and is thus useful for all FAB classes whereas PGM1 is monocyte restricted
Anti-calprotectin (previously calgranulin)	Mac387	Positive in most M4 and M5 AML; positive with both granulocyte and monocyte lineages
Anti-lysozyme	Anti-lysozyme (Pc)	Positive in granulocyte and monocyte lineages
CD61	Y2/51	Megakaryocytes and blasts of M7 AML
CD42b	MM2/174	Megakaryocytes and blasts of M7 AML
Anti-von Willebrand factor	F8/86 or Pc	Megakaryocytes and blasts of M7 AML
Anti-glycophorin A	JC159	Erythroid cells
Anti-glycophorin C	ret40f	Erythroid cells

*Although immature haemopoietic cells are positive for CD117 by flow cytometry, the antibody is not sufficiently sensitive to detect leukaemic blast cells in fixed decalcified trephine biopsy specimens; however mast cell expression is detected.

Table 2.7 EGIL classifications of B-lineage acute lymphoblastic leukaemia [11].

(All categories are positive for CD19 and/or CD79a and/or CD22; most cases, except mature B, are TdT positive)	
B-I (pro-B)	CD10−, cμ−, SmIg−
B-II (common)	CD10+, SmIg−, cμ−
B-III (pre-B)	cμ+
B-IV (mature B)	c or Sm κ or λ

c, cytoplasmic; CD, cluster of differentiation; Ig, immunoglobulin; Sm, surface membrane; TdT, terminal deoxynucleotidyl transferase.

Table 2.8 EGIL classifications of T-lineage acute lymphoblastic leukaemia [11].

(All cases are positive for c or Sm CD3; some cases are CD10 positive)	
T-I (pro-T)	CD7+, CD2−, CD5−, CD8−, CD1a−
T-II (pre-T)	CD2+ and/or CD5+ and/or CD8+, CD1a−
T-III (cortical T)	CD1a+, membrane CD3+ or −
T-IV (mature T)	Membrane CD3+, CD1a−
Group a	Anti-TCR αβ+
Group b	Anti-TCR γδ+

c, cytoplasmic; CD, cluster of differentiation; Sm, surface membrane; TCR, T-cell receptor.

The use of wider panels of antibodies permits the further separation of T-lineage and B-lineage ALL into categories that are believed to reflect the normal maturation within these lineages. More importantly, these categories show some correlation with cytogenetic subsets of ALL and consequently indicate differences in prognosis. A number of classifications and terminologies have been proposed, that of the EGIL group being shown in Tables 2.7 [11] and 2.8 [11]. Among B-lineage cases, common and pre-B ALL have a similar prognosis whereas the prognosis of early-B ALL is worse, even if the poor-risk group of infants less than a year of age are excluded [54]. Among T-lineage cases, the precise immunophenotype is of less significance. It should be noted that HLA-DR is expressed in the great majority of cases of B-lineage ALL, regardless of the maturity of the cell, whereas, among cases of T-lineage ALL, HLA-DR expression correlates with an immature immunophenotype.

Classifications of B-lineage ALL reflect a putative normal sequence of B-cell maturation in which early cells express only HLA-DR, TdT and pan-B antigens such as CD19, CD22 and CD79a. Subsequently there is expression of CD24 and CD10 followed by the appearance of cytoplasmic μ chain (cμ) and CD79b, then cytoplasmic κ and λ chain and, finally, SmIg. CD34 is usually expressed in pro-B and common ALL but not pre-B or mature B-cell ALL [7]. TdT is usually positive in pro-B and common ALL but may be negative in pre-B-ALL and is usually negative in mature B-ALL [7]. Co-expression of myeloid antigens, CD13 and CD33, is more common in early B precursor (pro-B) ALL but has not been found to be of any prognostic significance [54]. It should be noted that the category 'common ALL' does not necessarily include all cases expressing the common ALL antigen (CD10). Cases that also express SmIg are always excluded from this category and are classified as mature B-ALL, B-ALL or B-lineage non-Hodgkin's lymphoma. Depending on the classification used, cases expressing cytoplasmic μ chain or cytoplasmic κ or λ chain may also be excluded. The recognition of mature B-ALL is of considerable importance because of the need for alternative treatment regimens. The recognition of early precursor or pro-B-ALL may likewise be important since the prognosis is generally worse than that of common ALL. The identification of pre-B cases was at one stage considered important since such cases included a cytogenetic subgroup, t(1;19)(q23;p13), which was previously associated with an unfavourable prognosis (see page 119); since the prognosis of this subtype is greatly improved with current treatment, identification of pre-B cases that may have a t(1;19) is no longer important for determining prognosis and choice of treatment. It has been suggested that a category of transitional pre-B-ALL should also be recognized in which there is expression of surface and cytoplasmic μ chains without expression of κ or λ light chains [55]. This subtype, which is not associated with any specific karyotypic abnormality, has a good prognosis with standard therapy. As cytogenetic and molecular genetic investigation of cases of ALL becomes more widespread the importance of immunophenotyping in identifying unfavourable prognostic categories of B-lineage ALL is likely to lessen.

Immunophenotyping has a role in distinguishing leukaemic lymphoblasts of B lineage from immature reactive cells, known as haematogones. A proportion of haematogones may express markers of immaturity such as CD34, TdT and CD10. However they differ from leukaemic lymphoblasts in that the population

Table 2.9 A comparison of the immunophenotypic characteristics of haematogones and leukaemic lymphoblasts of B lineage.

Haematogones	Leukaemic lymphoblasts
Spectrum of cells from immature to mature	Cells apparently arrested at one stage of maturation
Surface membrane antigens expressed synchronously and with strength of expression appropriate to stage of maturation	Surface membrane antigens expressed asynchronously (e.g. co-expression of CD34 and CD20, co-expression of CD10 and strong CD22) or inappropriately weakly or strongly (e.g. absent CD45, absent CD20, absent CD22, weak CD38, weak CD10, weak CD19)
No aberrant antigen expression	Frequent aberrant expression of myeloid antigens (most often CD13, CD15, CD33) or CD7

CD, cluster of differentiation.

of cells ranges from immature to mature, in contrast to the more consistently immature and often aberrant immunophenotype of leukaemic lymphoblasts [56]. Recognition of these differences is best achieved with four-colour immunophenotyping; merely measuring the percentage of cells expressing different antigens may be misleading. Scatter plots show that leukaemic lymphoblasts form a much more compact cluster. The differences are summarized in Table 2.9.

Classifications of T-lineage ALL essentially divide cases into two groups with immunophenotypes analogous to those of early and cortical (or common) thymocytes, respectively, and a third group analogous to mature thymocytes or to T cells. In some classifications the first two categories are amalgamated [2] and in others the categories are increased to four [11]. HLA-DR and TdT expression are less likely with the more mature immunophenotypes. Overall, about 95% of cases express TdT. The various categories of T-lineage ALL have been found to show some prognostic differences but these are less marked than in the case of B-lineage ALL. In one study, using a classification proposed by the Pediatric Oncology Study Group, children whose lymphoblasts had an early thymocyte phenotype had an appreciably lower remission rate than those whose lymphoblasts had an intermediate or late phenotype, but there was no difference in event-free survival [57]. In another childhood study, using the same classification, CD3 positivity and CD10 negativity were associated with a worse prognosis but only CD10 negativity was an independent prognostic variable [58]. In a German multicentre study in adults, cases classified as pre-T (E-rosette forming cells (ERFC) negative) had a worse prognosis than T-cell cases (ERFC positive) [59]. In a further study of adults and children those

with an 'early' phenotype (SmCD3–CD1–) were more likely to be adults and although they had a lower mean white cell count the prognosis for survival was worse than in other cases [60]. Although there is a consensus that the immunophenotype in T-lineage ALL correlates with disease characteristics, with the more immature immunophenotypes probably being associated with a worse prognosis, this is not generally regarded as an indication for an alteration of management. Further categorization of T-lineage cases is thus of less importance than further categorization of B-lineage cases. In T-lineage cases, in contrast to B-lineage, there is little relationship between immunophenotype and specific chromosomal abnormalities, although a higher frequency of normal karyotype in cases with an immature phenotype has been reported [61].

It should be noted that a third or more of cases of ALL fail to express the common leucocyte antigen, CD45, an antigen, which is expressed on all normal T and B lymphocytes [62]. This must be remembered if a gating protocol uses CD45.

If immunophenotyping is to be used for the detection of minimal residual disease in ALL, it is necessary to use an appropriate panel of antibodies to recognize a leukaemia-associated immunophenotype [63]. Characteristics sought are either asynchronous expression of antigens (either co-expression of markers that are normally expressed on mature and immature cells respectively or failure to express a marker that is usually expressed at the same stage of maturation as another marker), aberrant expression of antigens, inappropriately weak or strong expression of antigens or expression of a marker or combination of markers on bone marrow or blood lymphoid cells that is normally expressed only by thymic cells.

Table 2.10 Typical antibody combinations for the identification of a leukaemia-related immunophenotype that can be used for detection of minimal residual disease.

Antibody combination	Abnormality detected
B-lineage ALL	
TdT and CD10 co-expressed with CD13, CD15, CD33, CD65, CD66c **or** 7.1/NG.2	Aberrant expression of a myeloid antigen
CD34 and CD19 co-expressed with CD13, CD15, CD33, CD65, CD66c **or** 7.1/NG.2	Aberrant expression of a myeloid antigen
CD19 and CD10 co-expressed with CD13, CD15, CD33, CD65, CD66c **or** 7.1/NG.2	Aberrant expression of a myeloid antigen
TdT and CD10 co-expressed with CD56 **or** CD34 and CD19 co-expressed with CD56	Aberrant expression of a natural killer/myeloid antigen
TdT and CD10 co-expressed with strong CD19, CD21 **or** CD22	Asynchronous expression
CD34 and CD10 co-expressed with strong CD19, CD21 **or** CD22	Asynchronous expression
CD34 and CD10 and CD19 co-expressed with strong CD58	Asynchronous expression
TdT and CD34 co-expressed with μ	Asynchronous expression
T-lineage ALL	
TdT or CD34 on peripheral blood or bone marrow CD3-positive T cells	Normally expressed only on thymic cells
CD1a	Normally expressed only on thymocytes, not on peripheral blood or bone marrow cells
CD4 and CD8 coexpressed	Normally only co-expressed on thymic cells
AML	
CD33 overexpressed	Stronger expression than on normal cells
CD34 and TdT and CD65	Asynchronous expression
CD34 and CD11b, CD14, CD15, strong CD33 or CD56	Asynchronous expression
CD117 and CD11b or CD15	Asynchronous expression
CD13-positive, CD33-negative	Lack of synchronous expression
CD13-negative, CD33-positive	Lack of synchronous expression
CD13-negative, CD15-positive	Lack of synchronous expression
HLA-DR-positive, CD15-positive	Asynchronous expression
CD34-positive, CD33-positive, HLA-DR-negative	Lack of synchronous expression
CD34-positive, CD117-positive, HLA-DR-negative	Lack of synchronous expression
CD117-positive, CD33-positive, HLA-DR-negative	Lack of synchronous expression
Co-expression of myeloid markers with CD2, CD3, CD5 or CD7	Aberrant expression of a T-lymphoid marker
Co-expression of myeloid markers with CD19 or CD20	Aberrant expression of a B-lymphoid marker
Expression of myeloid markers on blasts showing light scatter characteristics more typical of lymphoid cells or vice versa	Expression of markers on cells showing an inappropriate light scatter pattern

Abbreviations: c, cytoplasmic; CD, cluster of differentiation; ALL, acute lymphoblastic leukaemia; AML, acute myeloid leukaemia; TdT, terminal deoxynucleotidyl transferase; 7.1/NG.2, a monoclonal antibody recognizing chondroitin sulfate.

Expression of aberrant myeloid markers is common in T-lineage ALL, both at diagnosis and at relapse [64]. Such expression is uncommon at presentation of B-lineage ALL but at relapse it is significantly more common [64]. In general, at least three antigens need to be studied simultaneously for effective detection of minimal residual disease. Some of the range of abnormalities that have been used are shown in Table 2.10.

Immunophenotyping and biphenotypic leukaemia

A biphenotypic leukaemia is one in which a single clone of leukaemic cells expresses markers of two lineages, usually lymphoid and myeloid lineages. Some cases of biphenotypic leukaemia may be suspected on morphological grounds when there appear to be two different populations of blasts, but many cases have blasts that are cytologically uniform. Lymphoid and myeloid markers may be expressed simultaneously or a case may present with ALL and relapse as AML (with the same or an evolved karyotypic abnormality), or vice versa. Immunophenotyping is essential for the diagnosis of biphenotypic leukaemia, but assessment of cytological and cytochemical features is also necessary. It may be inferred that a leukaemia is biphenotypic if the percentage of cells having myeloid markers overlaps with the percentage of cells having lymphoid markers (e.g. totalling more than 120% [11]) but the diagnosis is more firmly based if a double-labelling technique is employed, combining either two immunological markers or cytochemistry and an immunological marker.

Cases should not be classified as biphenotypic on the basis of the expression of a single inappropriate marker. A scoring system, as initially suggested by Mirro and Kitchingman [65] is useful, with features being scored for their specificity for a certain lineage. The scoring system proposed by the WHO expert group [66], which is a modification of the EGIL scoring system [11], is shown in Table 2.11 and its use is recommended. Lineage-specific features such as Auer rods and MPO activity score highly whereas those which are lineage-associated rather than lineage-specific, such as CD7 expression and TdT activity, score fewer points. A minimum number of points for each of two lineages is required before a case is classified as biphenotypic. Cases not meeting these criteria are classified as AML with aberrant lymphoid antigen expression or ALL with aberrant myeloid antigen expression. Most cases of biphenotypic leukaemia express myeloid markers together with either B-lineage or T-lineage markers. Some of the latter also express natural killer markers [67]. The possibility of a biphenotypic leukaemia expressing markers of T- and B-lineage lymphocytes is acknowledged in some classifications [65, 66, 68] but not in all [11].

A further subtype of acute leukaemia, expressing both myeloid markers and the natural killer cell antigen CD56, could be regarded as biphenotypic,

Table 2.11 WHO modification of EGIL criteria for the diagnosis of biphenotypic leukaemia [11, 66].

Score	B lineage	T lineage	Myeloid
2	cCD79a cIgM cCD22	CD3 (c or Sm) anti-TCR (αβ or γδ)	MPO
1	CD19 CD10 CD20	CD2 CD5 CD8 CD10	CD117 CD13 CD33 CD65
0.5	TdT CD24	TdT CD7 CD1a	CD14 CD15 CD64

If >2 points is scored for both myeloid and one of the lymphoid lineages the case is classified as biphenotypic; in the original EGIL recommendations CD117 scored 0.5 rather than 1.
c, cytoplasmic; CD, cluster of differentiation; Ig, immunoglobulin; MPO, myeloperoxidase; Sm, surface membrane; TdT, terminal deoxynucleotidyl transferase.

although these cases do not generally meet the above criteria. An immature type with features of M0 AML but with expression of CD56 and weak expression of cytoplasmic CD3 has been described [69] together with a more mature type with azurophilic granules, MPO activity and CD56 positivity [70]. Weak expression of cytoplasmic CD3 in some cases (detected with polyclonal antibodies) is compatible with natural killer cell lineage since natural killer cells have truncated CD3ε messenger RNA (mRNA) [69]. Since other subtypes of AML have also been found to express CD56 it is not yet clear whether classification of these cases as biphenotypic is appropriate.

Cases that present with ALL and subsequently develop a secondary therapy-induced leukaemia, usually AML, should be distinguished from biphenotypic leukaemia. In the former case the two episodes of leukaemia have a different clonal origin whereas in the latter cases relapse is associated with phenotypic switch in the initial leukaemic clone. Distinction between these two possibilities is not possible on the basis of cytology and immunophenotype but requires cytogenetic or molecular genetic evidence.

Biphenotypic acute leukaemia in adults is associated with adverse cytogenetic abnormalities and with a prognosis that is worse than that of either ALL or AML [71]. In children, the prognosis appears to be less adverse. If alternative therapeutic regimens are found to improve the prognosis of biphenotypic acute leukaemia it may become necessary to apply immunophenotyping to virtually all cases of acute leukaemia in order to ensure that all such cases are recognized.

The WHO classification distinguished biphenotypic acute leukaemia (markers of different lineages expressed on the same cells) from bilineal acute leukaemia (two apparently distinct populations of blast cells) [66]. Since bilineal acute leukaemia has been observed to evolve into biphenotypic acute leukaemia [66], this distinction may be artificial.

Cytogenetic abnormalities differ somewhat between myeloid/B-lineage acute leukaemia and myeloid/T-lineage acute leukaemia (see page 113).

Immunophenotyping and undifferentiated stem cell leukaemia

With current immunophenotyping techniques, there are fewer than 1% of cases of acute leukaemia that cannot be classified as AML, ALL or acute biphenotypic leukaemia. However, there are cases where leukaemic cells have no lineage-specific markers, i.e. there is no clear evidence of myeloid or lymphoid differentiation, which can be designated 'unclassified acute leukaemia', 'acute stem cell leukaemia' or 'undifferentiated acute leukaemia' [11, 66, 72, 73]. Such cases often express CD34, CD38 and HLA-DR and may express TdT. They do not express markers regarded as specific for the myeloid lineage (such as CD13, CD33, MPO, CD65, CD117, CD41, CD61 and glycophorin) nor markers specific for either lymphoid lineage (such as CD19, CD22, CD10, CD79a and CD3). Expression of CD7 is not specific for the T lineage so does not exclude a diagnosis of undifferentiated acute leukaemia. Similarly, rearrangement of immunoglobulin heavy-chain genes or T-cell receptor genes does not exclude this diagnosis since such rearrangement can be seen in AML as well as ALL. A rigorous definition of a case as undifferentiated or stem cell leukaemia requires testing with the most sensitive techniques including testing for cCD79a, cCD22, cCD3 and cMPO [66]. The cytogenetic abnormalities observed (e.g. 5q– and trisomy 13) and the observation of myelodysplastic features in some cases suggests that acute undifferentiated leukaemia may be more closely related to AML than to ALL [73]. Although complete remission may occur, survival is poor.

Cytogenetic and molecular genetic abnormalities and the classification of acute leukaemia

In both acute leukaemia and MDS, normal polyclonal haemopoietic cells are largely replaced by abnormal cells, which are the progeny of a single cell and are therefore designated a clone. In AML, the abnormal clone of cells may include the granulocyte/monocyte, erythroid and megakaryocyte lineages or be restricted to the granulocytic/monocytic lineage.

In many instances the abnormal clone has an acquired chromosomal abnormality that can be detected by examination of the chromosomes of cells arrested in metaphase. The bone marrow cells may be examined directly or after a period in culture with or without various mitogens and synchronizing agents. All of a population of leukaemic cells may show the same chromosomal abnormality or further clonal evolution may have occurred so that there are cells with an additional abnormality, which represent a daughter clone or subclone. In cytogenetic terminology, subclones are referred to as sidelines derived from the stemline. Residual normal haemopoietic cells are karyotypically normal unless the patient happens to have a constitutional chromosomal abnormality. When the bone marrow of a patient with acute leukaemia is examined all cells may be found to have the same karyotypic abnormality (AA), indicating that they all belong to the same clone, or all cells may be karyotypically normal (NN) or there may be a mixture of normal and abnormal metaphases (AN). The latter situation almost always represents a mixture of normal and leukaemic cells. In AML supervening in MDS it can also represent an evolved daughter clone. If only normal metaphases are present the leukaemic clone may not have a chromosomal abnormality that is detectable by microscopy. However, all metaphases may be normal despite the presence of a karyotypically abnormal clone if only residual normal cells are entering mitosis *in vitro*. Initial failure of some centres to detect the characteristic chromosomal abnormality of AML M3 was subsequently found to be due to the use of a technique of direct examination so that only karyotypically normal erythroid cells were detected [74, 75], M3 being one of the types of leukaemia in which the erythroid and megakaryocyte lineages are not part of the leukaemic clone. Other centres, where cells were cultured before examination, detected the characteristic abnormality since the culture conditions selected for leukaemic cells. Successful cytogenetic analysis is more often possible on a bone marrow aspirate than on peripheral blood cells. Bone marrow aspiration is therefore recommended for this purpose, even if it is obvious from the peripheral blood that the patient has acute leukaemia.

Occasionally karyotypic evidence suggests the presence of two independent clones. Although this may occur, particularly when the bone marrow has been exposed to mutagenic influences, evidence from analysis of glucose-6-phosphate dehydrogenase (G6PD) alloenzymes and from DNA analysis suggests that in some patients apparently independent clones are subclones derived from a single parent clone that was cytogenetically normal. Similarly, a mixture of normal and abnormal metaphases can occur because only a subclone is cytogenetically abnormal.

When the karyotype of bone marrow cells is studied, some cells show random abnormalities, which

need to be distinguished from a non-random or consistent abnormality that indicates the presence of an abnormal clone. For this reason, according to the International System of Nomenclature [76], a clone is considered to be present if two cells show the same structural change or additional chromosomes or if three cells show the same missing chromosome. Various terms and abbreviations used in describing chromosomes and their abnormalities are shown in Table 2.12. Translocations are described as reciprocal if material is exchanged between chromosomes and as non-reciprocal when material from one chromosome is transferred to another. A balanced translocation is one in which there is no net gain or loss of chromosomal material, whereas an unbalanced translocation is one in which translocation is associated with loss or duplication of all or part of a chromosome. Translocations are described by international agreement [76] as follows: t(15;17)(q22;q21) indicates that there is a reciprocal translocation between chromosomes 15 and 17; the breakpoints are at band q22 on chromosome 15 and at band q21 on chromosome 17. This is the translocation found in M3 and M3V AML, the first specific abnormality to be linked to a morphologically recognizable subtype of acute leukaemia. In describing translocations, the chromosomes are listed in numerical order. In describing insertions, the chromosome into which material is inserted is listed first followed by the chromosome from which material has been derived.

Cytogenetic analysis provides some of the evidence that acute myeloid leukaemia can be divided into two broad groups. Cases associated with balanced translocations show a 3- to 4-fold increase in incidence with increasing age whereas cases associated with complex abnormal karyotypes (defined in this study as having at least 3 numeric or structural abnormalities) show an almost 30-fold increase [77]. The former group comprises mainly cases of *de novo* leukaemia whereas the latter group includes myelodysplasia-related AML.

The role of cytogenetic analysis in AML is summarized in Table 2.13 and will be discussed in more detail in the pages that follow.

Increasingly, patients with leukaemia are investigated by molecular genetic as well as cytogenetic techniques [80]. Some techniques, based on *in situ* hybridization, bridge conventional cytogenetic and purely molecular techniques while others bridge

Table 2.12 Abbreviations and terminology used in describing chromosomes and their abnormalities.

p	Short arm of a chromosome
q	Long arm of a chromosome
p+, q+	Addition of chromosomal material to the short arm or long arm, respectively
p−, q−	Loss of chromosomal material from the short arm or long arm, respectively
+	Addition of a chromosome
−	Loss of a chromosome
add	Additional material of unknown origin
band	Chromosomal region that, after staining, is distinguished from adjoining regions by appearing lighter or darker
c	Constitutional anomaly
del	Deletion
der	Derivative chromosome, an abnormal chromosome derived from two or more chromosomes; it takes its number from the chromosome which contributes the centromere
dic	Dicentric, a chromosome with two centromeres
dm	Double minute (see minute)
dup	Duplication, extra copy of a segment of a chromosome
hsr	Homogeneously staining region, indicative of amplification (multiple copies) of a small segment of a chromosome
inv	Inversion, i.e. a segment of a chromosome has been inverted
ins	Insertion, movement of a segment of a chromosome to a new position on the same or another chromosome; may be direct (dir) or inverted (inv)
iso or i	Isochromosome, a chromosome formed by duplication of the long arm or the short arm
mar	Marker chromosome, an abnormal chromosome that cannot be characterized and is therefore of unknown origin
min	Minute, an acentric fragment smaller than the width of a single chromatid; may be single or double
r	Ring chromosome
t	Translocation, movement of a segment of one chromosome to form part of another chromosome; a translocation is often reciprocal; a translocation may be described as balanced (no loss of chromosomal material detected on microscopic examination of metaphase spreads) or unbalanced (a segment of chromosome is seen to have been lost)
aneuploid	Cells having an abnormal number of chromosomes that is neither half nor a multiple of 46
centromere	The junction of the short arm (p) and the long arm (q)
diploid	Cells having the normal complement of 46 chromosomes (23 pairs)
haploid	Cells with 23 (unpaired) chromosomes; near haploid = 23–34 chromosomes
hypodiploid	Cells having fewer than 46 chromosomes, usually 35–45
karyotype	Written description of the chromosomal make-up of a cell and by extension of a clone of cells (or an individual)
karyogram	Systematized array of the chromosomes of a cell and by extension of a clone of cells (or an individual); chromosomes are displayed in decreasing order of size, which corresponds to increasing chromosome number; the sex chromosomes, X and Y, are displayed last
monosomy	Loss of an entire chromosome so that there is only a single copy, indicated by a '−' before the chromosome number, e.g. −7
paracentric inversion	Inversion of a segment of a chromosome confined to one arm
pericentric inversion	Inversion of a segment of a chromosome composed of part of both arms and the centromere
pseudodiploid	Cells having 46 chromosomes but with structural abnormalities being present
tetraploid	Cells having 92 chromosomes (four sets); near tetraploid = 81–103 chromosomes
triploid	Cells having 69 chromosomes (three sets); near triploid = 58–80 chromosomes
trisomy	Three copies of a chromosome, indicated by a '+' before the chromosome number, e.g. +8

Table 2.13 The role of cytogenetic analysis in acute myeloid leukaemia.

Recognition of an underlying constitutional abnormality that predisposes to AML such as Down's syndrome (trisomy 21 or equivalent), Fanconi's anaemia (susceptibility to clastogenic agents), familial monosomy 7 syndrome, familial t(7;20)(p?;p?) [78], familial t(3;6)(p14;p11) [79]

Recognition of subtypes of AML with differing prognosis requiring differing therapeutic approaches, including confirmation of AML of M3 or M3 variant subtype by demonstration of t(15;17)(q22;q21)

Confirmation of AML rather than MDS in patients with a low blast percentage, e.g. in patients with t(8;21)(q22;q22) and inv(16)(p13q22)

Identification of specific chromosomal rearrangements known to be associated with specific fusion genes, in order to indicate which molecular techniques are likely to be useful for assessing minimal residual disease

Recognition of therapy-related AML, following either alkylating agents or topoisomerase II-interactive drugs

Furthering knowledge of leukaemogenesis, e.g. by identifying sites of possible oncogenes, demonstration of the leukaemic nature of transient abnormal myelopoiesis of Down's syndrome

histological and molecular techniques. Techniques initially employed only in research rapidly find their way into diagnostic practice. Molecular techniques applicable to the investigation of leukaemia are summarized in Table 2.14. If molecular genetic techniques are to be used for the detection of minimal residual disease it is important that they are applied to the diagnostic sample in each patient to ensure the validity of a specific test in an individual patient. The role of molecular genetic analysis in AML is summarized in Table 2.15. Some applications will be discussed in detail in the following pages.

It is possible that in the future the diagnosis of acute myeloid leukaemia and of B-lineage and T-lineage acute lymphoblastic leukaemia will be made by DNA microarray analysis, which permits analysis of the expression of large numbers of genes; gene expression differs considerably between these three broad categories of leukaemia and also appears to differ from expression in other tumours [81]. It could also be envisaged that subtypes of acute leukaemia might be recognizable by the same means.

The recurrent cytogenetic abnormalities associated with specific subtypes of acute leukaemia can be detected by *in situ* hybridization techniques, particularly FISH, which can be performed on metaphase or interphase cells. Labelled probes used can be: (i) centromeric probes, which specifically identify each chromosome by means of sequences at its centromere; (ii) probes for specific DNA sequences, e.g. those at the breakpoints of recurring translocations; or (iii) 'whole chromosome paints', which hybridize to sequences extending over the whole chromosome.

Translocations can be recognized either by single-colour FISH using a probe that spans the entire breakpoint region and is therefore always split in a given translocation or, alternatively, by two-colour FISH using probes for sequences at the breakpoints on the two chromosomes involved, which are brought together on a single chromosome as a result of a translocation.

The genomic alteration resulting from a cytogenetic rearrangement can be identified by direct analysis of DNA amplified by the PCR technique or, alternatively, by analysis of mRNA transcribed from a fusion gene, using the technique of reverse transcriptase PCR (RT-PCR) to produce and amplify complementary DNA (cDNA). These two techniques will also detect relevant genomic alterations in some cases in which the karyotype is complex and ambiguous or apparently normal or in which cytogenetic analysis has failed. Multiplex-PCR is a useful way to screen cases for the most important translocations by using multiple pairs of primers for the identification of specific rearrangements. For example, cases of ALL can be simultaneously screened for t(9;22), t(4;11) and t(1;19) and cases of AML can be simultaneously screened for inv/t(16), t(15;17) and t(8;21).

Molecular genetic analysis can be used not only to identify specific subtypes of AML but also to detect mutations such as those in *RAS* or *FLT3* genes that are unrelated to subtype but may be of prognostic significance. Internal tandem duplications of *FLT3* are found in more than a quarter of patients with AML and are indicative of a considerably worse prognosis [82].

Table 2.14 A summary of molecular genetic techniques used in the investigation of leukaemia.

Technique	Principle	Application
Molecular cytogenetic techniques		
Fluorescence *in situ* hybridization (FISH)	Chromosomes or specific DNA sequences are identified by a probe bound to a fluorochrome; applicable to chromosomes in metaphase and, to a lesser extent in interphase	Detection of numerical abnormalities (monosomies, trisomies, hyperdiploidy); identification of translocations, detection of amplification of oncogenes or loss of either tumour suppressor genes or the normal allele corresponding to a gene contributing to a fusion gene (e.g. loss of *ETV6* in t(12;21)-associated ALL)
M-FISH	Multicolour FISH using five fluorochromes so that all individual chromosomes can be identified; five separate fluorochrome images are captured	Clarification of complex karyotypes
Spectral karyotyping (SKY)	Multicolour FISH using five fluorochromes and capturing a single image; combinations of fluorochromes are recognized by their spectral signature	Clarification of complex karyotypes
Comparative genomic hybridization (CGH)	Labelled patient and normal DNA, differentially labelled with fluorochromes, is hybridized to normal metaphases	Identification of the region of a chromosome where there is a gain or a loss can be used for indicating the likely nature of amplified oncogenes, e.g. in double minute chromosomes
Molecular genetic techniques		
Southern blot	DNA is digested by restriction endonucleases; the restriction fragments created are separated by gel electrophoresis following which they are blotted onto a membrane; a radioactive probe is then used to identify the DNA sequence of interest on a fragment of a specific size	Detection of rearrangement of a gene, e.g. an immunoglobulin or T-cell receptor gene (for demonstration of clonality) or rearrangement of an oncogene such as *MLL* which has multiple partners
PCR	A method of *in vitro* amplification of a defined DNA target that is flanked by regions of known sequence; to distinguish it from RT-PCR, this technique may be referred to as genomic PCR or DNA PCR	Detection of rearrangement of a gene, e.g. an immunoglobulin or T-cell receptor gene (for demonstration of clonality) or an oncogene—a much more sensitive technique than Southern blot analysis
RT-PCR	An *in vitro* method for reverse transcription of RNA followed by amplification of complementary DNA	Analysis of genes that are too long for analysis by a standard genomic PCR
Multiplex PCR	Simultaneous application of a number of pairs of primers so that any of a number of possible mutations can be identified	Simultaneous screening for a number of leukaemia-related mutations
Real-time PCR (RQ-PCR)	A quantitative PCR technique in which there is displacement of a fluorogenic product-specific probe which is degraded during the reaction, generating a fluorescent signal	Quantification of the amount of a specific DNA sequence present—useful for monitoring minimal residual disease
Primed *in situ* hybridization (PRINS)	A technique for identifying specific chromosomes by means of primers that are annealed to target α satellite chromosome-specific repetitive DNA sequences, followed by *in situ* primer extension using Taq DNA polymerase and incorporating fluorochrome-labelled dUTP	Applicable to the detection of monosomy 7 or trisomy 8
Molecular histological techniques		
In situ hybridization for detection of messenger RNA (mRNA)	A labelled probe detects specific mRNA, e.g. mRNA of κ or λ or mRNA of an oncogene such as cyclin D1 (*BCL1*)	Establishment of clonality or confirmation that an oncogene is expressed
Immunohisto-chemistry for detection of a gene product	An antibody (polyclonal or monoclonal) is raised to the protein product of a specific, gene, e.g. an oncogene or tumour suppressor gene	Demonstration that a normal or mutant oncogene or a tumour suppressor gene has a protein product in a specific cell (e.g. ALK or p53) or that a protein product has an abnormal distribution (e.g. PML protein in acute promyelocytic leukaemia)

Table 2.15 The role of molecular genetic analysis in acute myeloid leukaemia.

Recognition of subtypes of AML with differing prognosis requiring differing therapeutic approaches, including confirmation of AML of M3 or M3 variant subtype by demonstration of *PML-RARA* fusion gene, detection of the good prognosis *AML1-ETO* and *CBFB-MYH11* fusion genes and detection of the poor prognosis *BCR-ABL* fusion gene

Confirmation of AML rather than MDS in patients with a low blast percentage, e.g. in patients with *AML1-ETO* and *CBFB-MYH11* fusion genes

Recognition of therapy-related AML, e.g. by demonstration of *MLL* rearrangement following exposure to topoisomerase II-interactive drugs

Monitoring of minimal residual disease, either by detection of the product of a fusion gene or by detection of overexpression of a gene, e.g. *WT1*, which is often overexpressed in AML

Furthering knowledge of leukaemogenesis and of normal haemopoiesis, e.g. by identification of oncogenes and by demonstration of their role in normal haemopoiesis; identification of the mechanism of leukaemogenesis; demonstration of the intrauterine origin of some cases of AML in infants and children

---

Molecular genetic analysis not only aids the classification of acute leukaemia but is also of use in monitoring for minimal residual disease after remission has been induced by therapy. Cytogenetic analysis is of much less use for the latter purpose since it is possible to examine only a relatively small number of metaphases. For technical reasons, FISH is also relatively insensitive in the monitoring of minimal residual disease. When a fusion transcript is present it can be used for monitoring but in patients lacking a detectable fusion gene an alternative technique is needed. The *WT1* gene, which is expressed at only a low level in normal bone marrow, is over-expressed in the majority of patients with AML. Detection of such over-expression by real-time quantitative PCR (RQ-PCR) is potentially of use in these patients.

There is now a need for an MIC–M classification, adding molecular genetic analysis (M) to morphology (M), immunophenotype (I) and cytogenetics (C) to provide a more complete description of biological entities among the heterogeneous group of disorders classified as acute leukaemia [4]. When there is a characteristic cytogenetic abnormality but the molecular mechanism of leukaemogenesis has not been clarified, e.g. in common ALL associated with hyperdiploidy, only an MIC classification is possible, but more fully characterized subtypes can be recognized as MIC–M categories. The WHO expert group has now recommended that patients with 20% or more blast cells in either the peripheral blood or bone marrow should be categorized as AML and that myeloid neoplasms with certain cytogenetic abnormalities should be regarded as AML, regardless of the blast

count [83]. It is therefore recommended that the MIC–M classification be modified to conform with this advice. Three of the suggested MIC–M categories are identical with WHO categories but others, those with an 11q23 breakpoint, have been included in a single category by the WHO despite the fact that there are important biological differences between them.

Cytogenetic and molecular genetic abnormalities and the MIC–M classification of AML

With current techniques, 70–80% [84, 85] of patients with AML are found to have non-random (clonal) cytogenetic abnormalities, many of which are recurrent. Overall the commonest cytogenetic abnormality is trisomy 8 with anomalies of chromosome 7 in second place. Some chromosomal anomalies, such as trisomy 8 and trisomy 21, are found in all FAB subtypes and in both secondary and *de novo* leukaemia; they are not related to any readily apparent morphological or clinical features. Other anomalies, including t(15;17), t(8;21) and t or inv(16), have a strong association with a particular FAB type and are associated with specific morphological features; they rarely occur in secondary leukaemia and erythroid and megakaryocyte dysplasia are not usually a feature. It is possible that, in this group of anomalies, the leukaemia has arisen in a lineage-restricted stem cell. Other anomalies such as t(6;9), t(1;7), t(3;3) and inv(3) occur in multiple FAB subtypes and in myelodysplasia as well as in both *de novo* and secondary (irradiation or cytotoxic-drug-related) leukaemias;

it is likely that the association of such translocations with bi- or trilineage myelodysplasia and with multiple FAB categories indicates that the leukaemia has arisen in a multipotent stem cell, which has preserved its capacity to differentiate into cells of various lineages. Other anomalies involving predominantly loss of chromosomal material (such as –5, 5q–, –7, 7q–) show a similar lack of relationship to FAB types but an association with myelodysplastic features and with therapy-related MDS and secondary AML. Many patients with AML have more than one karyotypic abnormality. Complex abnormalities are particularly characteristic of M6 AML, secondary AML and AML arising in patients with previous MDS. Chromosomal abnormalities that are strongly associated with characteristic clinical and morphological features are often termed specific, whereas those that are not are termed non-specific.

Chromosomal abnormalities have been found to have independent prognostic significance in AML although the prognostic ranking has not been identical in different series of patients [84, 86–90]. In general, the best prognosis is seen with inv(16), t(8;21), t(15;17) and the worst with deletions or monosomies of chromosomes 5, 7 or both, t(1;7), t(6;9), inv(3), t(3;3) and complex karyotypic abnormalities. An intermediate prognosis is seen with trisomy 8 and translocations involving 11q23. Several very large clinical trials, under the auspices of the UK Medical Research Council, have established and validated prognostic grouping on the basis of cytogenetic abnormalities. In children and adults under the age of 55 years, a favourable prognosis was associated with

inv(16), t(8;21) and t(15;17) whereas an adverse prognosis was associated with –5, –7, 5q–, 3q abnormalities and a complex karyotype (five or more unrelated abnormalities); 7q– was not prognostically adverse unless it was part of a complex karyotype [90]. Patients not falling into either the favourable or the adverse group were assigned to an intermediate category. In older patients (median age 66 years), observations were similar except that the complex karyotype group has a significantly worse outcome than patients with –5, –7, 5q– or 3q abnormalities and the latter group were therefore re-assigned to the intermediate prognosis group. This prognostic categorization now determines treatment selection in UK trials.

The MIC Cooperative Study Group [3] proposed that cases of AML should be studied by morphological, immunological and cytogenetic techniques. They defined 10 categories but the classification was open-ended and new categories could be added once they had been clearly defined. A larger number of MIC–M categories can now be defined.

M2/t(8;21)(q22;q22)/*AML1-ETO* fusion

t(8;21)(q22;q22) [91–95] (Fig. 2.4) is one of the two most common specific translocations in AML, the other being t(15;17). Overall, cases of M2/t(8;21) comprise 4–9% of AML in different series of patients [77, 96, 97]; the frequency is higher in children (12–14% of AML) than in adults (6% of AML) [96, 98]. In elderly adults, the prevalence falls to 2% of cases [90]. Adult cases are usually young and more

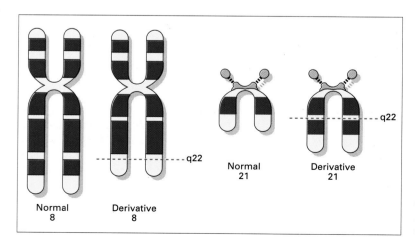

Fig. 2.4 A diagrammatic representation of the t(8;21)(q22;q22) abnormality. The breakpoints in the two derivative chromosomes are indicated (modified from [3]).

often male than female. In around half of childhood cases the translocation appears to have occurred *in utero* [99]; a second mutation occurring in extra-uterine life may be necessary for the leukaemic phenotype. The geographical distribution appears to be uneven with a higher percentage of cases showing this abnormality in Japan, among non-whites in South Africa [93] and in China [100].

Clinical and haematological features. t(8;21) is strongly associated with M2 AML, with a minority of cases being M1 or, less often, M4. The great majority of cases are de novo but abnormalities of 21q22, including t(8;21)(q22;q22), are found among cases of secondary AML with prior exposure to topoisomerase II-interactive drugs including etoposide and the anthracyclines [101, 102]. This subtype of leukaemia may also be linked to prior exposure to benzene [103]. Formation of chloromas, solid tumours of leukaemic cells, is not uncommon [104]. The complete remission rate and median survival are relatively favourable [89, 90, 105]. Prognosis is significantly better in those with a presenting white cell count (WBC) of 20×10^9/l or less [106]. Worse prognosis is also indicated by a higher value for the product of the WBC and the bone marrow blast percentage, with cut-off points of 2.5 and 20 dividing patients into three prognostic groups [107]. Survival is worse in secondary cases than in *de novo*, with a 5-year survival of about 30% [103].

Characteristic cytological features are observed [94, 95, 108, 109] (Figs 2.5–2.9, see also Fig. 1.3, page 5). There is maturation of leukaemic cells to neutrophils and consequently severe neutropenia is uncommon. Some patients have neutrophilia. The blasts are very heterogeneous, variable in size but often large and with a high nucleocytoplasmic ratio. Nuclei

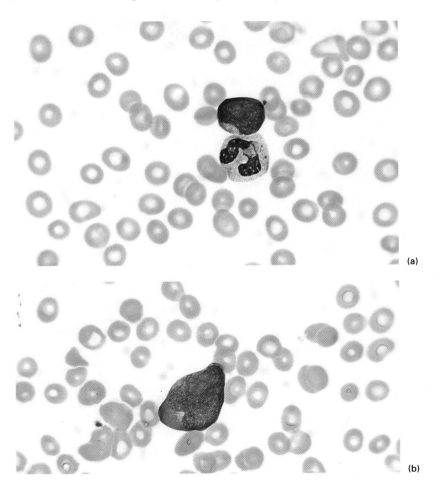

(a)

(b)

Fig. 2.5 PB and bone marrow (BM) films of a patient with AML M2/t(8;21). (a) PB showing a blast cell and an abnormal neutrophil. MGG × 870. (b) PB showing a strongly basophilic blast with a paranuclear hof representing the Golgi zone. MGG × 870.

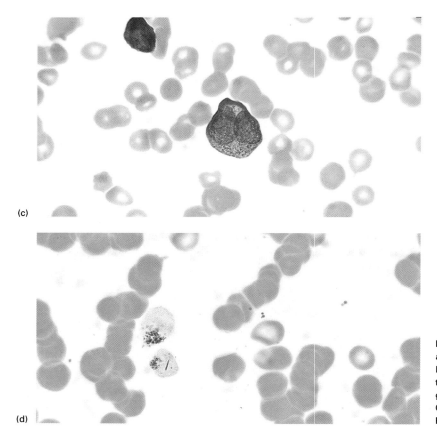

(c)

(d)

Fig. 2.5 (*Continued*) (c) PB showing an abnormal promyelocyte with peripheral basophilia. MGG × 870. (d) BM showing two blasts with peroxidase-positive granules in the hof of the nucleus. One blast also contains an Auer rod. Peroxidase × 870.

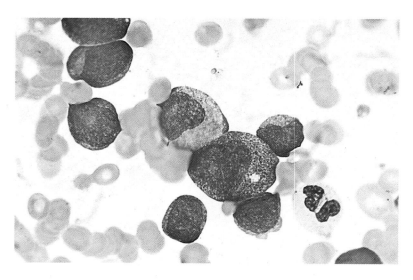

Fig. 2.6 BM film from a patient with AML M2/t(8;21) showing blasts and maturing granulocytic cells including a hypogranular neutrophil. MGG × 870.

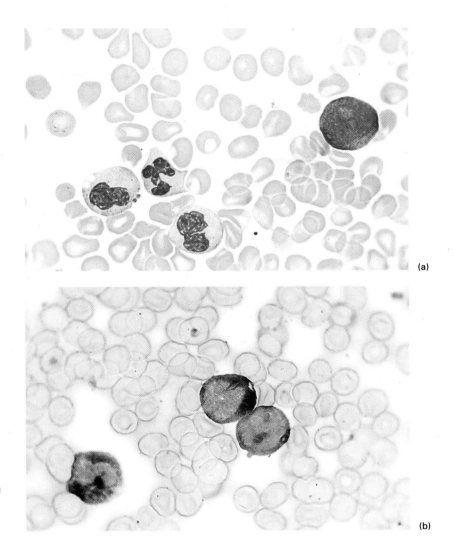

Fig. 2.7 BM film of a patient with AML M2/t(8;21). (a) A blast and three abnormal neutrophils. MGG × 870. (b) Sudan black B (SBB) stain showing strongly positive cells in one of which an Auer rod with a hollow core can be seen. SBB × 870.

are commonly indented or cleft with large nucleoli. Cytoplasm may be basophilic (Fig. 2.5b), sometimes vacuolated. Basophilia is sometimes confined to the periphery of the cytoplasm (Fig. 2.5c). Auer rods are common, often with a single slender Auer rod per cell. Some blasts may contain giant granules as may maturing cells. In individual cases, blasts may contain Auer rods, giant granules, both or neither. Binucleated myeloblasts, promyelocytes, myelocytes and metamyelocytes are seen [91]. Neutrophils often show hypogranularity, bizarre-shaped nuclei and the acquired Pelger–Huët anomaly. Homogeneous pink cytoplasm of mature neutrophils is character-

istic [109]. Maturing granulocytes may contain Auer rods, which are sometimes even found in metamyelocytes and neutrophils (Fig. 2.8a). Auer rods may also be observed in macrophages (Fig. 2.8b). An unusual feature, striking haemophagocytosis by neutrophils, has been described in a single case [110]. Bone marrow eosinophilia occurs in a proportion of patients who may be classified as having M2Eo AML (Fig. 2.9). Eosinophil granules vary in their staining characteristics, appearing orange, green/grey or blue [111]. Although some may have granules which are basophilic this feature is much less marked than in inv(16)/M4Eo (see below) [92]. Most patients do not

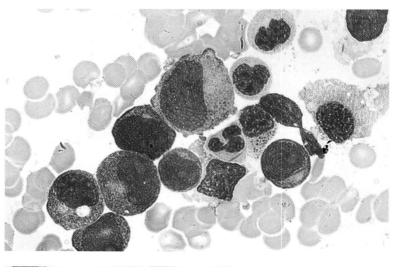

(a)

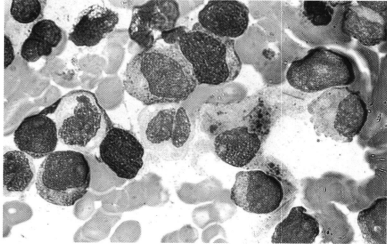

(b)

Fig. 2.8 BM film from a patient with AML M2/t(8;21). (a) A spectrum of maturing cells of granulocyte lineage—a blast cell and a neutrophil contain long thin Auer rods. (b) A macrophage containing an Auer rod. MGG × 870.

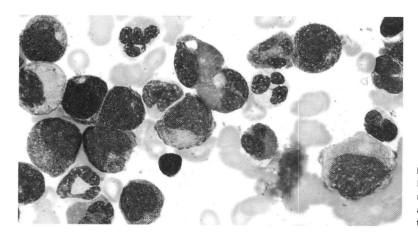

Fig. 2.9 BM film of a patient with AML M2Eo/t(8;21) showing maturing cells of neutrophil and eosinophil lineage; there are three eosinophil myelocytes and two mature eosinophils. MGG × 870.

have a peripheral blood eosinophilia but occasional patients have had a markedly elevated eosinophil count [112, 113] sometimes with an associated hypereosinophilic syndrome [113]. An increase of bone marrow basophils or mast cells occurs in a significant proportion of cases [108] and sometimes this is striking [114]. Although maturing granulocytes usually show dysplasia, other lineages usually do not; myelodysplastic features in erythroid and megakaryocyte lineages have been reported as uncommon in some series [95] and not present in others [94, 109]. Secondary cases may have a preceding myelodysplastic phase and show trilineage myelodysplasia. There may be a discrepancy in blast numbers between the bone marrow and the blood. Occasional cases present with bone marrow blast cells below 30%. If untreated, such cases evolve rapidly into AML [115]. A diagnosis of AML and treatment as such is therefore appropriate despite the low blast percentage. In the WHO classification (see below), such cases are categorized as AML even if the blast cells are less than 20% [116].

Cytochemical stains [94, 117] show localized Sudan black B (SBB) and MPO positivity in the blasts, often confined to the cleft or hof of the nucleus (Fig. 2.4d). Chloroacetate esterase (CAE) is strongly positive. There may also be Golgi zone positivity for α-naphthyl acetate esterase [95]. An MPO reaction may show Auer rods to be multiple and occasionally they are revealed in eosinophils as well as in the neutrophil series; Auer rods are sometimes positive for CAE and PAS as well as for MPO and SBB. Auer rods may have a non-staining core (Fig. 2.7b). The eosinophils in t(8;21)/M2 do not show the aberrant positivity for CAE, which is a feature of eosinophils in inv(16)/M4Eo AML [92]. The neutrophil alkaline phosphatase score is generally low [118] but neutrophils that are negative for SBB and MPO are uncommon [117]. Blasts are more commonly PAS positive than in AML in general; the pattern of staining is diffuse with some granules and rare blocks. PAS-positive erythroblasts are not a feature. Eosinophil granules may show aberrant PAS positivity but this is less a feature than for M4Eo/inv(16) AML (see below) [94].

This category of AML has a relatively good prognosis with 5-year survivals in adults of up to 70% being reported with chemotherapy alone [119, 120]. For this reason, stem cell transplantation in first remission is considered contraindicated. In one large series, survival was no better with stem cell transplantation [107]. Intensive treatment with high-dose cytosine arabinoside appears to be important in achieving long term survival [119]. The prognosis in children appears similarly good [120].

Immunophenotype. This category of AML has a characteristic immunophenotype (Fig. 2.10) [121]. Blast cells are characteristically positive for CD13, CD33, CD34, CD65, C117, MPO and HLA-DR [12]. Rare cases are negative for CD13, CD33 and CD14 but are positive for MPO [7]. Expression of CD34, HLA-DR and MPO is stronger than in other cases of AML whereas expression of CD13 and CD33 is more likely to be absent or weak [122]. CD11b and CD15 are expressed mainly on the maturing granulocytic cells [45]. There is usually positivity for the B-lineage marker CD19 and often for the natural killer cell marker CD56 [45, 123, 124]. Expression of CD56 may be indicative of a worse prognosis [125]. Co-expression of CD19 and CD34, which is uncommon in other subtypes of AML, suggests a diagnosis of AML with t(8;21) [126]. CD2, CD7, CD14, CD64 and TdT are usually negative [12, 45, 123] and, when TdT is positive, expression is usually weak [116].

Cytogenetic and molecular genetic features. The t(8;21)(q22;q22) rearrangement is shown in Fig. 2.11. Common secondary karyotypic abnormalities are loss of the Y chromosome in males, loss of the inactive X chromosome in females and del(9q). In one study, loss of a sex chromosome was found to be associated with a worse prognosis [127] and in another −Y was associated with a better prognosis but neither of these observations was confirmed in other studies [120]. MAC (morphology–antibody–chromosomes) techniques show the translocation is detectable in the granulocytic lineage but not in erythroid or megakaryocytic cells [128]. Eosinophils are also part of the neoplastic clone [92].

The molecular mechanism of leukaemogenesis is fusion of part of the *AML1* or *RUNX1* gene at 8q22 with part of the *ETO* (eight twenty-one) gene from 21q22 [129]. The normal *AML1* gene codes for one chain of a heterodimeric transcription factor (core binding factor—CBF) while the normal *ETO* gene is a putative transcription factor gene normally expressed in the brain. The fusion gene, *AML1-ETO* or *CBFA-ETO* (*CBFa-ETO*), which is formed on the derivative chromosome 8 as a result of the translocation, codes for a chimeric protein that is expressed in the leukaemic cells. The AML-ETO protein may exert its oncogenic effect by interfering with the transcription

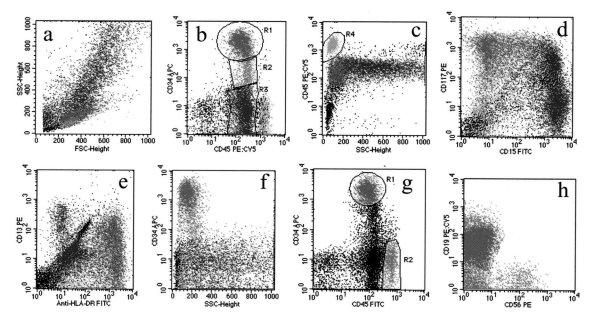

Fig. 2.10 Four-colour flow cytometry immunophenotyping in a patient with AML associated with t(8;21). Plots a, b and c show standard analysis regions set to delineate myeloid blast differentiation (compare with Fig. 2.3); plots d and e show CD117/CD15 and CD13/HLA-DR expression by these individual populations. The most immature blast cells (R1) are CD117+CD15–CD13+HLA–DR+. Maturing blasts (R2) are CD117+CD15+ and mature myeloid cells (R3) are CD15+CD117+/–HLA–DR weak. Plots g and h show CD19 expression by blast cells, though at levels weaker than on normal B cells (courtesy of Dr S Richards).

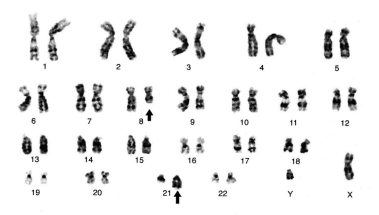

Fig. 2.11 Karyogram showing the translocation between chromosome 8 and chromosome 21 in a male patient with M2 AML and the karyotype t(8;21)(q22;q22) (courtesy of Professor Lorna Secker-Walker, London).

factor activity of normal AML1 protein. It should be noted that *RUNX1* is the internationally agreed designation of the gene still commonly called *AML1*; the approved designation refers to its homology with the Drosophila RUNT gene.

t(8;21) can be detected using dual-colour, dual-fusion FISH and probes for *AML1* and *ETO* [130] (Figs 2.12 and 2.13). The rearrangement can also be detected by RT-PCR in cytologically typical cases both with and without t(8;21). The cases with *AML1-ETO*

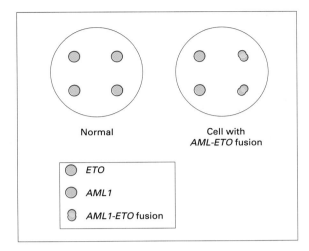

Fig. 2.12 Diagrammatic representation of dual-colour, dual-fusion FISH for the detection of *AML1-ETO*. The normal cell has two red *ETO* signals and two green *AML1* signals. The cell with a t(8;21) translocation has a normal green *AML1* signal, a normal red *ETO* signal and two yellow fusion signals representing *AML1-ETO* and *ETO-AML1*.

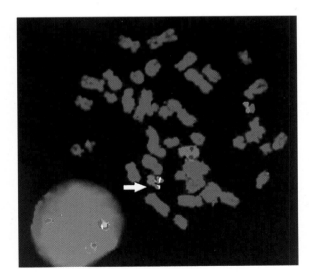

Fig. 2.13 Metaphase spread and interphase nucleus from a patient with M2 AML and t(8;21)(q22;q22) hybridized with probes to the genes *ETO* (green) and *AML1* (red). These are located at 8q22 and 21q22, respectively. Note one green signal (on the normal 8), one red signal (on the normal 21) and one yellow signal (on the derived chromosome 8) indicating the fusion of the two genes resulting from the translocation (courtesy of Dr Christine Harrison, Southampton).

rearrangement but without t(8;21) may be cytogenetically normal or may have complex chromosomal rearrangements (involving chromosomes 8 and 21 together with a third chromosome) or deletions or other abnormalities of chromosome 8 [108, 131]. Use of molecular techniques has been reported to increase the number of cases identified by up to 60% in comparison with cytogenetic analysis alone [132] but in another large study only 2 of 33 cases (6%) were not detected by cytogenetic analysis [97].

Minimal residual disease can be monitored by quantitative PCR but so far data are conflicting as to whether this gives prognostically useful information [133].

A c-*KIT* mutation is found in a significant proportion of patients with t(8;21), some of whom have aberrant bone marrow mast cells [134].

AML associated with t(16;21)(q24;q22) and *AML1-MTG16* fusion (see Table 2.19, p. 112) appears to be closely related to AML with t(8;21) with a similar molecular mechanism, M2 or M2Eo morphology and possible co-expression of CD19 and CD34 [135]. However cases with t(16;21) are usually therapy-related.

M3 or M3V/t(15;17)(q22;q21)/*PML-RARA* fusion

t(15;17)(q22;q21) (Fig. 2.14) is present in the great majority of patients with M3 and M3V AML and, with the exception of rare conditions such as hypergranular promyelocytic transformation of chronic granulocytic leukaemia or of polycythaemia rubra vera, is confined to this category of leukaemia. Overall, M3/M3V/t(15;17) constitutes 4–9% of cases of AML in different series of patients [77, 96]. In elderly adults, the prevalence falls to 4% of cases [90].

Clinical and haematological features. In the great majority of instances, M3 AML occurs *de novo* but a small proportion of cases follow therapy with topoisomerase II-interactive drugs and other agents [101, 102, 136]. The total white cell count is often normal or low in M3 AML but usually elevated in M3V AML. Disseminated intravascular coagulation with markedly increased fibrinolysis is common. M3/M3V AML has a particular sensitivity to differentiation therapy with all-*trans*-retinoic acid (ATRA). With modern treatment incorporating this agent, the prognosis is relatively good with reported remission rates as high as 85–90% and 5-year survivals as high as 50–60% [120]. Five-year survival in secondary cases also approaches 50% and is thus considerably

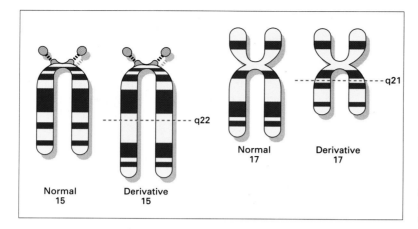

Fig. 2.14 A diagrammatic representation of the t(15;17)(q22;q21) abnormality (modified from [3]).

better than in most other types of therapy-related AML [136]. Arsenic trioxide (As_2O_3) and tetra-arsenic tetra-sulphide (As_4S_4) are also efficacious in M3/M3V AML [137]. Among chemotherapeutic agents, anthracyclines are of considerable importance whereas cytosine arabinoside may be of little or no importance [138, 139]. Prognosis is best in those with a lower presenting WBC (less than 2, 5 or 10×10^9/l in different trials [139, 140]) and a presenting platelet count greater than 40×10^9/l [141]; the worse prognosis in those with higher white cell counts is attributable to a higher early death rate. Overall the complete remission rate and median survival are relatively favourable [89, 90, 105].

The distinctive cytological and cytochemical features have been described on page 16.

Both ATRA and arsenic trioxide therapy lead to maturation of cells of the leukaemic clone, with sometimes a steep rise in the white cell count and with the appearance of maturing but cytologically abnormal cells. Tetra-arsenic tetra-sulphide may, however, lead to degeneration rather than differentiation of promyelocytes [137].

Immunophenotype. This category of AML has a characteristic immunophenotype (Fig. 2.15) [121], which can be useful in distinguishing M3 AML from other subtypes of AML. The immunophenotype of M3V AML is less distinctive [142, 143] but can be useful in helping to make a distinction from M5 AML. Flow cytometry in M3 AML shows, on light scatter measurements, a compact cluster with relatively high forward and sideways light scatter [144]. M3V tends to show more right-angle light scatter than M3 AML

[145]. M3 AML may show significant autofluorescence [145]. CD13, CD33 and MPO are characteristically positive but CD33 is more consistently positive than CD13 [116, 142]. CD33 expression is homogeneous [121] whereas CD13 expression tends to be heterogeneous [121, 146]. CD33 is characteristically more strongly expressed than in normal neutrophils [145]. HLA-DR and CD34, which are positive on early granulocytic lineage cells but negative on normal promyelocytes, are usually negative in M3 and M3V AML but expression is variable [145] and approaching a fifth of cases may be positive for CD34, particularly those with M3V cytological features [142, 143, 147, 148]. CD133, another marker of immaturity, was negative in a small number of patients tested [43]. CD7 is usually negative [42]. CD9 has been reported to be almost always positive whereas it is negative in most other subtypes of AML, but the usefulness of this is reduced by the fact that CD9 is rarely included in panels of McAb for typing of acute leukaemia. In addition, not all groups have found the same sensitivity and specificity of this marker [149]. Positive reactions with CD11b and CD14 McAb are seen in a minority of cases; these reactions, more typical of monocytes, do not correlate with anomalous expression of non-specific esterase by M3 cells [150]. CD64, which is also characteristic of the monocytic lineage, is usually positive whereas CD65 and CD117 have been reported to be more often negative [12]. Others have found CD117 to be sometimes positive [142, 143] or both CD117 and CD65 to be uniformly positive [146]. CD15 has been reported as negative [142, 146] or often positive [143]. CD11a, which is

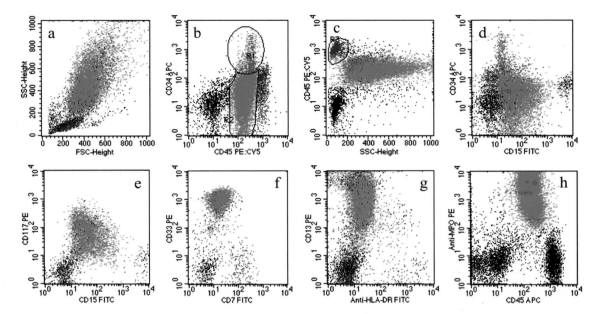

Fig. 2.15 Flour-colour flow cytometry immunophenotyping from a patient with AML associated with t(15;17) (*compare with* Fig. 2.3). Plots a, b and c show standard analysis regions, The blast cells in M3 AML are usually CD34–CD45+. Their key phenotypic features are shown in plots d–h. In plot d the blast cells have clearly lost CD34 expression but, in contrast to normal myeloid cells at this stage of differentiation, have not acquired CD15. Note the strong homogeneous CD33 expression (f), heterogeneous CD13 expression covering two log decades of fluorescence (g), the absence of HLA-DR expression (g) and the strong myeloperoxidase expression (h) (courtesy of Dr S. Richards).

often expressed in other categories of AML, is not expressed [151]. CD56 is usually negative [147] and when expressed has been correlated with a worse outcome [152]. CD2 and CD19 are positive in a significant minority of cases [45, 148]; expression of these antigens has been found to be more likely in M3 variant than in classical M3 AML [142, 147]. Cases of AML that are HLA-DR negative and CD2 positive are likely to be M3/M3V [7].

Cytogenetic and molecular genetic features. The frequency with which the specific t(15;17)(q22;q21) translocation (Fig. 2.16) is detected in AML M3/M3V is method dependent since direct examination without culture may result in only non-clonal erythroid cells entering mitosis [75]. MAC techniques show t(15;17) in the granulocytic lineage but not in erythroid or megakaryocyte lineages [128]. Typically, the translocation is detected by conventional cytogenetic techniques in about 90% of cases. Other patients have a *PML-RARA* fusion gene (or, less often, a *RARA-PML* fusion gene) formed by insertion. In addition to

the primary abnormality, 30–40% of cases show secondary karyotypic abnormalities. Among these the commonest are trisomy 8 (present in 12% of patients) and del(7q), del(9q) and +21 (each present in 1–2% of patients) [153]. An isochromosome of the long arm of the derivative 17, ider(17), which results in two copies of the *PML-RARA* fusion gene, is observed in fewer than 1% of patients [153]; in one study, the seven cases with ider(17)(q10)t(15;17)(q22;q21) were all M3 rather than M3 variant [147]. An adverse prognostic significance of secondary chromosomal anomalies was observed in one series of patients [154] but not in two others [153, 155]. Cases that lack Auer rods appear to be more likely to have additional chromosomal abnormalities [156].

The molecular mechanism of leukaemogenesis is fusion of part of the *PML* (promyelocytic leukaemia) gene at 15q22 with part of the *RARA* (retinoic acid receptor α, also designated *RARα*) gene from 17q21 [157] to form a fusion gene on the derivative chromosome 15. *PML* and *RARA* encode transcription

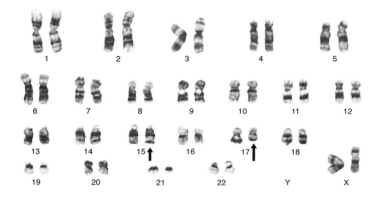

Fig. 2.16 Karyogram showing the translocation between chromosomes 15 and 17 in a female patient with M3 AML and the karyotype 46,XX,t(15;17)(q22;q21) (courtesy of Professor Lorna Secker-Walker).

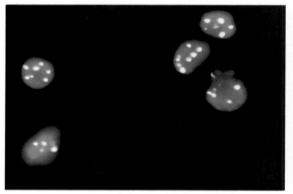

(a)

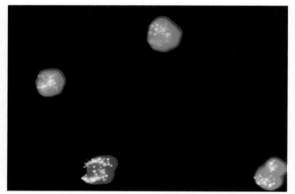

(b)

Fig. 2.17 Immunofluorescence technique using 5E10, a monoclonal antibody to promyelocytic leukaemia (PML) protein (green fluorescence); cells are counterstained with a blue fluorochrome (DAPI): (a) normal distribution of PML protein in relatively large nuclear bodies in a case of M2 AML; (b) abnormal microparticulate distribution of PML protein in a case of M3 AML (courtesy of Dr Sheila O'Connor, Leeds, and with permission of the British Journal of Haematology [159]).

factors. The PML-RARA fusion protein may be oncogenic because of its ability to sequester normal PML protein. In normal cells, immunofluorescence demonstrates that PML protein occurs in 10–30 discrete bodies within the nucleus (nuclear bodies) whereas in M3 AML there is a microparticulate or speckled distribution. Detection of this characteristic

pattern by immunocytochemistry has been found to be a reliable method of diagnosing M3 and M3V AML [158, 159] (Fig. 2.17); the necessary antibody is commercially available. The fusion gene *RARA-PML* on chromosome 17 is expressed in about 70% of cases of M3 AML and may also be oncogenic [160, 161]. In one study, expression of *PML-RARA* alone was found to produce both the phenotype of M3 AML and ATRA sensitivity whereas the expression of *RARA-PML* alone produced the cytological features of M3 AML but without the characteristic immunostaining pattern with anti-PML antibodies or ATRA sensitivity [162]. The precise breakpoints in *PML* and *RARA* differ between *de novo* and therapy-related cases [163].

Classical M3 AML may also be associated with complex variant translocations, simple variant trans-

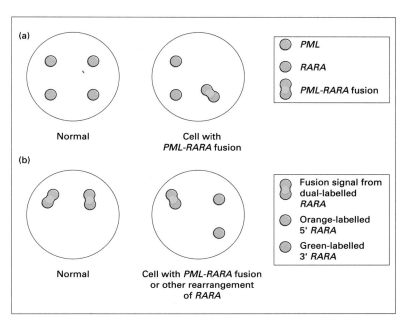

Fig. 2.18 Diagrammatic representation of two FISH strategies for the detection of *RARA* rearrangements: (a) dual-colour, single-fusion FISH technique in t(15;17)(q22;q21). The normal cell has two red *PML* signals and two green *RARA* signals. The abnormal cell has one normal red *PML* signal, one normal green *RARA* signal and a yellow *PML-RARA* fusion signal (b) dual-colour, break-apart FISH technique for the detection of *RARA* disruption in t(15;17)(q22;q21) or variant translocations such as t(11;17)(q23;q21). The normal cell has two similar signals each comprised of a red signal from 5′ *RARA* and a green signal from 3′ *RARA*. The abnormal cell has single normal red-green (yellow) signal and distinct smaller red and green signals resulting from disruption of the *RARA* gene.

locations and cryptic or masked translocations [161]. A complex translocation involves chromosomes 15 and 17 together with a third chromosome. A simple variant translocation involves either 15 or 17 (more often 17) and another chromosome; these cases should be included in the M3/t(15;17) MIC–M category if either *PML-RARA* or *RARA-PML* is expressed. In cryptic or masked translocations both chromosomes 15 and 17 appear normal, with the karyotype either being normal or showing an unrelated abnormality. In the majority of these cases, the same molecular mechanisms as have been described above are operating; in the case of simple variant and cryptic translocations there are submicroscopic translocations or insertions, which usually lead to *PML-RARA* expression but occasionally to expression only of *RARA-PML* [161]. *PML-RARA* fusion is very rare among cases of AML not recognized morphologically as M3 or M3 variant. In one study only a single instance was observed among 530 cases [164]; on morphological review, it was reclassified from M5 to M3 variant AML.

PML-RARA rearrangement can be detected by dual-colour, single-fusion FISH, using probes for *PML* and *RARA* (Fig. 2.18a) [130, 165]. Rearrangement of *RARA* can also be detected using dual-colour, break-apart FISH (Fig. 2.18b). *PML-RARA* fusion, *RARA-*

PML fusion or both can be detected by RT-PCR in the great majority of patients with a cytological diagnosis of M3 AML whether or not t(15;17) is detected by karyotypic analysis. The detection rate by PCR is higher if both fusion genes are sought [166].

Detection of minimal residual disease, by RT-PCR, after consolidation therapy is of prognostic significance [139, 167]. Treatment of molecular relapse may give superior results to waiting for haematological relapse [139]. In patients treated by stem cell transplantation, detection of minimal residual disease is of prognostic significance and directs the need for additional therapy post-transplant [167]. RQ-PCR is likely to prove to be the optimal technique for molecular detection of minimal residual disease.

M3 or M3-like/t(11;17)(q23;q21)/*PLZF-RARA* fusion and other leukaemias associated with rearrangement of the *RARA* gene

In addition to t(15;17)(q22;q21), there are three other translocations associated with rearrangement of the *RARA* gene with leukaemic cells having some features reminiscent of M3 AML. However, many of these cases show cytological, cytogenetic, molecular and clinical differences from M3/M3V AML and the designation 'M3-like' AML is therefore useful. These

Table 2.16 Characteristics of AML associated with rearrangement of the *RARA* gene [147, 160, 168–172].

Cytogenetics	Molecular genetics	Responsiveness to ATRA	Distribution of PML protein* [160, 171]	Frequency
t(15;17)(q22;q21)	*PML-RARA* fusion†	Yes	Microparticulate	About 99% of M3 and M3-like AML
t(11;17)(q23;q21)	*PLZF-RARA* fusion	No‡	Discrete nuclear bodies	0.5% of M3 and M3-like AML
t(11;17)(q13;q21)	*NuMA-RARA* fusion	Probably	Discrete nuclear bodies	Rare
t(5;17)(q32;q21)	*NPM-RARA* fusion	Probably	Discrete nuclear bodies	Even more rare
der(17)	*STAT5b-RARα* fusion	No	Microparticulate	Single case

*The normal distribution is as discrete nuclear bodies.
†Patients with *RARA-PML* but not *PML-RARA* fusion have PML distributed in discrete nuclear bodies and are resistant to ATRA [160].
‡Although lack of responsiveness is not absolute: also unresponsive to arsenic trioxide therapy [172].

types of AML are summarized and compared with M3/t(15;17)(q22;q21) in Table 2.16 [147, 160, 168–172]. As the mechanisms of leukaemogenesis differ and the responsiveness to specific treatments sometimes differs these should be regarded as distinct MIC–M subtypes of AML. Of the three, the most common is t(11;17)(q23;q21).

Clinical and haematological features. The WBC is usually not greatly elevated. The cytological features of AML associated with t(11;17)(q23;q21) differ somewhat from those of classical M3 AML, being in an intermediate position between M2 AML and M3 AML (Fig. 2.19); multiple Auer rods and 'faggots' are not often a feature and there may be a larger proportion of maturing granulocytes. Cells are generally more granular than those of M2 AML but less granular than classical M3 AML and granules do not show the red colouration characteristic of M3 AML; giant granules are sometimes present. The nucleus is usually round rather than irregular or bilobed, there is more chromatin condensation and maturing granulocytes may include Pelger–Huët forms [147]. In one patient with t(5;17) the cytological features were more similar to M3 but Auer rods were lacking [147] whereas two previously reported cases had been associated with M3 and M3V morphology respectively. The t(11;17)(q13;q21)/*NuMA-RARA* rearrangement has been described as associated with hypergranular blasts with irregular nuclei, together with Pelger-like cells. The single patient with AML associated with a *STAT5b-RARA* fusion gene was classified as M1 AML but a minority of bone marrow blasts were considered suggestive of M3 variant AML [171].

The prognosis of M3-like AML associated with t(11;17) is poor [120].

Immunophenotype. The immunophenotype of M3-like/t(11;17)(q23;q21)/*PLZF-RARA* AML differs from that of M3/t(15;17) AML [147]. There is usually expression of CD13 and CD33 and lack of expression of HLA-DR and CD34 but CD56 is much more often expressed than is classical M3/M3 variant [147].

Cytogenetic and molecular genetic features. All these categories of M3-like AML involve chromosome 17 and the *RARA* gene but the partner chromosome and the other gene involved differ. In t(11;17)(q23;q21) part of the *PLZF* (promyelocytic leukaemia zinc finger) gene at 11q23 fuses with the *RARA* gene [168, 170] to form a *PLZF-RARA* fusion gene on chromosome 11; there is a reciprocal *RARA-PLZF* fusion gene on chromosome 17. Both fusion genes are expressed and can be detected by RT-PCR [170]. Cases with a cryptic rearrangement leading to *PLZF-RARA* fusion are identical in other respects to those with t(11;17) [147]. Other fusion partners of RARA are *NPM* (**N**ucleo**p**hos**m**in), *NuMA* (**Nu**clear **M**itotic **A**pparatus) and *STAT5b* (see Table 2.16). Each of these rearrangements of RARA can be detected using dual-colour, break-apart FISH (see Fig. 2.18b).

M4Eo/inv(16)(p13q22) or t(16;16) (p13;q22)/*CBFB-MHY11* fusion

Inversion of chromosome 16 (Fig. 2.20a) and the less common reciprocal translocation between the chromosome 16 pair (Fig. 2.20) are associated with cases of AML with identical features. Such cases comprise 3–6% of AML with inv(16), being about five times as common at t(16;16). The frequency is slightly higher in children than in adults [98] and in elderly adults the prevalence falls to 1% of cases of AML.

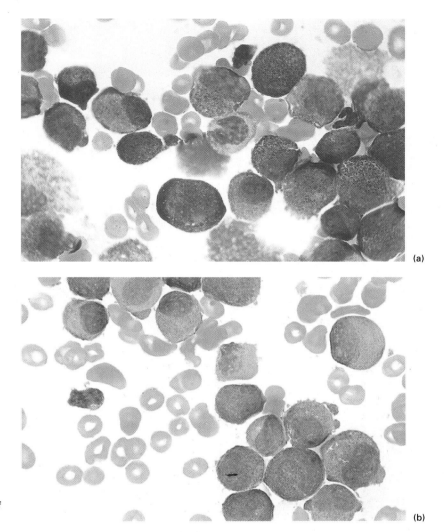

(a)

(b)

Fig. 2.19 BM film from a patient with M2/M3 AML with t(11;17)(q23;q21) showing: (a) more cells maturing beyond promyelocyte stage than is usual in classical M3 AML but with several hypergranular blasts being present; (b) several hypergranular promyelocytes and a cell with a single Auer rod (cells with multiple Auer rods were not seen). MGG × 870 (courtesy of Dr D.J. Culligan, Aberdeen).

Clinical and haematological features. This subtype of AML is associated with granulocytic and monocytic differentiation with cytologically abnormal eosinophils, which are often prominent, leading to a designation of M4Eo AML [75, 173, 174] (Figs 2.21 & 2.22), and see also Fig. 1.24, page 23). For convenience, the designation M4Eo will be used in the following paragraphs. However, it should be noted that a significant proportion of cases are classified as M1, M2, M2Eo, M4 or M5, i.e. they lack prominent eosinophilia, monocytic differentiation or both. Bone marrow eosinophils are less than 5% in more than

a quarter of patients [175]. Nevertheless, morphologically abnormal cells of eosinophil lineage are probably always present, although they may constitute as little as 0.2% of bone marrow cells [120, 175]. M4Eo AML is sometimes associated with meningeal leukaemia and with intracranial tumour formation by leukaemic cells. There have also been several reports of granulocytic sarcoma of the bowel occurring in advance of overt leukaemia. Patients are relatively young. The remission rate is high and prognosis is relatively good. The great majority of cases occur *de novo* but secondary cases are recognized following

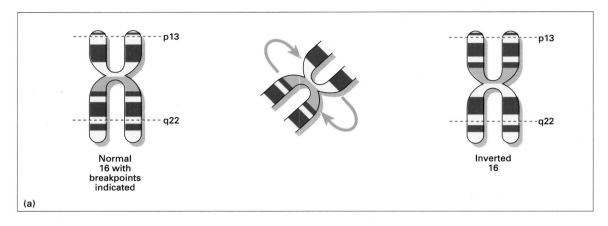

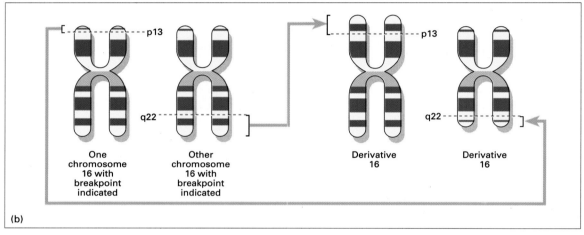

Fig. 2.20 (a) A diagrammatic representation of inv(16)(p13q22); this is an example of a pericentric inversion (modified from [3]). (b) A diagrammatic representation of t(16;16)(p13;q22).

exposure to topoisomerase II-interactive drugs and other agents [101, 102].

Blast cells are variable in size and shape with prominent cytoplasmic basophilia. Some are monoblasts and some are primitive cells with occasional eosinophil granules. Bone marrow blast cells are sometimes less than 20%; in the WHO classification (see below), such cases are nevertheless categorized as AML [116].

Auer rods are usually present although only in a minority of cells; they are sometimes present in mature neutrophils. Neutrophils may be cytologically abnormal [175]. Bone marrow eosinophils and to a greater extent eosinophil myelocytes show prominent pro-eosinophilic granules, which are basophilic in their staining characteristics (see Fig 2.21a and b). Mature eosinophils may be hypolobulated. In some cases the eosinophils have unusually large and folded nuclei. Eosinophils also show aberrant cytochemical reactions. Some have PAS-positive granules and some give positive reactions for CAE. PAS-positive granules are not specific for this subtype of leukaemia nor in fact for leukaemic eosinophils since they may be observed in t(8;21)/M2 [94] and sometimes in reactive eosinophilia [75]. Positivity for CAE may, however, indicate that eosinophils are part of a leukaemic process [75]. Despite the bone marrow eosinophilia, peripheral blood eosinophilia is unusual and blood eosinophils are usually morphologically normal. Cytogenetic analysis has confirmed that

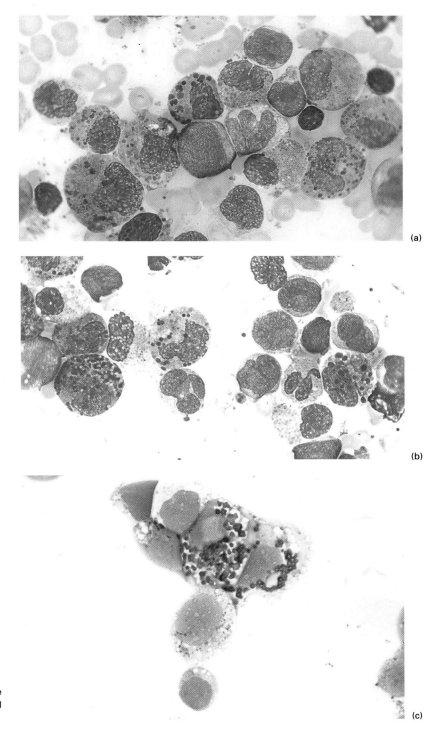

(a)

(b)

(c)

Fig. 2.21 BM film from a patient with AML M4Eo/inv(16). (a,b) MGG stain showing abnormal blasts, monocytes, mature eosinophils and eosinophil myelocytes with abnormally basophilic granules. MGG × 870. (c) SBB stain showing large abnormal granules in the eosinophil lineage and occasional small granules in monocytes. SBB × 870.

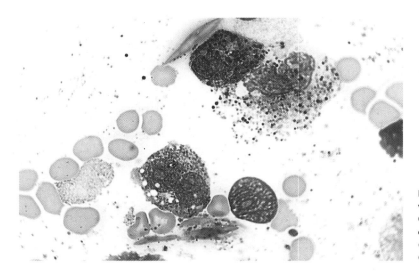

Fig. 2.22 BM film from a patient with AML M4Eo/inv(16) showing Charcot–Leyden crystals and abnormal cells of eosinophil lineage. MGG × 870 (courtesy of Dr R. Cobcroft and Dr D. Gill, Brisbane).

eosinophils are indeed part of the abnormal clone. Occasional patients with M4Eo/inv(16) have had increased bone marrow basophils and basophil precursors (confirmed by metachromasia with toluidine blue) [176] (see Fig. 1.24). Despite the monocytic differentiation, non-specific esterase reactions are often weak [175]. Dysplasia of erythroid and megakaryocyte lineages is not usual.

The prognosis of this category of AML is relatively good with 5-year survivals of up to 60% being reported [89, 90, 105]. Prognosis is significantly better in those with a presenting white cell count of 20 × 10^9/l or less [106]. The prognosis in children appears to be equally good [120]. In view of the relatively good prognosis, stem cell transplantation in first remission is generally considered contraindicated. Intensive post-remission intensification with high-dose cytosine arabinoside may contribute to improved survival [119]. Five-year survival in secondary cases approaches 50% and is thus considerably better than in most other types of therapy-related AML [136].

Immunophenotype. Flow cytometry immunophenotyping shows both granulocytic and monocytic differentiation (Fig. 2.23) [121]. The plot of sideways light scatter against forward light scatter may show a characteristic forked pattern [145]. Typically there is positivity for CD13, CD33, CD14, CD15, CD64, CD65, CD117, anti-MPO and HLA-DR while CD11b is positive in about a third of cases [177]. Antigen expression may show considerable heterogeneity with a population of blasts expressing CD34 but little

CD11b, CD14, CD15 or CD64, a population of maturing monocytes expressing CD33, CD11b, CD14 and CD64 and a population of granulocytes with considerable sideways light scatter and strong CD15 [145]. CD2 may be expressed and correlates with CD11b expression [151]. CD34 has been variously reported to be positive in about a third [177] or in the great majority [178, 179] of cases. CD34 and terminal deoxynucleotidyl transferase are more often positive than in AML in general [180]. CD7 is not usually expressed [179]. Strong expression of CD34 and CD13 and weak expression of CD33 has been reported to have a reasonably high sensitivity and specificity [180].

Cytogenetic and molecular genetic features. M4Eo AML is associated both with inv(16)(p13q22) (Fig 2.24) and, less often, t(16;16)(p13;q22) (Fig 2.25). The molecular mechanism of leukaemogenesis is the same. The commonest secondary chromosomal abnormalities are trisomy 8, trisomy 22 and 7q–, the latter two anomalies being uncommon in association with other specific chromosomal aberrations. The detection of trisomy 22 in a patient who appears to lack inv(16) is an indication for molecular analysis for the *CBFB-MYH11* fusion gene since a cryptic chromosomal rearrangement may be present [181]. M4Eo AML has also been described in association with a deletion of chromosome 16, del(16)(q22) [182]. Most such cases have been considered to show the same features as are seen with inv(16) but there have been reports suggesting that patients with del(16)(q22) have M4

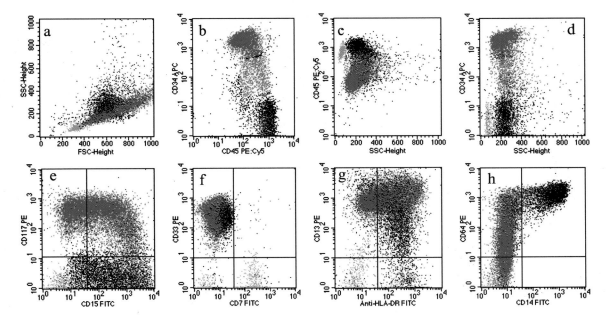

Fig. 2.23 Four-colour flow cytometry immunophenotyping in a patient with AML associated with inv(16) (*compare with* Fig. 2.3). Plots a–d show distinct CD34++, CD34 + and CD34– blast cell populations. Plots e and h show a spectrum of differentiation, with the most immature blast cell component (plot e) being CD34++CD117+CD15+/–. The mature monocytic component (CD34–) is CD14+CD64+CD15+ (plot h) with high levels of CD45 expression, comparable to that of normal lymphocytes. Blast cells show a continuous spectrum of maturation but at all stages of maturation there is evidence of monocytic differentiation (ranging from CD64+ to CD64+++CD14+). The blast cells continue to be CD33 and CD13 positive at all stages of differentiation (f and g) (courtesy of Dr S. Richards).

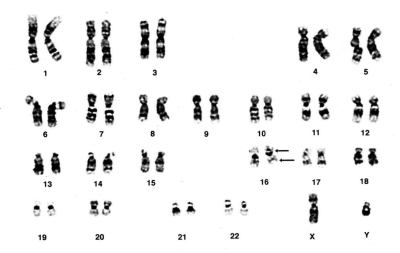

Fig. 2.24 A karyogram showing inv(16)(p13q22) (courtesy of Dr Fiona Ross, Salisbury).

AML without eosinophilia [75, 183] and with a high incidence of preceding MDS [183]. Both inv(16) and del(16) are relatively difficult to detect by conventional cytogenetic analysis and it can also be difficult to distinguish between the various abnormalities of chromosome 16 [75]. It may be that some of the cases reported as del(16) are actually examples of inv(16) while others, without the typical features of M4Eo

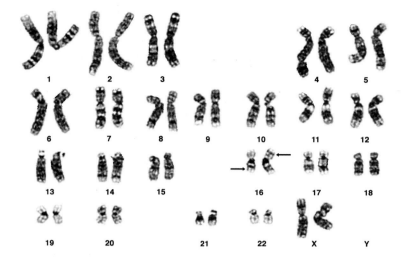

Fig. 2.25 A karyogram showing t(16;16)(p13;q22) (courtesy of Dr Fiona Ross).

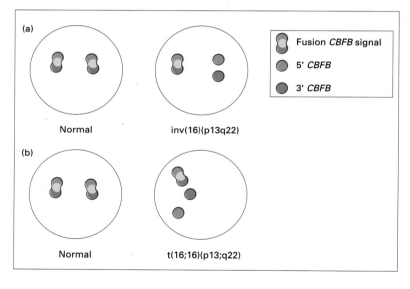

Fig. 2.26 Diagrammatic representation of a dual-colour, break-apart FISH technique for detecting the disruption of *CBFB* in inv(16)(p13q22) and t(16;16)(p13;q22), using a red-labelled probe for 5′ *CBFB* and a green-labelled probe for 3′ *CBFB*: (a) a normal cell has two yellow fusion signals whereas a cell with inv(16) has one normal fusion signal and separated red and green 5′ and 3′ *CBFB* signals on the two arms of the inverted chromosome; (b) a cell with a t(16;16) has one normal fusion signal on the q arm and a distinct green 3′ *CBFB* signal on the p arm of the same chromosome; the other chromosome 16 has a discrete red 5′ *CBFB* signal.

AML, may have a different mechanism of leukaemogenesis. M4Eo AML has also been associated with a variant translocation, t(5;16)(q33;q22).

The molecular mechanism of leukaemogenesis is fusion of part of the *CBFB* (core binding factor β, also designated *CBFβ*) gene at 16q22 with part of the *MYH11* (myosin heavy chain) gene at 16p13 to form a fusion gene, *CBFB-MYH11*, which codes for a protein that interferes with normal control of transcription [184]. The reciprocal fusion gene, *MYH11-CBFB*, is expressed in only a proportion of cases. *MYH11* is also referred to as *SMMHC* (smooth muscle myosin

heavy chain). The precise breakpoints differ at a molecular level between *de novo* and therapy-related cases [163]. A minority of patients have submicroscopic deletion of part of chromosome 16, telomeric to the *CBFB* gene [185]; this may be associated with a worse prognosis. A c-*KIT* mutation is found in a significant proportion of patients with inv(16), some of whom have aberrant bone marrow mast cells [134].

Inv(16)(p13q22) and t(16;16)(p13;q22) can be detected by two-colour FISH using probes for *CBFB* and *MYH11* (Fig. 2.26). FISH is useful for the detection of masked inv(16) in patients with simple variant translocations involving chromosome 16 and diverse partners. Both inv(16) and t(16;16) can also be detected by RT-PCR for *CBFB-MYH11*. A significant proportion of patients (up to a quarter) have been reported to have no detectable abnormality of chromosome 16 despite having the same molecular genetic abnormality demonstrable by RT-PCR. However this was not confirmed in a further large study in which all 27 cases were identified by conventional cytogenetic analysis [97]. When molecular techniques are employed the prevalence of this MIC–M subtype among cases of AML may be as high as 10% [174]. Cases that do not have the typical M4Eo cytological features are more likely to be missed on conventional cytogenetic analysis.

Detection of minimal residual disease above a certain level by RQ-PCR has been found predictive of relapse [133, 186].

M5/t(9;11)(p 21–22;q23)/*MLL-AF9* fusion

There is a strong association between monoblastic/ monocytic leukaemia and deletions or translocations with a breakpoint within the *MLL* gene at 11q23 [187]. Overall such cases comprise about 4% of cases of AML [96] but about 18% of childhood cases [98]. Some important subtypes of leukaemia with *MLL* rearrangement are shown in Table 2.17 and other less common subtypes in Table 2.18. Of the myeloid leukaemias in which there is a chromosomal rearrangement with an 11q23 breakpoint, that associated with t(9;11)(p21;q23) is the most common and will now be discussed.

Clinical and haematological features. The prevalence of AML with t(9;11)(p21;q23) is highest among children and infants (including babies with congenital leukaemia) but adult cases also occur. In one large series of children with AML, 7% were found to have t(9;11) [98]. A significant proportion of cases, about 8% in one series of patients [113], are secondary to topoisomerase II-interactive drugs. Soft tissue tumours of blast cells may be particularly common, t(9;11) being the most frequently observed karyotypic abnormality in one series of such patients [207]. The prognosis has varied considerably between different series of patients but in general has been poor in infants and children and intermediate in adults. In two studies the prognosis was found to be better than that of AML associated with other rearrangements with an 11q23 breakpoint [105, 208]. This was not so in a third series of childhood cases [98] although a fourth study found that in infants t(9;11) was a good prognostic factor [188]. In adults, AML associated with t(9;11) is favourable with regard to the probability of complete remission but intermediate with regard to overall survival [105]. Remission rate approaches 80% and 5-year-survival approaches 40% [120]. The prognosis of therapy-related cases is worse with less than 20% 5-year survival [209]. Most cases of AML with t(9;11) are M5a AML (Fig. 2.27) but some are M5b or M4 (Fig. 2.28) and occasional cases are M1, M2 or M7 [191]. Cases of ALL also occur. Auer rods are quite uncommon.

Table 2.17 Characteristics of acute leukaemia and related conditions associated with translocations and deletions involving 11q23 studied at the European 11q23 Workshop (percentages are shown in parentheses).

Translocation or other rearrangement	Total	Infants (less than 12 months)	Children (1–14 years)	ALL	AML	Main FAB category of AML	Other acute leukaemia*	t-AML/ MDS	t-MDS	Reference
t(4;11)(q21;q23)	183	63 (34)	36 (20)	173 (95)	6 (3)	M4	4 (2.2)	nil	10 (5.5)	[189]
t(6;11)(q27;q23)	30	2 (7)	6 (20)	3 (10)	27 (90)	M4/M5a	nil	nil	nil	[190]
t(9;11)(p21–22;q23)	125	21/123 (17)	46/123 (37)	9 (7)	108 (86)	M5a	3 (2)	5 (4)	10 (8)	[191]
t(10;11)(p12–22;q23)	20	6/19 (32)	10/19 (53)	4 (20)	15 (75)	M5a	1 (5)	nil	1 (5)	[192]
t(11;19)(q23;p13.1)	21	3 (14)	1 (5)	nil	19 (90)	M4	nil	2 (10)	7 (33)	[193]
t(11;19)(q23;p13.3)	32	13 (41)	7 (22)	21 (66)	7 (22)	M4 or M5a	4 (12)	nil	nil	[193]
del(11)(q23)	57	3 (5)	10 (33)	27 (47)	16 (28)	M4, M5a, M5b	2 (4)	12 (21)	1 (2)	[194]

ALL, acute lymphoblastic anaemia; AML, acute myeloid leukaemia; FAB, French–American–British classification; MDS, myelodysplastic syndrome; t-AML, therapy-related AML; t-MDS, therapy-related MDS.
*Other acute leukaemia = acute biphenotypic, acute stem cell and acute unclassified leukaemia.

Table 2.18 Some of the less common MIC–M categories of acute myeloid leukaemia* involving an 11q23 breakpoint and the *MLL* gene† [120, 188–206].

Translocation or other rearrangement	Type of leukaemia [195]	Molecular event
t(1;11)(p32;q23)	M5	*MLL-AF1p* fusion
t(1;11)(q21;q23)	M4	*MLL-AF1q* fusion
t(2;11)(p21;q23)‡		Not known
t(3;11)(p21;q23)	M5	*MLL-AF3p21* fusion
t(3;11)(q25;q23)	t-AML (M4)	*MLL-GMPS* fusion [196]
t(3;11)(q28;q23)	A case of M5 AML (t-AML)	*LPP-MLL* and *MLL-LPP* fusion genes [197]
t(4;11)(q21;q23)	M4 (more often ALL)	*MLL-AF4* fusion [189]
t(4;11)(q31;q23)‡		Not known
t(6;11)(q21;q23)		*MLL-AF6q21* fusion
t(6;11)(q27;q23)	M4 or M5	*MLL-AF6* fusion
t(8;11)(q24;q23)‡	M5	Not known [198]
t(9;11)(p21;q23)		*MLL-AF9*
t(9;11)(q21;q23)‡		Not known
t(9;11)(q22;q23)‡		Not known
t(10;11)(p12;q23)	M5a	*MLL-AF10* fusion [192]
t(10;11)(p11.2;q23)	AML	*MLL-ABI1* fusion
t(10;11)(q22;q23)‡	M4	Not known [199]
ins(10;11)(p11;q23q13–24)‡		Not known
ins(11;9)(q23;q34) inv(11) (q13q23)	A case of M4 AML	*MLL-FBP17* fusion [199]
t(11;11)(q13;q23)‡		Not known
inv(11)(p15q23)‡		Not known
inv(11)(q14.2q23.1)	A case of AML	*MLL-CALM* fusion [200]
t(11;12)(q23;p13)‡		Not known
t(11;14)(q23;q24)	A case of M5 AML	*MLL-gephyrin* fusion [201]
t(11;15)(q23;q12)‡		Not known
t(11;15)(q23;q14)	A case of AML	*MLL-AF15q14* fusion [202]
t(11;16)(q23;p13)		*MLL-CBP* fusion
cryptic t(11;17)(q23;p13)	A case of M4 AML (t-AML)	*MLL-GAS7* fusion [203]
t(11;17)(q23;q12–21)	M5 AML	*MLL-AF17* fusion
t(11;17)(q23;q25)		*MLL-MSF/AF17q* fusion
t(11;19)(q23;p13.1)	AML M5	*MLL-ELL* fusion [193]
t(11;19)(q23;p13.3)	AML M5 (also pro-B ALL)	*MLL-ENL* fusion [193]
t(11;19)(q23;q12 or q13)‡		Not known
t(11;21)(q23;q13)‡		Not known
t(11;22)(q23;q11)		*HCDCrel-MLL* fusion
t(11;22)(q23;q13)	AML	*MLL-P300* fusion [204]
t(X;11)(q13;q23)	M4 or M5	*MLL-AFX1* fusion
t(X;11)(q24;q23)—often complex	M2	*MLL-Septin 6/KIAA01* fusion [205]
Tandem partial duplication of *MLL*, with or without trisomy 11	AML (M0, M1, M2, M4, M7)	Partial tandem duplication of *MLL* [206]

*Some of these translocations are also associated with acute lymphoblastic leukaemia (ALL) or biphenotypic acute leukaemia suggesting that the mutation occurs in a pluripotent stem cell; in the case of t(4;11) the majority of cases are of ALL.
†Rearrangement of 11q23 may be detected by conventional cytogenetic analysis. Rearrangement of the *MLL* gene can be detected in a larger number of cases by fluorescent *in situ* hybridization (FISH); the reverse transcriptase polymerase chain reaction (RT-PCR) or Southern blotting; FISH with a dual colour *MLL* probe is particularly useful, the two signals being split when the gene is rearranged; this method is independent of prediction of the partner chromosome; deletion of chromosome 11, interpreted either as terminal or interstitial, has also been associated with M4 or M5 AML (and with MDS), but FISH analysis suggests that many apparent deletions are actually reciprocal translocations.
‡ Provisional MIC–M category as molecular event not fully elucidated.

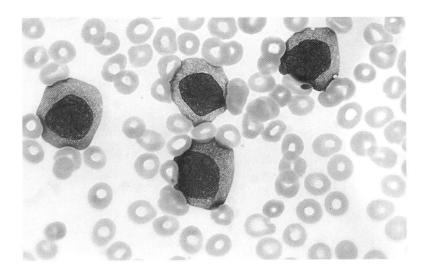

Fig. 2.27 PB film from a patient with M5a AML associated with t(9;11)(p21–22;q23). MGG × 870.

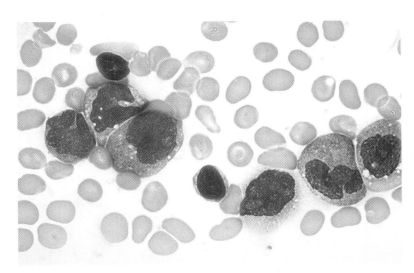

Fig. 2.28 BM film from a patient with M4 AML associated with t(9;11)(p21–22;q23). MGG × 870 (courtesy of the European 11q23 Workshop [191]).

Immunophenotype. The immunophenotype is characteristic of M5 AML. CD15, CD33, CD64, CD65 and HLA-DR are usually expressed. CD13 was found to be usually negative in one series [12] but positive in two-thirds of patients in another [191]. Similarly, CD14 was usually negative in one series [12] but positive in half the cases in another [191]. CD11b and 11c are often expressed [191]. CD34 and CD7 are positive in 40–50% of cases [191]. CD4, a marker of the monocytic lineage as well as of T lymphocytes, is sometimes expressed. NG2, a chondroitin sulphate proteoglycan is expressed. This immunophenotypic marker was initially reported to be expressed in AML associated with t(9;11) or other *MLL* rearrangement but not in AML without *MLL* rearrangement [210]. However, subsequently expression, together with CD56 expression, was demonstrated in cases with monocytic differentiation but without *MLL* rearrangement [211].

Cytogenetic and molecular genetic features. t(9;11)(p22; q23) is difficult to detect by conventional cytogenetic analysis since the alteration in the banding pattern is subtle (Fig. 2.29 & 2.30). Detection is facilitated by dual-colour, break-apart FISH, using probes for

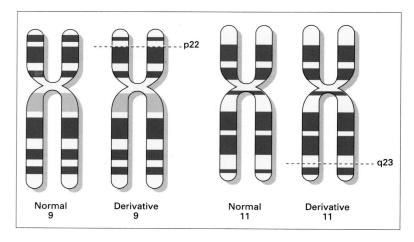

Fig. 2.29 Diagrammatic representation of t(9;11)(p22;q23) (modified from [3]); the 9p breakpoint is variable, p21–22.

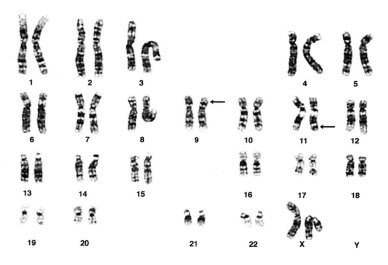

Fig. 2.30 A karyogram showing t(q;11)(p21–22;q23) (courtesy of Dr Fiona Ross).

5′ and 3′ *MLL* that are labelled with different fluorochromes; when the gene is rearranged the two colours are separated. The commonest secondary abnormalities associated with t(9;11) are trisomy 6, trisomy 8, trisomy 8q, trisomy 19 and duplication of the derivative chromosome 9 [191, 208, 212].

The molecular mechanism of leukaemogenesis is fusion of the *MLL* (mixed lineage leukaemia or myeloid lymphoid leukaemia) gene at 11q23 with the *AF9* gene at 9p21 to form an abnormal fusion gene, *MLL-AF9* [213]. The *MLL* gene, which is a homologue of the *Drosophila trithorax* gene, has been investigated by many independent groups and has also been designated *HRX*, *ALL-1* and *Htrx-1*. *MLL* rearrangements can be detected by Southern blotting

and *MLL-AF9* fusion by RT-PCR (providing a possible target for the detection of minimal residual disease). t(9;11) can also be detected by two-colour FISH using probes for the *MLL* and *AF9* genes [130]. Rearrangements of the *MLL* gene, including that present in t(9;11), can also be detected by dual-colour, break-apart FISH; the principle is the same as for detection of rearrangements of the *RARA* gene.

Other categories of AML with *MLL* rearrangement

Other categories of acute leukaemia with an 11q23 breakpoint have some characteristics in common with each other and with AML associated with t(9;11) but they differ in other important features. Molecular mechanisms of leukaemogenesis differ and, when the genetic abnormality is known, distinct MIC–M categories of acute leukaemia should be recognized.

Clinical and haematological features. Common characteristics include a predominance of M4 and M5 AML and a possible relationship to topoisomerase II-interactive drugs. Congenital cases have been reported in association with t(4;11)(q21;q23), t(10;11)(p13;q23) and t(11;19)(q23;p12–13) [214]. Features that differ between categories include the relative proportions of AML, ALL and biphenotypic leukaemia, the relative proportions of *de novo* and secondary cases, the proportion of patients presenting with MDS and the relative frequency of different FAB subtypes of AML [189, 194]. Prognosis also differs. Although prognosis is generally poor [105, 215]; the prognosis in cases with t(10;11)(p12;q23), as for cases with t(9;11)(p22;q23), appears to be intermediate or standard [216].

Immunophenotype. The immunophenotype is generally similar to that of AML associated with t(9;11). NG2 expression has been demonstrated in cases associated with *MLL* rearrangement associated with t(11;17)(q23;q21), t(11;19)(q23;p13), other chromosomal abnormality without cytogenetic evidence of an 11q23 abnormality and a normal karyotype [210].

Cytogenetic and molecular genetic features. Cytogenetic analysis underestimates the frequency of cases with 11q23 rearrangement [215]. FISH analysis, e.g. using dual-colour break-apart FISH, detects a higher proportion of cases but some are detected only by

Southern blot or other DNA analysis [215]. The *MLL-AF6*, *MLL-AF10* and *MLL-ENL* fusion genes can be detected by RT-PCR, providing a possible target for detection of minimal residual disease [133].

M1/t(9;22)(q34;q11)/*BCR-ABL* fusion

The reciprocal translocation t(9;22)(q34;q11) leads to the formation of the Philadelphia chromosome, an abbreviated chromosome 22 to which a small part of chromosome 9 has been translocated. The Philadelphia chromosome was initially designated by the abbreviation Ph[1], but it has been suggested that it is now more appropriate to omit the superscript [217]. The Ph chromosome was the first specific karyotypic abnormality to be recognized in relation to a human malignancy when its most characteristic association, with chronic granulocytic leukaemia (CGL), was described. It is also associated with ALL and, less often, AML and biphenotypic acute leukaemia. Ph-positive cases comprise fewer than 1% of cases of AML but are over-represented among M0 AML where they may represent more than a quarter of cases [218]. Most cases occur *de novo* but therapy-related cases are recognized [219].

With chemotherapy alone, prognosis is poor with only 30–40% of patients achieving a complete remission and median survival of less than a year [120]. The prognosis of therapy-related cases is, if anything, even worse [219].

Clinical and haematological features. Clinical features differ from those of Ph-negative AML in that hep-

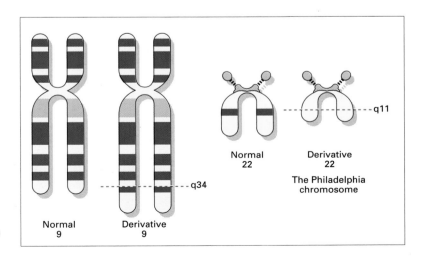

Fig. 2.31 Diagrammatic representation of t(9;22)(q34;q11) (modified from [3]).

Normal 9   Derivative 9   ----q34

Normal 22   Derivative 22   ----q11

The Philadelphia chromosome

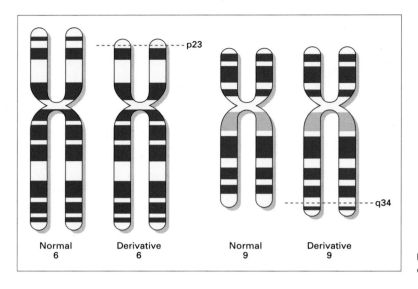

Normal 6   Derivative 6   Normal 9   Derivative 9

Fig. 2.32 Diagrammatic representation of t(6;9)(q23;q34.3) (modified from [3]).

atomegaly and splenomegaly are more common [220]. The WBC is, on average, higher and basophilia may be present. Cases are usually M0 or M1 and less often M2 or M4. Some are M0Baso. MPO activity may be weak or absent [75, 221]. Auer rods are uncommon. Most cases occur *de novo* but some have followed therapy with topoisomerase II-interactive drugs [222].

Immunophenotype. There are no specific immuno-phenotypic features. Lymphoid antigens such as CD19 are sometimes expressed.

Cytogenetic and molecular genetic features. The t(9;22) (q34;q11) rearrangement (Fig. 2.31) is the same as that seen in CGL (see page 182). The commonest associated chromosomal aberrations are monosomy 7, trisomy 8 and 19 and duplication of the derivative (22)t(9;22), the Ph chromosome [212].

The molecular mechanism is fusion of part of the *ABL* gene from chromosome 9 with part of the *BCR* gene on chromosome 22. The *BCR* breakpoint occurs equally frequently in the major breakpoint cluster region, as in CGL, and in the minor breakpoint cluster region, as in ALL. The fusion gene, *BCR-ABL*, codes for an abnormal tyrosine kinase, which is active in intracellular signal transduction. The chromosomal rearrangement is detectable by FISH (see page 184) and the *BCR-ABL* fusion gene by RT-PCR [195]. Minimal residual disease can be monitored by RQ-PCR.

M2Baso or M4Baso/t(6;9)(q23;q34)/*DEK-CAN* fusion

Leukaemia associated with t(6;9)(p23;q34.3) (Fig. 2.32) comprises fewer than 1% of cases of AML.

Clinical and haematological features. AML associated with t(6;9)(p23;q34.3) may be secondary or may develop *de novo*. Secondary cases can follow exposure to either topoisomerase II-interactive drugs [101] or alkylating agents. Prognosis is poor with regard to both the probability of complete remission and over-all survival [105]. Cases are usually M2 AML, less often M4 and least often M1 [223–225]. Myelodys-plastic features are quite common and an MDS may precede overt leukaemia. Bone marrow basophilia is common (Fig. 2.33) but not invariable and may also be present during the preceding myelodys-plastic phase [223]. Basophilic differentiation can be confirmed by metachromatic staining with toluidine blue (Fig. 2.33d). The peripheral blood basophil count is also often elevated [223]. Some cases have also had increased bone marrow eosinophils. Auer rods are often present [223, 225]. Patients tend to be young but, despite this, the prognosis is poor [223, 225]. It is likely that this leukaemia results from mutation in a multipotent stem cell, often in a myelodysplastic setting.

Immunophenotype. No specific immunophenotypic features have been recognized.

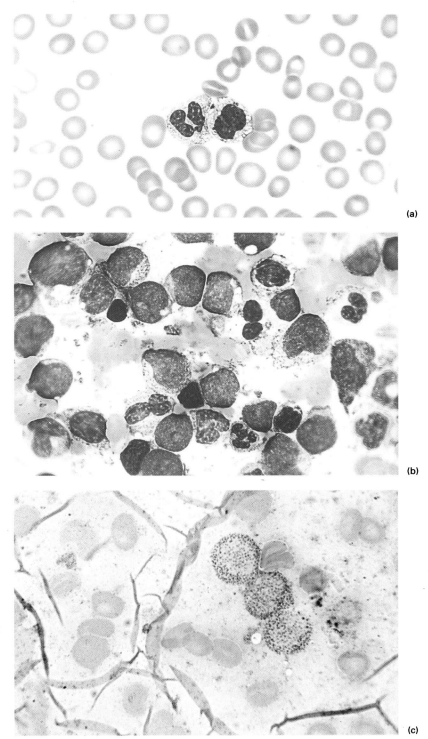

(a)

(b)

(c)

Fig. 2.33 PB and BM films from a patient with M2Baso AML associated with t(6;9)(p23;q34.3). (a) PB film showing abnormal basophils. MGG × 870.
(b) BM film showing neutrophilic and basophilic differentiation. MGG × 870.
(c) BM film showing positive reaction for chloroacetate esterase (CAE). CAE × 870. (*Continued on p. 104*)

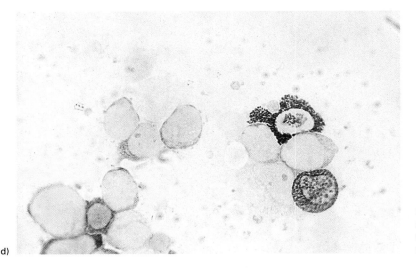

(d)

Fig. 2.33 (*Continued*) (d) BM film showing metachromatic staining with toluidine blue. Toluidine blue × 870 (courtesy of Dr D. Swirsky).

R.B. t(6;9)(p23;q34)

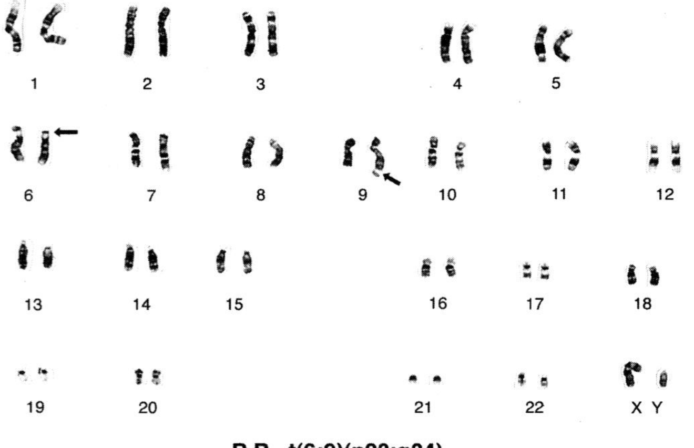

Fig. 2.34 Karyogram of the patient with M2Baso and t(6;9)(p23;q34.3) whose PB and BM films are shown in Fig. 2.33 (courtesy of Dr D. Swirsky and Miss Julie Bungey).

Cytogenetic and molecular genetic features. The t(6;9) (p23;q34.3) rearrangement is shown in Fig. 2.34. The frequent association of this translocation with basophilia and the close similarity of the breakpoint on chromosome 9 to that in CGL led to speculation that the *ABL* oncogene was implicated in leukaemogenesis. However, the breakpoint is not identical to that in CGL [224] and *ABL* is neither translocated nor rearranged. The molecular mechanism is a head-to-tail fusion of part of the *DEK* gene at 6p23 with part of the *CAN* gene at 9q34 (also known as *NUP214*) to form a fusion gene, *DEK-CAN* [226]. *CAN* codes for a nucleoporin, i.e. a protein belonging to the nuclear pore complex [227] while *DEK* codes for a

nuclear protein that appears to be a transcription factor [228]. *DEK-CAN* is detectable by RT-PCR, providing a potential target for monitoring of minimal residual disease.

The commonest secondary abnormalities associated with t(6;9) are trisomy 8 and trisomy 13.

AML/inv(3)(q21q26) or t(3;3)(q21;q26)/*EVI1* dysregulation

Inversions (Fig. 2.35) and translocations (Fig. 2.36) with 3q21 and 3q26 breakpoints are found in no more than 2% of haematological neoplasms including about 1% of cases of AML [96, 229]. This group of

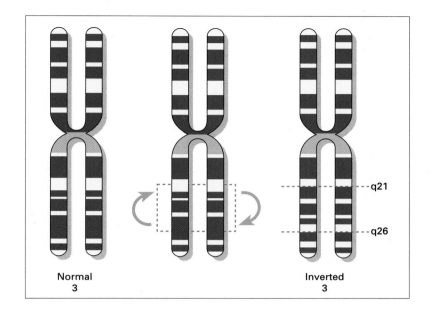

Fig. 2.35 A diagrammatic representation of inv(3)(q21q26); this is an example of a paracentric inversion (modified from [3]).

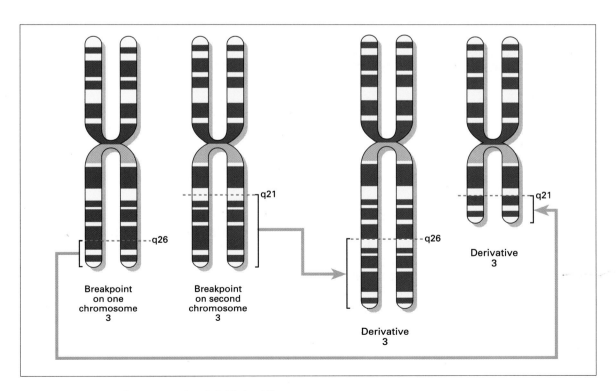

Fig. 2.36 A diagrammatic representation of t(3;3)(q21;q26).

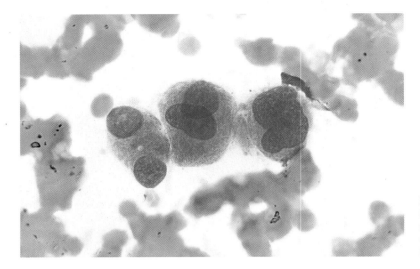

Fig. 2.37 BM film from a patient with inv(3)(q21q26) showing increased numbers of dysplastic megakaryocytes (by courtesy of Dr G. Lucas, Manchester). MGG × 870.

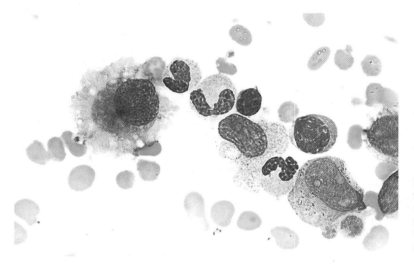

Fig. 2.38 BM film from a patient with t(3;3)(q21;q26) showing hypogranular neutrophils and a hypolobulated megakaryocyte (with thanks to the United Kingdom Cancer Cytogenetics Study Group [228]). MGG × 870.

disorders is sometimes referred to as the 3q21q26 syndrome. In addition to the association with AML there is an association with MDS and with myeloid blast crisis of Ph-positive CGL.

Clinical and haematological features. 3q21q26 abnormalities are associated with both *de novo* and therapy-related AML [219, 229]. Cases occur throughout adult life. An unusual clinical feature, described in three patients, is presentation with diabetes insipidus 1 to 3 months before diagnosis of AML [230]. The AML may be of any FAB category with the exception of M3 AML but cases of M7 AML are over-represented [229]. This subtype of AML is unusual

in that the platelet count is normal in about a third of cases and is elevated in some patients. Trilineage myelodysplasia is common. Dyserythropoietic features are non-specific but may include the presence of ring sideroblasts. The main dysplastic features seen in granulocytes are hypogranularity and the acquired Pelger–Huët anomaly. Auer rods are not a feature. Eosinophils and basophils are sometimes increased. Megakaryocytes are often increased in number as well as being dysplastic; both micromegakaryocytes and other dysplastic forms (e.g. multinucleated or large non-lobulated megakaryocytes) are seen (Figs 2.37 & 2.38) and there may be giant or hypogranular

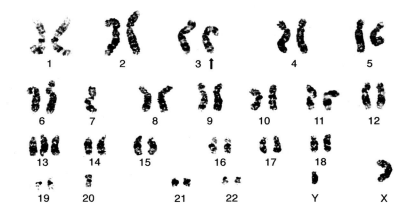

Fig. 2.39 Karyogram showing inv(3)(q21q26) (courtesy of Professor Lorna Secker-Walker).

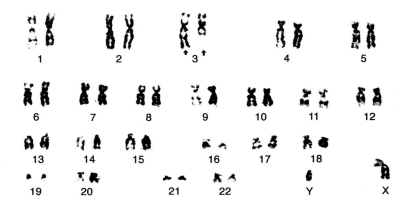

Fig. 2.40 Karyogram showing t(3;3)(q21;q26) (courtesy of Professor Lorna Secker-Walker).

platelets [229, 231]. There is sometimes associated bone marrow fibrosis.

The associated trilineage myelodysplasia indicates that this subtype of leukaemia results from a mutation in a multipotent stem cell. The prognosis is poor with the reported remission rate in a small number of patients being about 25% and the median survival being less than a year [120]. In two very large series of patients, prognosis was poor with regard to both complete remission [105] and overall survival [89, 90, 105].

Immunophenotype. No specific immunophenotypic features have been recognized.

Genetic and molecular features. Inv(3)(q21q26) (Fig. 2.39) is the commonest of this group of cytogenetic abnormalities but other rearrangements involving the same two breakpoints have also been observed including t(3;3)(q21;q26) (Fig. 2.40), ins(2;3)(p21;q21q26), ins(3;3)(q23–26;q21q26), ins(5;3)

(q14;q21q26) and ins(6;3)(q23;q21q26) [232]. Cases with either a 3q21 or a 3q26 breakpoint but not both share some features with the 3q21q26 syndrome, but there are also some differences. Such cases include t(1;3)(p36;q21) [229, 233], t(3;5)(q21;q31) [229, 234], t(3;6)(q21;p21) [235], t(3;12)(q26;p13) [229, 236], t(3;21)(q26;q22) [229, 237, 238] and del(3)(q12q21) [231] (see Table 2.19, page 112).

The commonest secondary cytogenetic abnormalities are monosomy 7, trisomy 8 and 5q– [212, 229].

The molecular mechanism of leukaemogenesis appears to be dysregulation of the *EVI1* (**E**cotropic **V**irus **I**ntegration **1**) gene at 3q26 when it is brought into proximity to the enhancer of the ribophorin gene at 3q21 [239]. Occasionally there is rearrangement and truncation of *EVI1* [240] but this is not usual [239]. *EVI1* is a transcription factor gene, which is expressed in the kidney and the ovary and in other tissues during embryogenesis but is not expressed

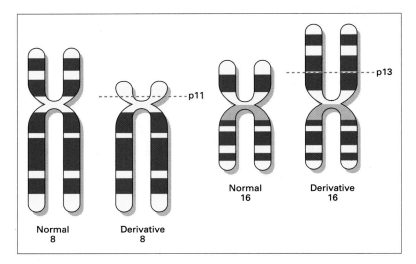

Normal
8

Derivative
8

Normal
16

Derivative
16

p11

p13

Fig. 2.41 Diagrammatic representation of t(8;16)(p11;p13) (modified from [3]).

in normal haemopoietic cells [239]; it is expressed in this subtype of AML but also in some other cases of AML and prognostically adverse subtypes of MDS lacking any cytogenetic abnormality of chromosome 3 [241].

This and other rearrangements of 3q26 can be detected by dual-colour, break-apart FISH [232]. Two probe pairs are necessary to cover two breakpoint cluster regions.

M5/t(8;16)(p11;p13)/*MOZ-CBP* fusion

AML associated with t(8;16)(p11;p13) (Fig. 2.41) is a rare variant of AML, comprising fewer than 1% of cases [96]. Most cases occur *de novo* but some are related to therapy with topoisomerase II-interactive drugs [163, 219].

Clinical and haematological features. t(8;16)(p11;p13) is associated with AML with monocytic differentiation [242–244]. More than half the reported cases have been M5, particularly M5a with the majority of the remainder being M4. AML may be secondary or occur *de novo*. Secondary cases have followed both radiotherapy and exposure to a variety of types of chemotherapeutic agent including alkylating agents and topoisomerase II-interactive drugs [101, 102]. There is a short latent period and usually no myelodysplastic phase. Many *de novo* cases have been in infants and children and if the secondary cases are excluded the median age is low. Spontaneously re-

mitting congenital leukaemia has occurred [214]. A prominent haemostatic abnormality, sometimes interpreted as disseminated intravascular coagulation and sometimes as increased fibrinolysis, is usual. Extramedullary disease, including skin infiltration, is common [244]. The prognosis appears to be relatively poor.

The majority of cases have shown haemophagocytosis by leukaemic cells (Fig. 2.42), particularly erythrophagocytosis, to the extent that the first case described was designated malignant histiocytosis. In other cases this was only a minor feature. Monoblasts are often granulated but Auer rods are not a feature.

Immunophenotype. The characteristic immunophenotype is positivity for HLA-DR, CD33 and CD15 [243, 244]. CD13 and CD14 are positive in about half of reported cases. CD34 and TdT are usually negative. As in other cases of M4 and M5 AML, there may be expression of the natural killer marker, CD56.

Cytogenetic and molecular genetic features. This translocation involves *CBP*. There is fusion of the *MOZ* gene on chromosome 8 with the *CBP* gene from 16p13 [245, 246].

Secondary chromosomal abnormalities include trisomy 1 and trisomy 8 [212].

AML with the same clinical and cytological features has also been associated with variant translocations involving chromosome 8, including t(6;8) (q27;p11), t(8;14)(p11;q11.1), t(8;19)(p11;q13), t(8;22) (p11;q13) and t(3;8;17)(q27;p11;q12) [244] and also

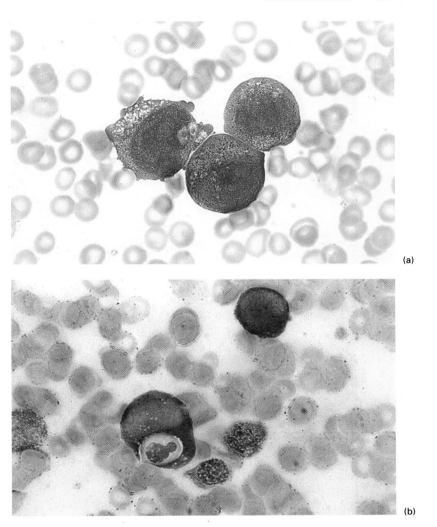

(a)

(b)

Fig. 2.42 BM aspirate from a patient with M5 AML associated with t(8;16)(p11;p13). (a) Three monoblasts. MGG × 870. (b) A neutrophil and two monoblasts, one of which has phagocytosed a neutrophil. Double esterase reaction: CAE, blue; α-naphthyl acetate esterase, brown × 870 (courtesy of Professor D. Catovsky).

with inversion of chromosome 8, inv(8)(p11q13) [247].

M7/t(1;22)(p13;q13)/*RBM15-MKL1* fusion

t(1;22)(p13;q13) is associated with acute megakaryoblastic leukaemia (Fig. 2.43) occurring in infants and young children. The median age of reported cases is under 6 months [248, 249]. Identical twins showing concordance for this subtype of AML have been described suggesting a possible intrauterine origin of the leukaemia [250] and one congenital case has been reported [214]. The sex incidence is equal. Hepato-

megaly and splenomegaly are common. Hyperdiploidy is a common association with extra chromosomes often including an extra der(1) and extra copies of chromosomes 2, 6, 7, 10, 19 and 21 [120, 212, 248, 251, 252]. CD45 expression may be weak and initial misdiagnosis as a non-haemopoietic tumour has been common among reported cases [212]. The bone marrow blast percentage is low with a series of 10 patients having a median of 22% blasts [249]; in 4 of the 10 patients, blasts were less than 20%. There is dysmegakaryopoiesis with some micromegakaryocytes. Prognosis is intermediate with a reported remission rate of 55% and 4-year survival of approximately 30%

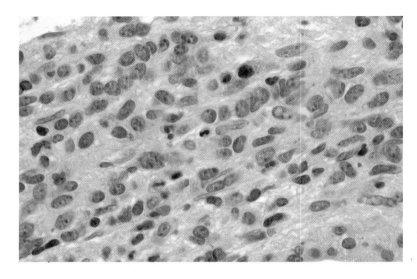

Fig. 2.43 Trephine biopsy section from a patient with M7 AML associated with t(1;22)(p12;q13) (courtesy of Dr R.D. Brunning, Minnesota). Haematoxylin and eosin (H & E) × 870.

[120]. The molecular mechanism is formation of an *RBM15-MKL1* fusion gene on chromosome 1 [253]; an *MKL1-RBM15* fusion gene is also formed but is not transcribed in all patients. The fusion gene on chromosome 1 has also been designated *OTT-MAL* [254].

M1-M2/t(16;21)(p11;q22)/*FUS-ERG* fusion

t(16;21)(p11;q22) is associated mainly M1 and M2 AML. Haemophagocytosis by leukaemic blasts is a common feature [255]. The most common secondary cytogenetic abnormality is trisomy 10. The mechanism of leukaemogenesis is formation of a *FUS-ERG* fusion gene. Despite a high rate of complete remission, prognosis is poor with the median survival being about a year [120]. The *FUS-ERG* fusion gene can be detected by RT-PCR.

M2Baso/12p–

Deletions and translocations involving 12p bands p11–13 such as del(12)(p11p13) (Fig. 2.44) are associated with AML M2 or M4 with basophilic differentiation. Such abnormalities occur in about 1.5% of AML cases [96]. Although this is a MIC category of AML it does not constitute a MIC–M category since the molecular mechanism of leukaemogenesis has not yet been defined. The blasts of M2Baso cases may be difficult to recognize as myeloid by light microscopy alone since they are generally agranular; electron

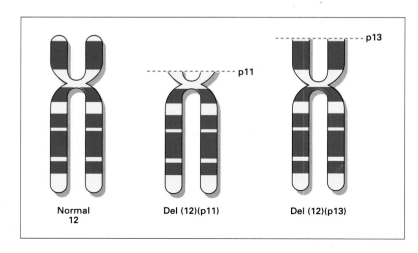

Fig. 2.44 A diagrammatic representation of del(12)(p) showing the range of breakpoints; del(12)(p11) and del(12)(p13) are illustrated (modified from [3]).

microscopy or the use of McAb may be necessary [3]. The blasts can also be identified by metachromatic staining with toluidine blue, astra blue or SBB. M2Baso/12p– may occur as a secondary or a *de novo* AML. The same chromosomal defect is seen in MDS secondary to chemotherapy/radiotherapy. Cases with del(12)(p11p13) have a relatively good prognosis but cases with a larger deletion, del(12)(p11.2), are more likely to have additional chromosomal abnormalities, particularly of chromosomes 5 and 7, and have a worse prognosis [256].

M4/trisomy 4

Trisomy 4 is particularly associated with M4 AML and also with M1 or M2 and occasionally M0 AML. This is a MIC but not a MIC–M category of AML, since the underlying molecular events responsible for leukaemogenesis have not yet been defined. The leukaemia may be secondary or *de novo* [257]. Such cases comprise well below 1% of AML cases. Double minute chromosomes are the commonest additional cytogenetic abnormality. Common clinical features are hepatomegaly, splenomegaly and lymphadenopathy. Four of 34 reported cases have also had soft tissue tumours [257].

M1/9q–

Del(9)(q13;q22) is mainly associated with M1 AML, although some cases have been M2 or M4 and one case was M6 [258, 259]. All such cases are rare, in most series comprising well below 1% of AML cases [71, 96]. This is a MIC but not a MIC–M category of AML. Typical morphological features include a preponderance of agranular blasts with marked variation in size and a high nucleocytoplasmic ratio. The blasts commonly have Auer rods, vacuoles or both.

M0/M1/trisomy 13

Cases of AML with trisomy 13 comprise well below 1% of cases of AML. This is a MIC but not a MIC–M category of AML. Patients are predominantly elderly males. Characteristically, there is AML with little maturation, particularly M0 and M1 AML [260]. Cytological features often include small blasts, which can be confused with lymphoblasts, and hand mirror blasts (Fig. 2.45). Auer rods are uncommon and dysplastic features are relatively uncommon. The prognosis is poor, even if intensive treatment is given. The commonest secondary abnormalities are trisomy 8 and 21, quadrosomy 13, del(7q) and tetraploidy [212, 260].

AML arising in germ cell tumour/i(12p)

A unique and rare type of AML is that which derives from a germ cell tumour, usually a mediastinal germ cell tumour with yolk sac elements occurring in males [261–263] but occasionally arising in an ovarian germ cell tumour [264]. An isochromosome of

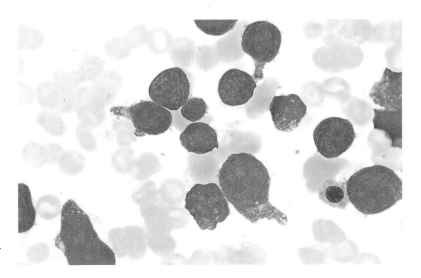

Fig. 2.45 BM film from a patient with M0 AML and trisomy 13. MGG × 870 (courtesy of the United Kingdom Cancer Cytogenetics Study Group [260]).

Table 2.19 Some of the less common MIC–M categories of acute myeloid leukaemia not involving 11q23 or the *MLL* gene [103, 135, 188, 220, 215, 229, 235–238, 256, 266–286].

Translocation	Type of leukaemia	Molecular event
t(1;3)(p36;q21)	t-AML and t-MDS	*MEL1* over-expressed, probably because of proximity to the ribophorin I gene [266]
t(1;11)(q23;p15)	M2 (t-AML)	*NUP98-PMX1* fusion [267]
t(1;12)(q21;p13)	A case of M2 AML	*TEL-ARNT* fusion [268]
t(1;21)(p36;q22)	t-AML	*AML1* rearranged [269]
t(2;11)(q31;p15)		*HOXD13-NUP98* fusion
t(3;5)(q25.1;q34)	AML or MDS	*NPM-MLF1* fusion [235]
t(3;12)(q26;p13)	MDS, AML, blast crisis of CGL	heterogeneous at 3q26, mainly *TEL* at 12p13; *MDS1/EVI1-TEL* fusion [236, 256]
t(3;21)(q26;q22)	AML, either t-AML or following MPD; blast crisis of CGL	heterogeneous (mainly *AML1-EAP, AML1-EVI1* and *AML1-MDS1* fusion genes) [229, 237, 238]
t(4;12)(q11–22; p13)	M0 and M2 AML	*BTL6-ETV6* [270]
Cryptic t(5;11)(q35;p15.5), and often with 5q– [271]	Childhood AML (M1, M2 or M4)	*NSD1-NUP98* *NUP98-NSD1* fusion
t(5;12)(q31;p13)	case of AML with eosinophilia	*ACS2-ETV6* [272]
t(7;11)(p15;p15)	M2 AML, in Chinese and Japanese	*NUP98-HOXA9* fusion or *NUP98-HOXA13* [273, 274]
t(7;12)(p15;p13)*		*ETV6* rearranged
t(7;12)(q36;p13), often cryptic	Infant AML	*HLXB9-ETV6* fusion [275]
t(8;11)(p11.2;p15)	M1 AML (1 case)	*NUP98-NSD3* [276]
t(8;22)(p11;q13)	M5 AML	*MOZ-P300* and *P300-MOZ* fusion genes [277]
t(9;11)(p22;p15)	AML	*LEDGF-NUP98* fusion [278]
t(9;12)(q34;p1?) (cryptic)	AML (2 cases)	*ETV6-ABL* fusion [279]
t(10;11)(p12–13; q14–21)	M0, M1, M2, M4 and M5 AML	*CALM-AF10* fusion, less often *AF10-CALM* fusion [200, 215, 280]
t(10;16)(q22;p13)	Childhood M5a AML	*MORF-CBP* fusion [281]
inv(11)(p15q11)		*NUP98-DDX10* fusion
t(11;20)(p15;q11)		*NUP98-TOP1* fusion
t/dic(12;13)(p11.2–13; p11–q14)	Various FAB categoaries (M1, M1, M2 and M5) and MDS	*ETV6-CDX2* fusion [256, 282]
t(12;15)(p13;q25)	A case of M2 AML	*ETV6-TRKC* fusion [283]
t/dic(12;20)(p12–13; p11.2–q13)*	AML or MDS	Not known [256]
t(12;22)(p13;q11)	Various FAB categories (M1, M4, M7)	*MN1-ETV6* fusion [284]
t(16;21)(p11;q22)	AML (M1, M2, M4, M5, M7) and MDS	*FUS/TLS-ERG* fusion [285]
t(16;21)(q24;q22)	t-AML, M2 or M2Eo; t-MDS; *de novo* MDS or AML	*AML1-MTG16* fusion [103, 135]
t(X;6)(p11;q23)	M0Baso in infants	Not known [286]
Normal	A case of M0 AML	*SET-CAN* fusion

AML, acute myeloid leukaemia; CGL, chronic granulocytic leukaemia; MDS, myelodysplastic syndrome; MPD, myeloproliferative disorder; t-AML, therapy-related acute myeloid leukaemia; t-MDS, therapy-related myelodysplastic syndrome.
*Provisional MIC–M category as exact molecular mechanism not determined.

12p is specifically associated with germ cell tumours and is also found in the leukaemic cells indicating a common clonal origin. This is a MIC but not a MIC–M category of AML since the molecular mechanism of leukaemogenesis has not yet been defined; however, the critical region appears to be 12p11.2–12.1. The commonest associated chromosomal abnormalities are +X (either acquired or as a constitutional abnormality in Klinefelter's syndrome) and trisomy 8 [265]. A variety of FAB types have been described. The commonest is M7 but M4, M5, M6, malignant his-tiocytosis and MDS (FAB RAEB category) have also been observed. AML and the germ cell tumour may present simultaneously or AML may appear after apparently successful treatment of the germ cell tumour.

Other cytogenetic subtypes of AML

Monosomy 5, monosomy 7 and deletions of the long arm of chromosome 7 (–5, –7, 7q–) and complex cytogenetic abnormalities are associated particularly with secondary AML and with trilineage myelodys-plasia (see below). Other recurrent chromosomal abnormalities include trisomy 22 (associated with M4 AML) and trisomy 11, i(17q), del(20q) and t(1;7)(p11;p11)—the latter four abnormalities all associated with multiple FAB subtypes and often also with myelodysplastic features or preceding MDS suggesting the abnormal clone has arisen from a multipotent stem cell. Trisomy 11 is often associated with tandem partial duplication of the *MLL* gene, which may be the primary lesion and the molecu-lar mechanism of leukaemogenesis [204]. Other cytogenetic abnormalities, each of which is associated with less than 1% of cases of AML, are shown in Table 2.19.

Secondary (therapy-related) acute myeloid leukaemia

Two broad groups of secondary (therapy-related) acute myeloid leukaemia (t-AML) are now recog-nized. In the first type, MDS and AML occur following exposure to either alkylating agents (e.g. chlorambucil, busulphan, melphalan) or nitrosoureas (e.g. BCNU and lomustine (CCNU)). MDS or acute leukaemia, the latter often evolving from MDS, usu-ally occurs 5–10 years after drug exposure. Cases of AML often show trilineage dysplasia. Auer rods are less common than in *de novo* AML whereas increased basophils, bone marrow hypocellularity and bone marrow fibrosis are more common. The leukaemia may be of any FAB type except M3 with M6 being over-represented. Cases of this type of t-AML can be difficult to assign to a FAB category. The prognosis is generally poor. Common and uncommon cytogenetic abnormalities in t-AML are shown in Table 2.20.

A second type of therapy-related acute leuk-aemia occurs following exposure to topoisomerase II-interactive drugs, both the topoisomerase II-inhibitors (epipodophyllotoxins such as etoposide and teniposide) and intercalating topoisomerase II-inhibitors such as the anthracyclines (daunorubucin, doxorubicin and epirubicin), mitoxantrone, dactino-mycin and dioxypiperazine derivatives such as bimolane. The interval between exposure to the drug and the development of leukaemia is shorter than with the alkylating agents, often only 2–5 years. Although MDS may occur it is less common than when therapy-related leukaemia follows alkylating agents. Characteristic chromosomal abnormalities are shown in Table 2.20. In the case of some of these chromosomal abnormalities, e.g. those with 11q23 breakpoints, quite a large proportion of cases are sec-ondary whereas in others, such as t(8;21)(q22;q22) and t(15;17)(q22;q12), the secondary cases are only a small proportion of total cases. In contrast to acute leukaemia following the alkylating agents, occasional cases following topoisomerase II-interactive drugs have been lymphoblastic (see page 126) or bipheno-typic rather than myeloid; these cases are related to translocations with an 11q23 breakpoint. The prog-nosis of secondary leukaemia following the topoiso-merase II-interactive drugs is not necessarily as bad as that following the alkylating agents but appears to be worse than that of *de novo* cases with the same cytogenetic abnormality. The uncommon cases of secondary leukaemia with t(8;21)(q22;q22) and t(15;17)(q22;q12) appear to have a similar complete remission rate to *de novo* cases; although little infor-mation is available on the long term prognosis it also appears to be worse than that of *de novo* cases [103, 136]. Cases involving the *MLL* gene certainly have a poor long term prognosis despite an initially high complete remission rate [163, 209].

These two types of therapy-related acute leukaemia are specifically recognized in the WHO classification [83] (see below) with cases being assigned to the category of t-AML/t-MDS rather than being categor-ized with other cases with the same cytogenetic abnormality.

Cytogenetic abnormalities and bilineage/biphenotypic leukaemia

About a third of biphenotypic leukaemias are Ph-positive [71, 291]. The second commonest group are a variety of abnormalities with an 11q23 break-point, particularly t(4;11) and del(11)(q23). Other

Table 2.20 Cytogenetic abnormalities associated with secondary (therapy-related) acute leukaemia [101–103, 136, 163, 209, 219, 287–290].

Following alkylating agents and nitrosoureas	Following topoisomerase II-interactive drugs
Drugs incriminated	*Drugs incriminated*
Chlorambucil, busulphan, cyclophosphamide, melphalan, carmustine (BCNU), lomustine (CCNU)	Etoposide, teniposide, doxorubicin, daunorubicin, epirubicin, mitozantrone, bimolane, razoxane, dactinomycin
Chromosomal rearrangements	*Chromosomal rearrangements*
Complex chromosomal abnormalities, often including −7, 7q−, −5 and 5q−; also 12p−, −17, 17p−, 13q−, −18, 20q−, der(1)t(1;7) (p11;p11) and other unbalanced translocations leading to loss of part of 5q or 7q and/or dup of (1q)	Chromosomal rearrangements with an 11q23 breakpoint (*MLL* gene often shown to be rearranged):
t(1;3)(p36;p21) [290]	t(1;11)(p32;q23)*
inv(3)(q21q26)	t(1;11)(q21;q23)
t(3;3)(q21;q26)	t(3;11)(p21;q23)
t(6;9)(p23;q34.3)	t(3;11)(q25;q23)
t(8;16)(p11;p13)	t(3;11)(q28;q23)
	t(4;11)(q21;q23)†
	t(5;11)(q35;q23)*
	t(6;11)(q27;q23)
	t(9;11)(p21;q23)
	t(10;11)(p11;q23)
	t(10;11)(p13;q23)
	inv(11)(p14q23)
	t(11;11)(p13–15;q23)
	t(11;16)(q23;p13)†
	t(11;17)(q23;p13) cryptic
	t(11;17)(q23;q25)
	t(11;19)(q23;p13.3)†
	t(11;19)(q23;p13.1)
	t(11;21)(q23;q22)
	Chromosomal rearrangements with a 21q22 breakpoint (*AML1* gene often shown to be rearranged):
	t(1;21)(p36;q22)
	t(3;21)(q26;q22)
	t(7;21)(q31;q22)
	t(8;21)(q22;q22)
	t(16;21)(q24;q22)
	Chromosomal rearrangements with an 11p15 breakpoint (*NUP98* gene often shown to be rearranged):
	t(1;11)(q23;p15)
	t(2;11)(q35;p15)
	t(7;11)(p15;p15) [219]
	t(10;11)(q22~23;p15) [219]
	inv(11)(p15q22 or q23)
	t(11;17)(p15;q21)
	t(11;20)(p15;q11)
	Other:
	t(6;9)(p23;q34.3)
	t(8;16)(p11;p13)
	t(9;22)(q34;q11)‡ [219]
	t(15;17)(q22;q12) [136]
	inv(16)(p13q22) [136]
	t(16;16)(p13;q22) [136]

*Therapy-related ALL [288].
†Including therapy-related ALL [288].
‡Therapy-related AML, ALL or CGL.

reported cases have had del(5)(q23q33), monosomy 7, complex abnormalities and a variety of miscellaneous abnormalities. Biphenotypic leukaemia generally appears to have a poor prognosis, possibly but probably not only because of the frequent association with an adverse karyotype.

Cytogenetic abnormalities differ somewhat between myeloid/B-lineage acute leukaemia, in which t(9;22) and t(4;11) may be found, and myeloid/T-lineage acute leukaemia in which these abnormalities are absent but complex chromosomal rearrangements may be observed [66].

L1 or L2/M0/t(9;22)/*BCR-ABL* fusion

t(9;22)(q34;q11) is associated with a variety of types of biphenotypic leukaemia, particularly with cases showing evidence of myeloid and B-lymphoid differentiation but also with occasional cases with B and T lymphoid or B, T and myeloid differentiation [291]. The majority of cases are adult; a minority are children. Morphologically, cells more often appear lymphoid but in some cases they appear myeloid. Presentation is with cells of the neoplastic clone showing simultaneous expression of lymphoid and myeloid antigens.

L1 or L2/M5/t(4;11)(q21;q23)/*MLL-AF4* fusion

t(4;11)(q21;q23) is associated with L1/L2 ALL with an early B-precursor phenotype, with M5a AML and with bilineage/biphenotypic leukaemia. In the bilineage/biphenotypic leukaemias the myeloid component is often of the monocytic lineage. Although the ALL component is usually early B precursor it is occasionally common or pre-B ALL. Some patients have either biphenotypic blasts or two blast populations at diagnosis while others present with ALL and either have blasts of myeloid phenotype emerging early during the course of treatment or subsequently relapse with a myeloid phenotype.

Leukaemias with the t(4;11) abnormality can be seen as forming a single entity since they share clinical and haematological features [292] and a common molecular mechanism. About a quarter of the cases described have been of congenital leukaemia and others have been in infants or young children but cases also occur in adults. The leukaemia usually develops *de novo* although occasional cases have followed therapy with topoisomerase II-interactive drugs.

Other translocations between chromosome 11 (with an 11q23 breakpoint) and a number of partner chromosomes have also been associated with biphenotypic leukaemia, as have cases with a deletion of chromosome 11 with an 11q23 breakpoint. The partner chromosomes in the translocations have included 9, 17 and 19 [191, 291, 293].

Cytogenetic abnormalities and the MIC–M classification of ALL

With techniques now available 70–90% of cases of ALL have a demonstrable cytogenetic abnormality. Some cytogenetic abnormalities (such as 6q– and 9p–) are associated with both B- and T-lineage ALL while others are confined to one lineage or are associated with a specific immunophenotype within a lineage. Translocations with breakpoints involving immunoglobulin genes (heavy chain, κ or λ) are generally B lineage and those involving *TCR* genes are largely confined to T-lineage ALL. Hyperdiploidy is commonly associated with B-lineage ALL and is rare in T-lineage ALL.

In ALL, chromosomal abnormalities correlate with other clinical and haematological factors of prognostic importance but they also have a considerable independent prognostic significance. This has been most clearly delineated for B-lineage ALL.

The MIC classification [2] integrated morphology, immunophenotype and cytogenetics. The classification was open-ended so that new categories could be added as recognized. There is now a need to incorporate molecular genetic data into an ALL classification as was proposed in the MIC–M classification. The more important of the provisional MIC–M categories of ALL will be discussed in detail. Less common B-lineage entities are shown in Table 2.21 (for less common T-lineage entities see Table 2.22).

B-lineage ALL

L1/high hyperdiploidy/common ALL/mechanism unknown

This is the commonest form of childhood ALL in developed countries, being responsible for the typical peak in incidence in early childhood.

Clinical and haematological features. This major MIC category accounts for about a quarter of childhood ALL [297, 298] but only about 7–8% of ALL in adults

Table 2.21 Some of the less common MIC–M categories of B-lineage ALL.

Translocation or other non-random abnormality	Type of leukaemia	Molecular event	Detection (in addition to conventional cytogenetic analysis)
ins(5;11)(q31;q13–q23)		*AF5q31-MLL*	
t(6;11)(q27;q23)	Early B-cell precursor ALL, AML, T-ALL	*MLL-AF6* fusion gene	RT-PCR, FISH [190]
t(9;11)(p21;q23)	Early B-cell precursor ALL, AML, biphenotypic AL	*MLL-AF9* fusion gene	RT-PCR, FISH [191]
t(10;11)(p12–22;q23)	Early B-cell precursor ALL	*MLL-AF10* fusion gene	RT-PCR, FISH [192]
t(11;19)(q23;p13.3)	Early B-cell precursor ALL, common and pre-B ALL, AML	*MLL-ENL* fusion gene	RT-PCR, FISH [193]
t(X;11)(q13;q23)	ALL	*MLL-AFX1* fusion gene	RT-PCR, FISH
dic(7;12)(p11;p12)	Common or pre-B ALL	Unknown	
t(8;14)(q11.2;q32)	Pre-B ALL	*IGH* gene rearranged	FISH [294]
dic(9;12)(p11;p12)	Common ALL	Unknown*	
dic(9;20)(p11–13;q11)	Common or pre-B ALL	Unknown	FISH
t(5;14)(q31;q32)	Common ALL with eosinophilia	*IL3* gene at 5q31 is dysregulated by being juxtaposed to part of the *IGH* gene at 14q32 leading to overexpression of IL3 and eosinophilia	
inv(19)(p13q13)(cryptic)		*E2A-FB1* fusion [295]	

IGH, immunoglobulin heavy chain; see Table 2.18 for other abbreviation definitions.
*An *ETV6/TEL-CBFA* transcript was detected in 4 of 4 cases tested suggesting that a cryptic t(12;21)(p13;q22) was also present [296].

[299, 300]. In developing countries, the incidence is lower than in developed countries. The prevalence, and probably the incidence, appears to be higher in children in Nordic countries than elsewhere with 33% and 46% of cases have been reported to have high hyperdiploidy (defined in these studies as a clone with at least 52 chromosomes) [301, 302]. The peak incidence is between 5 and 10 years. There is a female preponderance. The white cell count is relatively low. Cytological features are typically those of L1 ALL. PAS-block positivity is usual. The prognosis is good. Even in adults, who have a worse prognosis than children with high hyperdiploidy, there is a 50% 5-year survival [300]. In childhood cases, the leukaemic clone may arise during intrauterine life [303].

Immunophenotype. The immunophenotype is that of common ALL, i.e. the common ALL antigen (CD10)

is expressed and cytoplasmic and surface membrane immunoglobulin are not expressed. There is a correlation between weak or absent expression of CD45 and hyperdiploidy [304].

Genetic and molecular genetic features. The term 'high hyperdiploidy' indicates that leukaemic cells have more than 50 (but fewer than 66) chromosomes. Cases of ALL with 'low hyperdiploidy' (47–50 chromosomes) have somewhat different characteristics including a worse prognosis [298]. Near triploidy may be closely related to high hyperdiploidy and has a similarly good prognosis [298]. The molecular mechanism of leukaemogenesis in high hyperdiploidy is unknown and this should therefore be regarded as a MIC category of ALL but not a MIC–M category. The karyotypic abnormality can be demonstrated by conventional cytogenetic analysis (Fig. 2.46), by comparative genomic hybridization, by

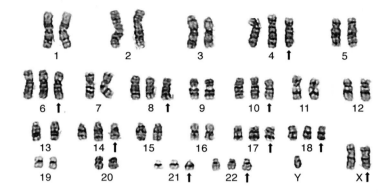

Fig. 2.46 Karyogram of a child with acute lymphoblastic leukaemia (ALL) and a high hyperdiploid clone, 56,XXY,+4,+6,+8,+10,+14,+17,+18,+21, +22; additional chromosomes are arrowed (by courtesy of Professor Lorna Secker-Walker and the LRF UKCCG karyotype data base).

flow cytometry to quantitate nuclear DNA and by multicolour FISH for combinations of the more frequent supernumerary chromosomes (X, 4, 6, 8, 10, 14, 16, 18, 20, 21) [305]. Because of the good prognosis, screening of all patients with failed or normal cytogenetic analysis for high hyperdiploidy is advised [294]. A good prognosis has been associated particularly with trisomy for chromosomes 4, 10 and 17 so an alternative approach is to screen specifically for these trisomies [306, 307]. Some prognostic differences have been found, related to the specific chromosomes gained [294]. Gain of chromosomes 4, 6, 10, 17 has been related to a better prognosis and gain of 5 or the presence of an i17(q10) has been related to a worse prognosis [294]. The presence of unfavourable cytogenetic rearrangements, such as t(9;22), can negate the otherwise good prognosis of high hyperdiploidy [294].

L1 or L2/t(12;21)(p12;q22)/early precursor or common ALL/*ETV6-AML1* fusion

This is one of the commonest subtypes of childhood ALL but was largely unrecognized until the late 1990s because the translocation is usually cryptic; this is because the involved portions of the two chromosomes are both small and have similar banding patterns.

Clinical and haematological features. When molecular techniques are used, t(12;21)(p12;q22) is found in 10–30% of cases of childhood B-lineage ALL [296, 308–311] but in only 2–4% of adult cases [294, 310, 312]. Affected children are aged mainly between 2 and 9 years [313] and adults are usually but

not always young adults [294]. When this type of leukaemia occurs in infants and children the translocation has often occurred in intra-uterine life [303, 314]. It is likely that a second post-natal event is required both because of the long latent period that is observed and because the prevalence of the translocation at birth is about 100-fold the prevalence of this type of leukaemia during childhood. Most cases have L1 cytological features. The remission rate is high. Long-term survival was initially reported to be good [311, 313] but in more recent studies has not differed from that of ALL in general [315, 316, 317]. Recognition of this MIC–M category of ALL may have therapeutic implications since the leukaemic cells appear to be particularly sensitive to asparaginase and results may be better with regimens containing high doses of this agent [318].

Immunophenotype. The immunophenotype may be early precursor B, common or pre-B ALL with the relative frequencies varying considerably between different reported series. Myeloid antigens such as CD13 and CD33 are co-expressed in a quarter to a half of cases [311, 319] and, conversely, t(12;21) is found in two thirds of patients in whom these myeloid antigens are expressed [319]. In comparison with other precursor-B ALL, there is higher expression of CD10, CD40 and HLA-DR and lower expression of CD9, CD20 and CD86 [320].

Cytogenetic and molecular genetic features. The translocation is difficult to detect by conventional cytogenetic analysis and may be misinterpreted as del(12)(p12). The above percentages relate to detection by *in situ* hybridization. The molecular mechanism of leukaemogenesis is fusion of two

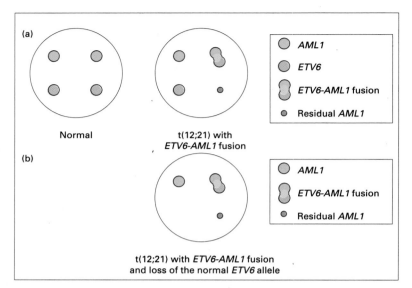

(a)

Normal

t(12;21) with
ETV6-AML1 fusion

○ AML1
○ ETV6
⬤ ETV6-AML1 fusion
• Residual AML1

(b)

○ AML1
⬤ ETV6-AML1 fusion
• Residual AML1

t(12;21) with ETV6-AML1 fusion
and loss of the normal ETV6 allele

Fig. 2.47 Diagrammatic representation of extra-signal, dual-colour FISH for detection of *ETV6-AML1* fusion in cryptic t(12;21)(p13;q22), using an orange *AML1* probe and a green *ETV6* probe; (a) in a normal cell there are two orange signals and two green signals whereas in a cell with t(12;21) there is one orange *AML1* signal, one green *ETV6* signal, a yellow fusion *ETV6-AML1* signal and an extra small orange residual *AML1* signal; (b) when a translocation is present and the normal allele of *ETV6* has been lost the normal green *ETV6* signal is lacking.

transcription factor genes, *ETV6* of the *ETS* family (previously known as *TEL*) and *AML1* (also known as *CBFA*), to form a fusion gene, *ETV6-AML1* (or *TEL-AML1* or *TEL-CBFA*) on the derivative chromosome 21. The fusion gene, *ETV6-AML1* on der(12) is less consistently transcribed and is thus less likely to be relevant to leukaemogenesis. The other allele of *ETV6* is usually deleted [313]. In a significant proportion of cases, leukaemic cells have a second copy of the *ETV6-AML1* fusion gene as a result of either +der(21)t(12;21) or ider(21)(q10)t(12;21) [301]. Girls may lose one copy of chromosome X as a secondary cytogenetic abnormality [321].

The genetic defect can be detected by RT-PCR and by FISH using a probe for the *ETV6* gene and a chromosome 21 paint (metaphase FISH) or probes for *ETV6* and *AML1* (metaphase or interphase FISH). If *ETV6* and *AML1* probes are used it is possible to detect not only the translocation but also the deletion of a normal *ETV6* allele (Fig. 2.47). The detection rate is higher with RT-PCR [301]. The detection rate by RT-PCR is somewhat higher when there is a detectable abnormality of chromosome 12 or chromosome 21 than when there is not—56% cf. 31% [315]. The amount of minimal residual disease at the end of induction therapy, as evaluated by a limiting dilution PCR assay, is of prognostic significance [316].

L1 or L2/t(1;19)(q23;p13)/pre-B ALL/*E2A-PBX* fusion

This subtype constitutes 2–5% of childhood ALL and 1–3% of adult cases [298, 300, 322].

Clinical and haematological features. Adult patients are relatively young [298]. In one series there was a correlation with a high white cell count, non-white ethnic origin and central nervous system disease [323]. However, in other series of adult cases the white cell counts were low [299, 300]. Cytological features are most often L1 but sometimes L2 and sometimes very similar to L3 (Fig. 2.48) [324]. The prognosis in childhood cases was previously poor but with current more intensive treatment has been found, in several series of patients, to be as good as, if not better than, that of ALL associated with high hyperdiploidy [298, 325]. A poor prognosis has been reported in adults [326]. In childhood cases the leukaemic clone may arise during intrauterine life [303].

Immunophenotype. The immunophenotype is often that of pre-B ALL, i.e. cytoplasmic μ chain is positive but not SmIg. About a quarter of cases with a pre-B immunophenotype are found to have this translocation. The typical immunophenotype is CD19, CD22, CD10 and CD9 positive and CD21 and CD34 negative. CD20 expression may be positive or negative [323]. A

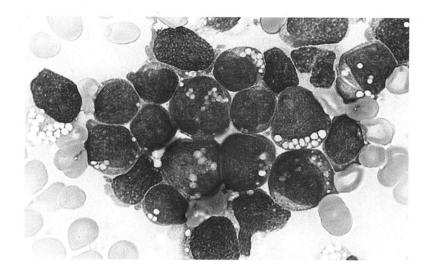

Fig. 2.48 BM film in ALL with t(1;19)(q23;p13) and L3 cytological features (by courtesy of Dr G. Flandrin, Paris). MGG × 870.

smaller number of cases have a common ALL phenotype (CD10 positive, cytoplasmic immunoglobulin negative) or express both surface and cytoplasmic immunoglobulin. If a smaller range of McAb is used, positivity for CD19 and CD10 with negativity for CD34 is suggestive of t(1;19) and can be taken as an indication for cytogenetic or molecular genetic analysis [6].

Cytogenetic and molecular genetic features. The molecular mechanism of leukaemogenesis is fusion of the *PBX1* gene from 1q23 with part of the transcription activator gene, *E2A*, at 19p13 to form a hybrid gene *E2A-PBX1* gene, which codes for an abnormal transcription factor [327].

t(1;19) may occur as a balanced or unbalanced translocation. A straightforward balanced translocation, t(1;19)(q23;p13), is the less common abnormality. More common is the unbalanced der(19) t(1;19)(q23;p13) in which the derivative chromosome 1 has been lost and has been replaced by a second copy of the normal chromosome 1 (Fig. 2.49). There is a prognostic difference between the balanced and the unbalanced translocation, the unbalanced cases having a better prognosis is three series of patients [325, 328, 329].

t(17;19)(q21–22;p13) is a variant of t(1;19), which leads to fusion of *E2A* with *HLF* (**H**epatic **L**eukaemia **F**actor). The fusion gene, *E2A-HLF* codes for an abnormal transcription factor.

The molecular defect of both t(1;19) and t(17;19) can be detected by RT-PCR. The fusion protein, E2A-PBX, can be detected with a McAb, applicable both to flow cytometry and immunohistochemistry [330].

L1 or L2/t(9;22)(q34;q11)/common ALL/*BCR-ABL* fusion

ALL associated with t(9;22)(q34;q11) is referred to as Philadelphia-positive ALL, the derivative chromosome 22 being known as the Philadelphia (Ph) chromosome. Most cases occur *de novo* but therapy-related cases are also recognized [163, 219].

Clinical and haematological features. The prevalence of Ph-positive ALL increases markedly with increasing age. About a 15–30% of adults fall into this category in comparison with only 1–2% of children. The white cell count and the peripheral blood blast percentage are higher than in other adults with ALL [331, 332]. The prognosis is poor, although it is better in children aged between 1 and 9 years than in adolescents and adults and in some but not all studies is improved with more intensive chemotherapy [331, 332]. The complete remission rate is lower than in other cases of ALL [332] and the subsequent relapse rate is subsequently higher so that overall and disease-free survival are considerably worse. It is possible that the prognosis in children is improved by stem cell transplantation in first remission [329].

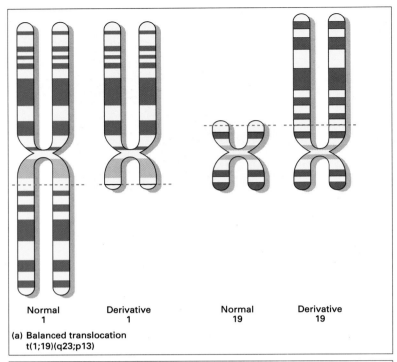

Normal
1

Derivative
1

Normal
19

Derivative
19

(a) Balanced translocation
t(1;19)(q23;p13)

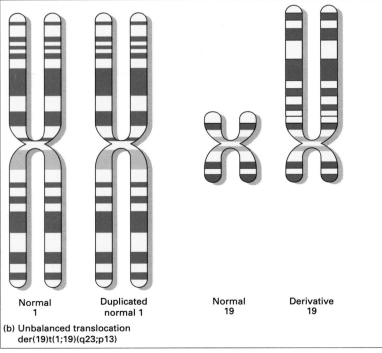

Normal
1

Duplicated
normal 1

Normal
19

Derivative
19

(b) Unbalanced translocation
der(19)t(1;19)(q23;p13)

Fig. 2.49 Diagrammatic representation of balanced and unbalanced forms of t(1;19)(q23;p13).

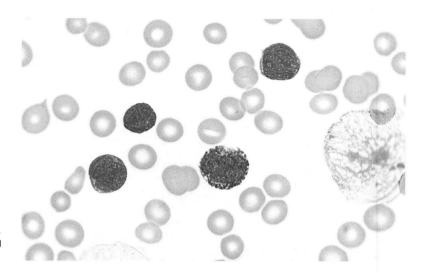

Fig. 2.50 PB film from a patient with L1, Ph-positive ALL showing blast cells and a basophil. MGG × 870.

Cases may be L1 or L2 but L2 cytological features are more common than in ALL in general. In two series 70% and 82% of cases respectively were classified as L2 [331, 333]. Occasional cases have an increased basophil count (Fig. 2.50). There is a significant association with the presence of micromegakaryocytes but this observation is not pathognomonic of Ph positivity [334].

Immunophenotype. The immunophenotype is usually that of common ALL (about 90% of cases) but a minority have a pre-B immunophenotype and a small minority are early precursor-B cell [299, 322, 332, 335]. Twenty to fifty per cent of cases express myeloid antigens [298, 331, 335]. In one series of patients CD34 was more often expressed than in ALL in general [333] but this was not so in another series [331]. Homogeneous expression of CD10 and CD34 with low but heterogeneous expression of CD38 and expression of CD13 has been found to be reasonably sensitive and specific for *BCR-ABL*-positive ALL; it has been suggested that this immunophenotype can be used to select patients for molecular analysis [336].

Cytogenetic and molecular genetic features. t(9;22) is also the characteristic cytogenetic abnormality of CGL. The translocations in ALL and CGL do not differ cytogenetically but at a molecular level the breakpoint on chromosome 22 may differ. About a quarter of cases of Ph-positive ALL have a breakpoint within the major breakpoint cluster region (M-BCR), i.e. they have the same molecular lesion as occurs in CGL.

However, the majority of cases, about three-quarters, have a breakpoint in the minor breakpoint cluster region (m-BCR), this abnormality being very rare in CGL.

The mechanism of leukaemogenesis is fusion of part of the *ABL* oncogene from chromosome 9 with part of the *BCR* gene on chromosome 22 to form a hybrid gene on chromosome 22 designated *BCR-ABL*. c-*ABL* is homologous with v-*abl*, a retroviral oncogene, which has a role in murine leukaemia. *BCR-ABL* codes for a chimeric protein with aberrant tyrosine kinase activity, which functions in intracellular signalling pathways. In the majority of cases of Ph-positive ALL, those with an m-BCR breakpoint on chromosome 22, the BCR-ABL protein has a molecular weight of 190 kD while in a minority, those with an M-BCR breakpoint, it has a molecular weight of 210 kD, as in CGL.

Characteristic secondary cytogenetic abnormalities in Ph-positive ALL are duplication of the Ph chromosome, abnormalities of 9p, monosomy 7 and hyperdiploidy [300, 335]. Monosomy 7 as a secondary abnormality is associated with an M-BCR breakpoint, with co-expression of myeloid antigens and with a particularly bad prognosis. Secondary abnormalities of 9p are associated with m-BCR breakpoints, with lack of expression of myeloid antigens and with a very bad prognosis. The prognosis may be somewhat better in cases with hyperdiploidy as an associated abnormality.

The cytogenetic defect is detectable by two-colour FISH using *BCR* and *ABL* probes (see page 184). The molecular defect can be detected by RT-PCR. FISH studies show that, as for CGL, there may be loss of chromosome 22 material and, particularly, chromosome 9 material from the der(9) in Ph-positive ALL but the prevalence is much lower than in CGL; this loss of chromosomal material can be seen in patients with an m-BCR breakpoint [337]. RT-PCR can be used to monitor minimal residual disease, the detection of which is of prognostic significance [338].

L1 or L2/t(4;11)(q21;q23)/early precursor-B ALL/*MLL-AF4* fusion

This subtype of ALL occurs at all ages but is particularly frequent among cases of congenital ALL and among cases occurring in young infants [189, 339]. It constitutes more than half of these cases. Cases occurring in infants often originate in intra-uterine life [303, 340]; intrauterine exposure to topoisomerase II-interactive agents is suspected as an aetiological factor. One percent of children with ALL above the age of 1 year have t(4;11) [294] whereas in adult ALL the prevalence is 3–5% and increases with age [300, 322].

Clinical and haematological features. Marked splenomegaly and a high white cell count are common as is central nervous system disease. Prognosisis very poor in infants and adults but somewhat better in children.

Among infants and adults, females are affected more than males, but in the age group 1–14 years males are more affected. Cytological features are of either L1 or L2 ALL but L2 morphology is more common than in ALL in general.

Immunophenotype. t(4;11)(q21;q23) is strongly associated with early B-precursor ALL, i.e. there is positivity for TdT and pan-B markers such as CD19 but with CD10 being negative. Aberrant expression of CD15 and CD65 is common and CD33 is sometimes positive [341]. Myeloid antigens are expressed in about half of cases [299]. At relapse the immunophenotype is sometimes that of biphenotypic acute leukaemia or of monoblastic AML. Positivity with a McAb to chondroitin sulphate proteoglycan, NG2, has been demonstrated [341]. CD133 was consistently expressed in a small number of patients tested whereas it was expressed in less than half of other patient with ALL [43].

Cytogenetic and molecular genetic features. The molecular mechanism of leukaemogenesis in association with t(4;11)(q21;q23) (Fig 2.51) is formation of a fusion gene, *MLL-AF4*, incorporating part of the *MLL* (**M**yeloid–**L**ymphoid **L**eukaemia) gene at 11q23 and part of the *AF4* from 4q21 [293]. *AF4* codes for a protein that is probably a transcription factor [342].

Rearrangement of the *MLL* gene, including that of t(4;11), can be detected by dual-colour break-apart FISH; the principle is the same as for detection of rearrangements of the *RARA* gene. *MLL-AF4* fusion

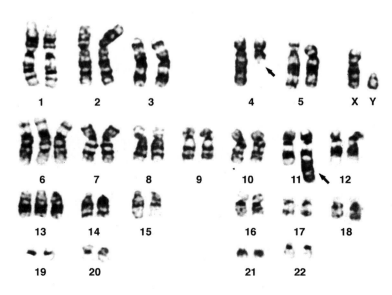

Fig. 2.51 A karyogram showing t(4;11)(q21;q23) (by courtesy of Professor H. Smith, Brisbane, Australia).

can be detected by RT-PCR. Minimal residual disease, which is of prognostic significance, can be monitored by RT-PCR [338]. Only about 50% of patients have rearrangements of antigen-receptor genes and such rearrangements are therefore often not useful for minimal residual disease monitoring [343].

L1 or L2/t(11;V)(q23;V)/early precursor-B ALL

Other translocations with 11q23 breakpoints and rearrangement of the *MLL* gene are also associated with B-lineage ALL and, sometimes, with biphenotypic leukaemia or AML. Some of these are shown in Tables 2.17 and 2.18. Among adults these cases comprise about 4% of cases of ALL [300] and in children 2–3% [298]. Although leukaemias associated with these translocations have some features in common they differ in other characteristics.

Clinical and haematological features. The clinical features resemble those of t(4;11)/ALL in that there is a preponderance of infants and children and an association with high white cell counts and central nervous system disease. One neonate with congenital leukaemia associated with t(11;19)(q23;p13) has been reported [214]. If the *MLL* gene is rearranged the prognosis is equally poor in all translocations with an 11q23 breakpoint [298, 344]. As for ALL associated with t(4;11), the prognosis may be better in those between the ages of 1 and 10 years than in infants or older children [329].

Immunophenotype. The immunophenotype is usually that of early B-precursor ALL. Positive reactions with a McAb to chondroitin sulphate proteoglycan show strong correlation with rearrangement of the *MLL* gene and are observed in cases with t(11;19) as well as cases with t(4;11) [341]. Cases with t(11;19)(q23;p13) may likewise show aberrant expression of CD15 and CD65 [341]. Homogeneous expression of CD4, expression of CD56 and lack of expression of CD34 shows a significant correlation with a rearranged *MLL* gene [345].

Cytogenetic and molecular genetic features. The molecular mechanism is the fusion of part of the *MLL* gene with one of a number of structurally different genes on a large number of partner chromosomes, some of which are shown in Tables 2.17 and 2.18. Partner chromosomes have included 1, 6, 9, 10, 12, 19, 20 and X [190–193, 293]. Rearrangement of the *MLL* gene is an essential feature of this type of ALL. Cases that have cytogenetic abnormalities with 11q23 breakpoints but without *MLL* rearrangement, e.g. many cases with del(11)(q23), have different disease characteristics including a better prognosis [344]. They should not be included in this subtype of ALL.

Rearrangements of the *MLL* gene can be detected by dual-colour, break-apart FISH; the principle is the same as for detection of rearrangements of the *RARA* gene.

Many of the molecular rearrangements resulting from translocations with an 11q23 breakpoint can be demonstrated by RT-PCR and rearrangement of the *MLL* gene can be demonstrated by Southern blotting.

L3/t(8;14)(q24;q32) or t(8;22)(q24;q11) or t(2;8)(p12;q24)/B ALL/*MYC* dysregulation

Translocations similar to those of Burkitt's lymphoma occur in 1–2% of cases of ALL, as defined by the FAB group. As already noted, in the WHO classification such cases are classified as non-Hodgkin's lymphoma.

Clinical and haematological features. Clinical and haematological features do not differ between cases with the commonest of these translocations, t(8;14), and those with the two variant translocations. All are associated very largely with L3 ALL cytology. Prognosis was previously very poor but has improved greatly with the introduction of specific, very intensive chemotherapy. This subtype of ALL has a high incidence in patients with human immunodeficiency virus (HIV) infection; in them the prognosis remains poor although with triple anti-retroviral therapy a successful outcome can sometimes be achieved.

Immunophenotype. The immunophenotype is usually of a mature B cell, i.e. there is expression of SmIg. Some cases express cytoplasmic μ chain. Rare cases do not express SmIg. CD10 may be expressed. In contrast to other cases of ALL, the majority of cases do not express nuclear TdT. The minority of cases that are atypical in not having L3 cytological features nevertheless have a mature B immunophenotype.

Cytogenetic and molecular genetic features. The mechanism of leukaemogenesis is dysregulation of c-*MYC*, a transcription factor gene, as a consequence of its being brought into proximity to positive regulatory elements of the immunoglobulin heavy chain (*IGH*) gene at 14q32, the κ gene (*IGK*) at 2p12 or the λ gene (*IGL*) at 22q11. There is often mutation of the *MYC* gene as well as translocation. Dysregulation of *MYC* is associated with a very high proliferative rate.

On conventional cytogenetics the translocations do not differ from those seen in Burkitt's lymphoma but at a molecular level the breakpoints of endemic and sporadic cases differ. As in the case of Burkitt's lymphoma, t(8;14)(q24;q32) is by far the commonest of these abnormalities, followed by t(8;22)(q24;q11) and t(2;8)(p12;q24). The commonest associated karyotypic abnormality is dup(1)(p12–31).

In t(8;14), c-*MYC* is translocated to chromosome 14 whereas in t(2;8) and t(8;22) c-*MYC* remains on chromosome 8 but part of the κ and λ genes, respectively, is translocated to chromosome 8.

The cytogenetic abnormality is detectable by FISH using either a chromosome 8 paint (which will not show breakpoints) or probes for *MYC* and *IGH*, with or without a centromeric chromosome 8 probe. The latter technique employs a green probe for *IGH*, a red probe for *MYC* and a blue probe for the centromere of chromosome 8; in a normal cell there are two red, two green and two blue signals with the red and blue signals being close together whereas a cell with a t(8;14) has single red and green signals, two blue signals and two fusion yellow signals (Fig. 2.52). Rearrangement of *MYC*, both in t(8;14) and the variant translocations, can be detected by dual-colour, break-apart FISH using a red probe for 5′ *MYC* and a green probe for 3′ *MYC*; the principle is the same as for detection of rearrangements of the *RARA* gene. The t(8;14) translocation can be detected by RT-PCR and LD-PCR (long distance-PCR) [338].

L2/L3/t(14;18)(q32;q21)/*MYC* dysregulation

The translocation that characterizes follicular lymphoma can also occur in *de novo* B-lineage ALL [346].

Clinical and haematological features. Cytological features are of either L2 or L3 ALL. Bone, soft tissue and CNS involvement are common. Prognosis is poor.

Immunophenotype. The immunophenotype may be that of a mature B cell or of pre-B or common ALL. Cells express CD10, CD19 and CD20.

Cytogenetic and molecular genetic features. Complex cytogenetic and molecular genetic abnormalities are usual. A leukaemogenic mechanism shared by all cases is dysregulation of *BCL2* by proximity to positive regulatory elements of the immunoglobulin heavy chain (*IGH*) gene at 14q32. There is often also *MYC* rearrangement and involvement of *BCL6*. The translocation can be detected by a dual-colour, dual-

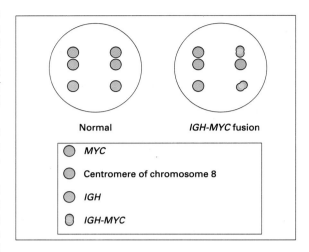

Fig. 2.52 Diagrammatic representation of tricolour, dual-fusion FISH for detection of *IGH-MYC* juxtaposition, using an orange *MYC* probe, a green *IGH* probe and a blue probe for the centromere of chromosome 8. The normal cell has two pairs of orange *MYC* and centromeric blue signals and two green *IGH* signals. The cell with *IGH-MYC* juxtaposition as a result of t(8;14) has a normal pair of orange *MYC* and blue centromeric signals, a normal green *IGH* signal, two fusion *IGH-MYC* signals and a second blue centromeric signal adjacent to one of the fusion signals.

Rearrangements In the *MYC* region can also be detected using a dual-colour, break-apart FISH technique In which *MYC* Is Identified with a dual-colour, orange-green (yellow) probe; when rearrangement has occurred, two distinct orange and green signals are seen. This second strategy will detect rearrangements In the *MYC* region occurring with t(8;22)(q24;q11) and t(2;8)(p11;q24) as well as with the more common t(8;14)(q24;q32).

fusion FISH technique using a green probe for *IGH* and a red probe for *BCL2*.

Other cytogenetic categories of B-lineage ALL

B-lineage ALL may also be associated with hypodiploidy and near haploidy. Hypodiploidy with 33 to 44 chromosomes has been associated with a worse prognosis than ALL in general [347] and near haploidy (variously defined as 24 to 28 or 23 to 29 chromosomes) with an even worse prognosis [317, 347]. Near haploid metaphases usually retain both sex chromosomes and preferentially gain chromosomes 10, 14, 18 and 21 into the haploid chromosome set [348]. Because of the poor prognosis, screening of all patients with failed or normal cytogenetic analysis for near haploidy is advised [348]. For other MIC–M categories of B-lineage ALL see Table 2.21.

T-lineage ALL

In T-lineage ALL there is only a weak relationship between immunological phenotype and specific cytogenetic abnormalities and neither correlates with the FAB type. About a quarter of cases of T-lineage ALL are associated with a variety of translocations involving *TCR* genes, particularly the *TCR* α and δ

genes at 14q11–13 and the *TCR* β gene at 7q32–36 but occasionally the *TCR* γ gene at 7p13. Examples of such translocations are shown in Table 2.22 [245] and two representative abnormalities will be discussed in more detail.

L1 or L2/t(10;14)(q24;q11)/T-lineage/*HOX11* dysregulation

This category of ALL comprises about 5% of childhood T-lineage ALL and about 14% of adult T-lineage ALL [298].

Table 2.22 Some of the MIC–M categories of T-lineage ALL. (Derived from references 245 and 349 and other sources.)

Cytogenetic abnormality	Mechanisms of leukaemogenesis	Approximate frequency
t(1;7)(p34;q34)	*LCK* gene at 1p34 dysregulated by proximity to the *TCRB* gene	
t(1;14)(p32;q11)	*TAL1* (*SCL*) gene at 1p32, a gene for a TF, is dysregulated	3%
t(1;7)(p32;q35)	by proximity to the *TCRAD* locus at 14q11 or the *TCRB* gene at 7q35	<1%
t(5;14)(q35;q32) (cryptic)	*HOX11L2* is transcriptionally activated, probably by proximity to the transcription regulatory elements of *CTIP2* at 14q32 [349]	15–20%
t(7;9)(q34;q34.3)	*TAN1*, a gene coding for a transmembrane protein active in signal transduction, is disrupted and the truncated protein produced is located in the nucleus	3–5%
t(7;9)(q35;p13)	*TAL2* gene, a TF gene at 9p13, is dysregulated by proximity to the *TCRB* gene	<1%
t(7;10)(q35;q24) t(10;14)(q24;q11)	*HOX11* gene at 10q24 dysregulated by proximity to the *TCRB* at 7q35 or the *TCRAD* locus at 14q11	10%
t(7;11)(q35;p13)	Rhombotin-2 (*RBTN2*) or *LMO2* gene at 11p13, a TF gene, is dysregulated by proximity to the *TCRB* gene at 7q35	2–7%
t(7;19)(q35;p13)	*LYL1* gene, a TF gene at 19p13, is dysregulated by proximity to the *TCRB* gene (*LYL* = lymphoid leukaemia gene)	<1%
t(8;14)(q24;q11)	*MYC* at 8q24 is dysregulated by proximity to the *TCRAD* locus at 14q11	1–2%
t(11;14)(p15;q11)	*LMO1* gene (previously known as rhombotin-1, *RBTN1* gene) at 11p15, a TF gene, is dysregulated, by proximity to the *TCRAD* locus	3–7%
t(11;14)(p13;q11)	*LMO2* gene (previously known as rhombotin-2, *RBTN2* gene) at 11p13, a TF gene, is dysregulated, by proximity to the *TCRAD* locus	<1%
inv(14)(q11q32)	*TCL1* at 14q11 is dysregulated by proximity to the *IGH* gene	
t(14;14)(q11;q32)	*TCL1* at 14q11 is dysregulated by proximity to the *IGH* gene	

TF, transcription factor, see Table 2.18 for other factor abbreviation definitions.

Clinical and haematological features. The majority of cases have L1 ALL cytological features. Prognosis is relatively good.

Immunophenotype. The majority of cases have an intermediate or common thymocyte phenotype, i.e. CD1, CD4 and CD8 are expressed in addition to CD5 and CD7. About a quarter express CD10 [298].

Cytogenetic and molecular genetic features. The mechanism of leukaemogenesis is dysregulation of *HOX11*, a transcription factor gene, as a consequence of proximity to the αδ *TCR* gene cluster at 14q11. A similar mechanism of leukaemogenesis is operative in T-lineage ALL with t(7;10)(q35;q24) when the *HOX11* gene is dysregulated by proximity to the *TCR* β gene at 7q35.

Both rearrangements are detectable by PCR.

L1 or L2/*TAL*ᵈ deletion/T-lineage/*TAL* dysregulation

This is one of the commoner subtypes of T-lineage ALL, accounting for up to a third of cases. It is more frequent among children and adolescents than adults [350]. The genetic abnormality, a small deletion on chromosome 1, is detectable only by molecular techniques.

Clinical and haematological features. Clinical and haematological features do not differ from other cases of T-lineage ALL [245].

Immunophenotype. No specific immunophenotype has been recognized except that this subtype of T-lineage ALL occurs preferentially among cases expressing TCR αβ and CD10 is usually expressed.

Cytogenetic and molecular genetic features. The mechanism of leukaemogenesis is that a small deletion leads to the fusion of most of the sequences of a transcription factor gene on chromosome 1, *TAL1* (also known as *SCL*), with the promoter of an upstream gene, *SIL*. This leads to dysregulation of the *TAL1* gene (which is normally expressed in haemopoietic precursors and endothelial cells but is not expressed in normal T cells). Breakpoints in both the *SIL* gene and the *TAL1* gene differ. The *TAL1* gene can also be dysregulated by translocations (Table 2.22) but this is much less common than dysregulation as a consequence of a microdeletion.

Submicroscopic deletion involving 1q32, *TAL*ᵈ, can be detected by PCR or RT-PCR [350]. RT-PCR detects a higher proportion of cases than genomic PCR.

Secondary (therapy-related) acute lymphoblastic leukaemia

Therapy-related ALL, although rare, is being increasingly recognized. Such cases are usually either Ph-positive or associated with balanced translocations with an 11q23 breakpoint (see Table 2.20); they follow administration of topisomerase-II interactive drugs. The latent period is short, usually less than 2 years. Cases associated with 11q23 breakpoints and rearrangement of the *MLL* gene have included t(1;11)(p32;q23), t(4;11)(q21;q23), t(5;11)(q35;q23), t(11;16)(q23;p13) and t(11;19)(q23;p13) [288]. The great majority of cases are of B lineage but one case of T-lineage ALL has been reported associated with *MLL* rearrangement [288].

The WHO classification of acute leukaemia

The WHO classifications of acute leukaemia are part of a broader classification of tumours of haemopoietic and lymphoid tissues published in outline form in 1999 and in definitive form in 2001 (Table 2.23) [5].

Table 2.23 The WHO classification of AML.

Therapy-related AML and MDS
Alkylating agent-related
Topoisomerase II-inhibitor-related
Other types

AML with recurrent cytogenetic abnormalities*
AML with t(8;21)(q22;q22) and *AML1-ETO* fusion
AML with abnormal bone marrow eosinophils with
   inv(16)(p13q22) or t(16;16)(p13;q22) and *CBFB-MYH11* fusion
Acute promyelocytic leukaemia with t(15;17)(q22;q12) and
   variants
AML with 11q23 *(MLL)* abnormalities

AML with multilineage dysplasia†
Following MDS or MDS/MPD
Without antecedent MDS

AML not otherwise categorized

---

*If therapy-related cases are found to have these recurrent cytogenetic abnormalities this should be noted but such cases are categorized as therapy-related AML or MDS, not as AML with recurrent cytogenetic abnormalities.
†Defined as having at least 50% of cells dysplastic in at least 2 lineages.

Table 2.24 The WHO classification of AML—AML not otherwise categorized.

Category*	Criteria
AML, minimally differentiated	Similar to FAB M0 category except that cases with 20–30% PB or BM blasts are included
AML without maturation	Similar to FAB M1 category except that cases with 20–30% PB or BM blasts are included
AML with maturation	Similar to FAB M2 category except that cases with 20–30% PB or BM blasts are included
Acute myelomonocytic leukaemia	Similar to FAB M4 category except that cases with 20–30% PB or BM blasts are included
Acute monoblastic and monocytic leukaemia	Similar to FAB M5 category except that cases with 20–30% PB or BM blasts are included and the WHO classification recognizes the existence of monoblasts that lack non-specific esterase activity but can be recognized by immunophenotyping
Acute erythroid leukaemia { Erythroleukaemia / Pure erythroid leukaemia	Similar to FAB M6 category except that cases with 20–30% PB or BM blasts are included / A category nor recognized in the FAB classification (*see* text)
Acute megakaryoblastic leukaemia	Similar to FAB M7 category except that it is more precisely defined (at least 50% of blasts are megakaryoblasts) and cases with 20–30% PB or BM blasts are included; some but not all cases have prominent fibrosis; AML and transient myeloproliferative disorders of Down's syndrome are a recognized variant
Acute basophilic leukaemia	Differentiation is primarily to basophils but there may be blasts with granules characteristic of mast cells as well as basophil-type granules
Acute panmyelosis with myelofibrosis	Trilineage hyperplasia with increased blasts; increased reticulin deposition with or without collagen fibrosis
Myeloid sarcoma	Granulocytic or monocytic sarcoma

*By definition, cases do not meet the criteria for any other category of AML.

The working parties that drew up these classifications sought to incorporate immunophenotypic analysis and, for some major categories of acute leukaemia, the results of cytogenetic and molecular genetic analysis were also incorporated.

The WHO classification of AML

The WHO criteria for regarding a patient as having AML differ from the FAB criteria in that cases with at 20–30% bone marrow or peripheral blood blasts are categorized as AML rather than MDS; the blast count also includes promonocytes and abnormal promyelocytes [83].

The WHO classification of AML is summarized in Tables 2.23 and 2.24 [83, 116, 351]. Classification is hierarchical, with cases with certain recurrent cytogenetic abnormalities being categorized first, followed by cases with multilineage dysplasia then therapy-related cases. Finally, the remaining cases are assigned on the basis of cytological features to categories that have many similarities to the FAB categories of AML. The method of assigning patients to the different diagnostic categories is summarized in Fig. 2.53.

The WHO categories associated with t(8;21) and inv(16)/t(16;16) are identical to the MIC–M categories described above [116]. However, the WHO classification includes within the same category of acute promyelocytic leukaemia, not only classical and variant cases associated with t(15;17) but also cases of AML with t(11;17)(q23;q21) and *PMZF-RARA* fusion, t(5;17)(q23;q12) with *NPM-RARA* fusion and t(11;17)(q13;q21) with *NuMA-RARA* fusion (although cases with *NPM-RARA* are noted to be 'usually classified as atypical acute promyelocytic leukaemia') [116]. In view of the differing therapeutic respons-

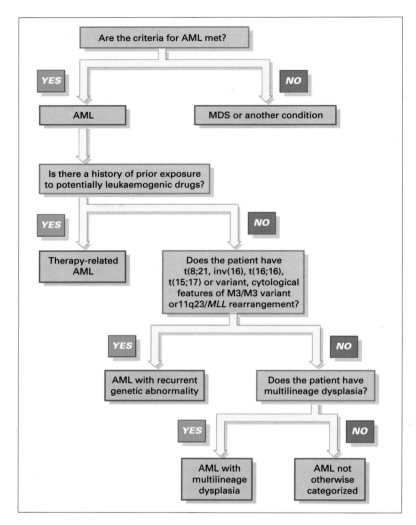

Fig. 2.53 A flow chart showing how individual patients are categorized in the WHO classification.

iveness of cases with fusion genes other than *PML-RARA* (see page 89), grouping of these cases with those having a *PML-RARA* fusion gene may be criticized. Similarly, the WHO classification has, in the interests of simplicity, grouped together all cases with rearrangements of 11q23 involving the *MLL* gene [116]. This may obscure the very real differences between cases with different fusion genes.

The WHO category of AML, not otherwise categorized [351], is a default category for cases that do not meet the criteria for other categories of AML. Many of the sub-types of this category are equivalent to FAB categories, except that a lower blast percentage is accepted. Others differ in their criteria or describe

entities not specifically recognized in the FAB descriptions. Within the group designated 'acute erythroid leukaemias' the WHO classification recognizes an 'erythroleukaemia' (erythroid/myeloid), which is similar to the FAB category of M6 AML, and a 'pure erythroid leukaemia', in which more than 80% of BM cells are erythroid and there is no evidence of a significant myeloblastic component. The latter, a rare condition, was recognized in 1923 by Giovanni Di Guglielmo, who suggested the name 'acute erythremic myelosis' [352]. The designation 'M6 variant AML' has also been proposed [353]. Pure erythroid leukaemia is characterized by the dominance of cells that are either medium or large erythroid cells, rec-

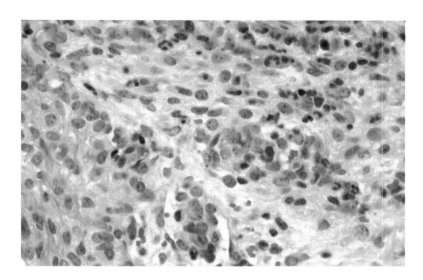

Fig. 2.54 Trephine biopsy section from a patient with acute panmyelosis (courtesy of Dr R.D. Brunning).

ognizable by conventional cytological features, or blast-like cells that can be shown to be erythroid by specialized techniques, such as transmission electron microscopy [351]. A further condition newly recognized in the WHO classification is acute panmyelosis with myelofibrosis [351]. These patients usually have pancytopenia with a hypercellular bone marrow showing trilineage hyperplasia but with increased immature cells; there is increased reticulin deposition and sometimes collagen fibrosis (Fig. 2.54). The condition previously described as acute myelofibrosis includes some cases that meet the WHO criteria for acute panmyelosis with myelofibrosis but other cases represent acute megakaryoblastic leukaemia with fibrosis [354].

Some patients designated AML, not otherwise categorized, have recurrent cytogenetic abnormalities other than those that the WHO classification recognizes as defining specific categories. These may, nevertheless, be discrete entities, as recognized in the MIC–M classification. Such recurrent abnormalities include t(6;9)(p23;q24) and t(8;16)(p11;p13), the latter mentioned in association with three different WHO sub-types of AML, not otherwise categorized [355].

The WHO includes under the designation acute leukaemias of ambiguous lineage, biphenotypic and bilineal leukaemia and undifferentiated acute leukaemia [66] (see pages 71 and 72).

In the WHO classification, ALL is designated precursor B lymphoblastic leukaemia/lymphoblastic lymphoma (precursor B-cell acute lymphoblastic leukaemia) [355] or precursor T lymphoblastic leukaemia/lymphoblastic lymphoma (precursor T-cell acute lymphoblastic leukaemia) [356], the distinction between lymphoblastic leukaemia and lymphoblastic lymphoma being regarded as arbitrary. The prognostic significance of certain cytogenetic and molecular genetic abnormalities is emphasized although they do not contribute to classification.

References

1 Kristensen JS, Ellegaard J, Hansen KB, Clausen N and Hokland P (1988) First-line diagnosis based on immunological phenotyping in suspected acute leukaemia: a prospective study. *Leuk Res,* **12**, 773–782.
2 First MIC Cooperative Study Group (1986) Morphologic, immunologic, and cytogenetic (MIC) working classification of acute lymphoblastic leukaemias. *Cancer Genet Cytogenet,* **23**, 189–197.
3 Second MIC Cooperative Study Group (1988) Morphologic, immunologic and cytogenetic (MIC) working classification of the acute myeloid leukaemias. *Br J Haematol,* **68**, 487–494.
4 Bain BJ (1998) The classification of acute leukaemia: the necessity for incorporating cytogenetic and molecular genetic information. *J Clin Pathol,* **51**, 420–423.
5 Jaffe ES, Harris NL, Stein H and Vardiman JW (2001) *World Health Organization Classification of Tumours: Pathology and Genetics of Tumours of Haematopoietic and Lymphoid Tissues,* IARC Press, Lyon.
6 Farahat N, van der Plas D, Praxedes M, Morilla R, Matutes E and Catovsky D (1994) Demonstration of cytoplasmic and nuclear antigens in acute leukaemia using flow cytometry. *J Clin Pathol,* **47**, 843–849.

7 Jennings CD and Foon KA (1997) Recent advances in flow cytometry: applications to the diagnosis of hematologic malignancy. *Blood*, **90**, 2863–2892.

8 Janossy G, Coustan-Smith E and Campana D (1989) The reliability of cytoplasmic CD3 and CD22 antigen expression in the immunodiagnosis of acute leukemia: a study of 500 cases. *Leukemia*, **3**, 170–181.

9 del Vecchio L, Schiavone EM, Ferrara F, Pace E, Lo Pardo C, Pacetti M *et al.* (1989) Immunodiagnosis of acute leukemia displaying ectopic antigens: proposal for a classification of promiscuous phenotypes. *Am J Hematol*, **31**, 173–180.

10 The General Haematology Task Force of the BCSH (1995) Immunophenotyping in the diagnosis of acute leukaemias. *J Clin Pathol*, **47**, 777–781.

11 Bene MC, Castoldi G, Knapp W, Ludwig WD, Matutes E, Orao A and van't Veer MB; European Group for the Immunological Characterization of Leukemias (EGIL) (1995) Proposals for the immunological classification of acute leukemias. *Leukemia*, **9**, 1783–1786.

12 Rothe G and Schmitz G for the Working Group on Flow Cytometry and Image Analysis (1996) Consensus protocol for the flow cytometric immunophenotyping of hematopoietic malignancies. *Leukemia*, **10**, 877–895.

13 Stewart CC, Behm FG, Carey JL, Cornbleet J, Duque RE, Hudnall SD *et al.* (1997) U.S.-Canadian consensus recommendations on the immunophenotypic analysis of hematologic neoplasia by flow cytometry: selection of antibody combinations. *Cytometry*, **30**, 231–235.

14 Bain BJ, Barnett D, Linch D, Matutes E and Reilly JT (2002) Revised guideline on immunophenotyping in acute leukaemias and chronic lymphoproliferative disorders. *Clin Lab Haematol*, **24**, 1–13.

15 Bain BJ and Gupta R (2003) *A to Z of Haematology*, Blackwell Publishing, Oxford.

16 Coustan-Smith E, Sancho J, Hancock ML, Boyett JM, Behm FG, Raimondi SC *et al.* (2000) Clinical importance of minimal residual disease in childhood acute lymphoblastic leukemia. *Blood*, **96**, 2691–2696.

17 Dworzak MN, Fröschl G, Printz D, Mann G, Pötschger U, Fritsch G *et al.* (2002) Prognostic significance and modalities of flow cytometric minimal residual disease detection in childhood acute lymphoblastic leukemia. *Blood*, **99**, 1952–1958.

18 Pombo de Oliveira M, Matutes E, Rani S, Morilla R and Catovsky D (1988) Early expression of MCS2 (CD13) in the cytoplasm of blast cells from acute myeloid leukaemia. *Acta Haematol*, **80**, 61–64.

19 Matutes E, Rodriguez B, Polli N, Tavares de Castro J, Parreira A, Andrews C *et al.* (1985) Characterization of myeloid leukemias with monoclonal antibodies 3C5 and My9. *Haematol Oncol*, **3**, 179–186.

20 Neame PB, Soamboonsrup P, Browman GP, Meyer RM, Benger A, Wilson WEDC *et al.* (1986) Classifying acute leukaemia by immunophenotyping; a combined FAB–immunologic classification of AML. *Blood*, **68**, 1355–1362.

21 San Miguel JF, Gonzalez M, Canizo MC, Anta JP, Zola H and Lopez Borrasca A (1986) Surface marker analysis in acute myeloid leukaemia and correlation with the FAB classification. *Br J Haematol*, **64**, 547–560.

22 Griffin JD, Davis R, Nelson DA, Davey FR, Mayer RJ, Schiffer C *et al.* (1986) Use of surface marker analysis to predict outcome of adult acute myeloblastic leukemia. *Blood*, **68**, 1232–1241.

23 Vainchenker W, Villeval JL, Tabilio A, Matamis H, Karianakis G, Guichard J *et al.* (1988) Immunophenotype of leukemic blast cells with small peroxidase-positive granules detected by electron microscopy. *Leukemia*, **2**, 274–281.

24 Campos L, Guyotat D, Archimbaud E, Devaux Y, Treille D, Larise A *et al.* (1989) Surface marker expression in adult acute myeloid leukaemia: correlations with initial characteristics, morphology and response to therapy. *Br J Haematol*, **72**, 161–166.

25 Urbano-Ispizua A, Matutes E, Villamor N, Sierra J, Pujades A, Reverter J-C *et al.* (1992) The value of detecting surface and cytoplasmic antigens in acute myeloid leukaemia. *Br J Haematol*, **81**, 178–183.

26 Traweek ST (1993) Immunophenotypic analysis of acute leukemia. *Am J Clin Pathol*, **99**, 504–512.

27 del Poeta G, Stasi R, Venditti A, Suppo G, Aronica G, Bruno A *et al.* (1994) Prognostic value of cell marker analysis in *de novo* acute myeloid leukemia. *Leukemia*, **8**, 388–394.

28 Larson RS and McCurley TL (1995) CD4 predicts nonlymphocytic lineage in acute leukemia: insights from analysis of 125 cases using two-color flow cytometry. *Am J Clin Pathol*, **104**, 204–211.

29 Wang JCY, Beauregard P, Soamboonsrup P and Neame PB (1995) Monoclonal antibodies in the management of acute leukemia. *Am J Hematol*, **50**, 188–199.

30 Di Noto R, lo Pardo C, Schiavone EM, Manzo C, Vacca C, Ferrara F and del Vecchio L (1996) Stem cell factor receptor (c-kit, CD117) is expressed on blast cells from most immature types of acute myeloid malignancies but is also a characteristic of a subset of acute promyelocytic leukaemia. *Br J Haematol*, **92**, 562–564.

31 Sanz MA and Sempere A (1996) Immunophenotyping of AML and MDS and detection of residual disease. *Bailliére's Clin Haematol*, **9**, 35–55.

32 Cohen PL, Hoyer JD, Kurtin PJ, Dewald GW and Hanson CA (1997) Acute myeloid leukemia with minimal differentiation: a multiparameter study. *Am J Clin Pathol*, **109**, 32–38.

33 Linch DC, Allen C, Beverley PCL, Bynoe AG, Scott CS and Hogg N (1983) Monoclonal antibodies differentiating between monocytic and myelomonocytic variants of AML. *Blood*, **63**, 566–573.

34 Imamura N, Inada T, Mtasiwa DM and Kuramoto A (1989) Demonstration of thrombospondin (TSP) receptor on the cell surface of acute megakaryoblastic leukemia. *Am J Hematol*, **31**, 142–143.

35 Villeval JL, Testa U, Vinci G, Tonthat H, Bettaieb A, Titeux M *et al.* (1985) Carbonic anhydrase I is an early

marker of normal human erythroid differentiation. *Blood*, **66**, 1162–1170.

36 Erber WN, Breton-Gorius J, Villeval JL, Oscier DG, Bai Y and Mason DY (1987) Detection of cells of megakaryocyte lineage in haematological malignancies by immunoalkaline phosphatase labelling cell smears with a panel of monoclonal antibodies. *Br J Haematol*, **65**, 87–94.

37 Athale UH, Razzouk BI, Raimondi SC, Tong X, Behm FG, Head DR *et al.* (2001) Biology and outcome of childhood acute megakaryoblastic leukemia: a single institution's experience. *Blood*, **87**, 3727–3732.

38 Karandikar NJ, Aquino DB, McKenna RW and Kroft SH (2001) Transient myeloproliferative disorder and acute myeloid leukemia in Down syndrome. *Am J Clin Pathol*, **116**, 204–210.

39 Sperr WR, Horny H-P, Lechner K and Valent P (2000) Clinical and biological diversity of leukemias occurring in patients with mastocytosis. *Leuk Lymphoma*, **37**, 473–486.

40 Farahat N, Lens D, Morilla R, Matutes E and Catovsky D (1995) Differential TdT expression in acute leukemia by flow cytometry: a quantitative study. *Leukemia*, **9**, 583–587.

41 Huh YO, Smith TL, Collins P, Bueso-Ramos C, Albitar M, Kantarjian HM *et al.* (2000) Terminal deoxynucleotidyl transferase expression in acute myelogenous leukemia and myelodysplasia as determined by flow cytometry. *Leuk Lymphoma*, **37**, 319–331.

42 del Poeta G, Stasi R, Venditti A, Cox C, Aronica G, Masi M *et al.* (1995) CD7 expression in acute myeloid leukemia. *Leuk Lymphoma*, **17**, 111–119.

43 Wuchter C, Ratei R, Spahn G, Schoch C, Harbott J, Schnittger S *et al.* (2001) Impact of CD133 (AC133) and CD90 expression analysis for acute leukemia immunophenotyping. *Haematologica*, **86**, 154–161.

44 Raife TJ, Lager DJ, Kemp JD and Dick FR (1994) Expression of CD24 (BA-1) predicts monocytic lineage in acute myeloid leukemia. *Am J Clin Pathol*, **101**, 296–299.

45 Kita K, Shirakawa S, Kamada N and the Japanese Cooperative Group of leukemia/lymphoma (1994) Cellular characteristics of acute myeloblastic leukemia associated with t(8;21)(q22;q22). *Leuk Lymphoma*, **13**, 229–234.

46 Vidriales MB, Orfao A, González M, Hernández JM, López-Berges MC, Garcia MA *et al.* (1993) Expression of NK and lymphoid-associated antigens in blast cells in acute myeloblastic leukaemia. *Leukemia*, **7**, 2026–2029.

47 Legrand O, Perrot J-Y, Baudard M, Cordier A, Lautier R, Simonin G *et al.* (2000) The immunophenotype of 177 adults with acute myeloid leukemia: proposal of a prognostic score. *Blood*, **96**, 870–877.

48 Raspadori D, Damiani D, Lenoci M, Rondelli D, Testoni N, Nardi G *et al.* (2001) CD56 antigenic expression in acute myeloid leukemia identifies patients with poor clinical prognosis. *Leukemia*, **15**, 1161–1164.

49 Ogata K, Yokose N, Shioi Y, Ishida Y, Tomiyama J, Hamaguchi H *et al.* (2001) Reappraisal of the clinical significance of CD7 expression in association with cytogenetics in de novo acute myeloid leukaemia. *Br J Haematol*, **115**, 612–615.

50 Bain BJ, Clark DC, Lampert IL and Wilkins BS (2001) *Bone Marrow Pathology*, Third Edition, Blackwell Science, Oxford.

51 Arber DA and Jenkins KA (1996) Paraffin section immunophenotyping of acute leukemia in bone marrow specimens. *Br J Haematol*, **106**, 462–468.

52 Bain BJ (2001) Bone marrow trephine biopsy. *J Clin Pathol*, **54**, 737–742.

53 Budde R (1995) Enzyme and immunohistochemical studies on acute monocytic leukemia (FAB M5): proposal for a new immunohistochemical subclassification. *Acta Haematol*, **95**, 102–106.

54 Hann I, Richards SM, Eden OB and Hill FGH on behalf of the Medical Research Council Childhood Leukaemia Working Party. (1998) Analysis of the immunophenotype of children treated in the Medical Research Council United Kingdom Acute Lymphoblastic Leukaemia XI (MRC UKALLXI) Medical Research Council Childhood Leukaemia Working party. *Leukemia*, **12**, 1249–1255.

55 Koehler M, Behm FG, Shuster J, Crist W, Borowitz M, Look AT *et al.* (1993) Transitional pre-B-cell acute lymphoblastic leukemia of childhood is associated with favourable prognostic clinical features and an excellent outcome: a Pediatric Oncology Group Study. *Leukemia*, **7**, 2064–2068.

56 McKenna RW, Washington LT, Aquino DB, Picker LJ and Kroft SH (2001) Immunophenotypic analysis of hematogones (B-lymphocyte precursors) in 662 consecutive bone marrow specimens by 4-color flow cytometry). *Blood*, **98**, 2498–2507.

57 Crist WM, Shuster JJ, Falletta J, Pullen DJ, Berard CW, Vietta TJ *et al.* (1988) Clinical features and outcome in childhood T-cell leukemia-lymphoma according to the stage of thymocyte differentiation: a pediatric oncology group study. *Blood*, **72**, 1891–1897.

58 Pui C-H, Williams DL, Roberson PK, Raimondi SC, Behm FG, Lewis SH *et al.* (1988) Correlation of karyotype and immunotype in childhood acute lymphoblastic leukemia. *J Clin Oncol*, **6**, 56–61.

59 Thiel E, Kranz BR, Raghavachar A, Bartram CR, Löffler H, Messerer D *et al.* (1989) Prethymic phenotype and genotype of pre-T(CD7+/ER−)-cell leukemia and its clinical significance within adult acute lymphoblastic leukemia. *Blood*, **73**, 1247–1258.

60 Cascavilla N, Musto P, D'Arena G, Ladogana S, Melillo L, Carella AM *et al.* (1996) Are 'early' and 'late' T-acute lymphoblastic leukemias different diseases? A single centre study of 34 patients. *Leuk Lymphoma*, **21**, 437–442.

61 Raimondi SC, Behm FG, Roberson PK, Pui C-H, Rivera GK, Murphy SB and Williams DL (1988) Cytogenetics of childhood T-cell leukemia. *Blood*, **72**, 1560–1566.

62 Paulus U, Couzens S, Jenny M, English M and Poynton C (2001) CD45 negative acute lymphoblastic leukaemia in children. *Br J Haematol*, **113**, Suppl. 1, 45.

63 Campana D and Coustan-Smith E (2002) Advances in the immunologic monitoring of childhood acute lymphoblastic leukaemia. *Best Practice Research Clin Haematol*, **15**, 1–19.

64 Hur M, Chang YH, Lee DS, Park MH and Cho HI (2001) Immunophenotypic and cytogenetic changes in acute leukaemia at relapse. *Clin Lab Haematol*, **23**, 173–179.

65 Mirro J and Kitchingman GR (1989) The morphology, cytochemistry, molecular characteristics and clinical significance of acute mixed-lineage leukaemia. In Scott CS (Ed), *Leukaemia Cytochemistry: Principles and Practice*, Ellis Horwood Limited, Chichester, 1989.

66 Brunning RD, Matutes E, Borowitz M, Flandrin G, Head D, Vardiman J and Bennett J (2001) Acute leukaemias of ambiguous lineage. In Jaffe ES, Harris NL, Stein H and Vardiman JW (Eds), *World Health Organization Classification of Tumours: Pathology and Genetics of Tumours of Haematopoietic and Lymphoid Tissues*, IARC Press, Lyon, pp. 106–107.

67 Dunphy CH, Gregowicz AJ and Rodriguez G (1995) Natural killer cell leukemia with myeloid antigen expression: a previously undescribed form of acute leukaemia. *Am J Clin Pathol*, **104**, 212–215.

68 Matutes E, Morilla R, Farahat N, Carbonell F, Swansbury J and Dyer M (1997) Definition of biphenotypic leukemia. *Haematologica*, **82**, 64–66.

69 Suzuki R, Yamamoto K, Seto M, Kagami Y, Ogura M, Yatabe Y *et al.* (1997) CD7+ and CD56+ myeloid/ natural killer cell precursor acute leukemia: a distinct hematolymphoid disease entity. *Blood*, **90**, 2417–2428.

70 Scott AA, Head DR, Kopecky KJ. Appelbaum FR, Theil KS, Grever MR *et al.* (1994) HLA-DR–, CD33+, CD56+, CD16– myeloid/natural killer cell acute leukemia: a previously unrecognized form of acute leukemia potentially misdiagnosed as French–American–British acute myeloid leukemia-M3. *Blood*, **84**, 244–255.

71 Legrand O, Perrot J-Y, Simonin G, Baudard M, Cadiou M, Blanc C *et al.* (1998) Adult biphenotypic acute leukaemia: an entity with poor prognosis which is related to unfavourable cytogenetics and P-glycoprotein overexpression. *Br J Haematol*, **100**, 147–155.

72 Brito-Babapulle F, Pullon H, Layton DM, Etches A, Huxtable A, Mangi M *et al.* (1990) Clinicopathological features of acute undifferentiated leukaemia with a stem cell phenotype. *Br J Haematol*, **76**, 210–214.

73 Cuneo A, Ferrant A, Michaux J-L, Bosly A, Chatelain B, Stul M *et al.* (1996) Cytogenetic and clinicobiological features of acute leukemia with stem cell phenotype: study of nine cases. *Cancer Genet Cytogenet*, **93**, 31–36.

74 Berger R, Bernheim A, Daniel M-T, Valensi F and Flandrin G (1981a) Karyotype and cell phenotypes in primary acute leukemias. *Blood Cells*, **7**, 287–292.

75 Bitter MA, Le Beau MM, Rowley JD, Larson RA, Golomb HM and Vardiman JW (1987) Associations between morphology, karyotype, and clinical features in myeloid leukemias. *Hum Pathol*, **18**, 211–225.

76 Standing Committee on Human Cytogenetic Nomenclature (1978) An international system for human cytogenetic nomenclature. *Cytogenet Cell Genet*, **21**, 309–404.

77 Schoch C, Kern W, Krawitz P, Dugas M, Schnittger S, Haferlacj T and Hiddemann W (2001) Dependence of age-specific incidence of acute myeloid leukemia on karyotype. *Blood*, **98**, 3500.

78 Riccardi VM, Humber TJ and Peakman D (1975) Familial cancer reciprocal translocation [t(7p;20p)] and trisomy 8. *Am J Hum Genet*, **27**, 76A.

79 Markkanen A, Ruutu T, Rasi V. Franssila K, Knuutila S and de la Chapelle A (1987) Constitutional translocation t(3;6)(p14;p11) in a family with hematologic malignancies. *Cancer Genet Cytogenet*, **25**, 87–95.

80 Kearney L (2001) Molecular cytogenetics. *Bailliere's Clin Haematol*, **14**, 645–658.

81 Golub TR, Slonim DK, Tamayo P, Huard C, Gaasenbeek M, Mesirov JP *et al.* (1999) Molecular classification of cancer: class discovery and class prediction by gene expression monitoring. *Science*, **286**, 531–537.

82 Kottaridis PD, Gale RE, Frew ME, Harrison G, Langabeere SE, Belton AA *et al.* (2001) The presence of FLT3 internal tandem duplication in patients with acute myeloid leukemia (AML) adds important prognostic information to cytogenetic risk group and response to the first cycle of chemotherapy: analysis of 854 patients from the United Kingdom Medical Research Council AML 10 and 12 trials. *Blood*, **98**, 1752–1759.

83 Brunning RD, Matutes E, Harris NL, Flandrin G, Vardiman J, Bennett J and Head D (2001) Acute myeloid leukaemia: introduction. In Jaffe ES, Harris NL, Stein H and Vardiman JW (Eds), *World Health Organization Classification of Tumours: Pathology and Genetics of Tumours of Haematopoietic and Lymphoid Tissues*, IARC Press, Lyon, pp. 77–80.

84 Yunis JJ, Lobell M, Arnesen MA, Oken MM, Mayer MG, Rydell RE and Brunning RD (1988) Refined chromosome study helps define prognostic subgroups in most patients with primary myelodysplastic syndrome and acute myelogenous leukaemia. *Br J Haematol*, **68**, 189–194.

85 Mitelman F. *Catolog of Chromosome Aberrations in Cancer*. Sixth edition. (CD-Rom) Wiley-Liss, New York, 1998.

86 Fourth International Workshop on Chromosomes in Leukemia, 1982 (1984) Clinical significance of chromosome abnormalities in acute nonlymphoblastic leukemia. *Cancer Genet Cytogenet*, **11**, 332–350.

87 Schiffer CA, Lee EJ, Tomiyasu T, Wiernik PH and Testa JR (1989) Prognostic impact of cytogenetic abnormalities in patients with *de novo* acute nonlymphocytic leukemia. *Blood*, **73**, 263–270.

88 Fenaux P, Preudhomme CV, Laï JL, Morel P, Beuscart R and Bauters F (1989b) Cytogenetics and their prognostic value in *de novo* acute myeloid leukaemia: a report on 283 cases. *Br J Haematol*, **73**, 61–67.

89 Grimwade D, Walker H, Oliver F, Wheatley K, Harrison C, Harrison G *et al.* (1998) The importance of diagnostic cytogenetics on outcome in AML: analysis of

1,612 patients entered into the MRC AML 10 trial. The Medical Research Council Adult and Children's Leukaemia Working Parties. *Blood*, **92**, 2322–2333.

90 Grimwade D, Walker H, Harrison G, Oliver F, Chatters S, Harrison CJ et al. on behalf of the Medical Research Council Adult Acute Leukaemia Working Party (2001) The predictive value of hierarchical cytogenetic classification in older adults with acute myeloid leukemia (AML): analysis of 1065 patients entered into the United Kingdom Medical Research Council AML11 trial. *Blood*, **98**, 1312–1320.

91 Trujillo JM, Cork A, Ahearn MJ, Youness EL and McCredie KB (1979) Hematologic and cytologic characterization of 8/21 translocation acute granulocytic leukaemia. *Blood*, **53**, 695–706.

92 Berger R, Bernheim A, Daniel M-T, Valensi F, Sigaux F and Flandrin G (1982) Cytological characterization and significance of normal karyotypes in t(8;21) acute myeloblastic leukaemia. *Blood*, **59**, 171–178.

93 Fourth International Workshop on Chromosomes in Leukemia, 1982 (1984) Translocation (8;21)(q22;q22) in acute nonlymphocytic leukemia. *Cancer Genet Cytogenet*, **11**, 284–287.

94 Swirsky DM, Li YS, Matthews JG, Flemans RJ, Rees JHK and Hayhoe FGJ (1984) 8;21 translocation in acute granulocytic leukaemia: cytological, cytochemical and clinical features. *Br J Haematol*, **56**, 199–213.

95 Haferlach T, Bennett JM, Löffler H, Gassmann W, Andersen JW, Tuzuner N et al. for the AML Cooperative Group and ECOG (1996) Acute myeloid leukemia with translocation (8;21). Cytomorphology, dysplasia and prognostic factors in 41 cases. *Leuk Lymphoma*, **23**, 227–234.

96 Berger R, Flandrin G, Bernheim A, Le Coniat M, Vecchione D, Pacot A et al. (1987) Cytogenetic studies on 519 consecutive de novo acute nonlymphocytic leukemias. *Cancer Genet Cytogenet*, **29**, 9–21.

97 Rowe D, Cotterill SJ, Ross FM, Bunyan DJ, Vickers SJ, McMullan DJ et al. (2000) Cytogenetically cryptic AML1-ETO and CBFβ-MYH11 gene rearrangements: incidence in 412 vases of acute myeloid leukaemia. *Br J Haematol*, **111**, 1053–1056.

98 Raimondi SC, Chang MN, Ravindranath Y, Behm FG, Gresik MV, Steuber CP et al. for the Pediatric Oncology Group (1999) Chromosomal abnormalities in 478 children with acute myeloid leukemia: clinical characteristics and treatment outcome in a Cooperative Pediatric Oncology Group study—POG 8821. *Blood*, **94**, 3707–3718.

99 Wiemels JL, Xiao Z, Buffler PA, Maia AT, Ma X, Dicks BM et al. (2002) In utero origin of t(8;21) *AML1-ETO* translocations in childhood acute myeloid leukemia. *Blood*, **99**, 3801–3805.

100 Li Y-S and Yang C-L (1987) Consistent chromosomal changes in Chinese patients with acute nonlymphocytic leukemia. *Cancer Genet Cytogenet*, **26**, 379–380.

101 Pedersen-Bjergaard J and Rowley JD (1994) The balanced and the unbalanced chromosome aberrations of acute myeloid leukemia may develop in different ways and may contribute differently to malignant transformation. *Blood*, **83**, 2780–2787.

102 Thirman MJ and Larson RA (1996) Therapy-related myeloid leukemia. *Hematol Oncol Clin North Am*, **10**, 293–320.

103 Slovak MK, Bedell V, Popplewell L, Arber DA, Schoch C and Slater R (2002) 21q22 balanced chromosome aberrations in therapy-related hematopoietic disorders: report from an international workshop. *Genes Chromosomes Cancer*, **33**, 379–394.

104 Luckit J, Bain B, Matutes E, Min T, Pinkerton R and Catovsky D (1998) An orbital mass in a young girl. *Leuk Lymphoma*, **28**, 621–622.

105 Byrd JC, Mrozek K, Dodge R, Carroll AJ, Edwards C, Pettenati MJ et al. (2001) Pre-treatment cytogenetics predict initial induction success and overall survival in adult patients with de novo acute myeloid leukemia: results from CALGB 8461. *Blood*, **98**, 457a.

106 Löwenberg B (2001) Prognostic factors in acute myeloid leukaemia. *Bailliére's Clin Haematol*, **14**, 65–75.

107 Nguyen S, Leblanc T, Fenaux P, Witz F, Blaise D, Pigneux A et al. (2002) A white blood cell index is the main prognostic factor in t(8;21) acute myeloid leukemia (AML): a survey if 161 cases from the French AML Intergroup. *Blood*, **99**, 3517–3523.

108 Andrieu V, Radford-Weiss I, Troussard X, Chane C, Valensi F, Guesnu M et al. (1996) Molecular detection of t(8;21)/AML1-ETO in AML M1/M2: correlation with cytogenetics, morphology and immunophenotype. *Br J Haematol*, **92**, 853–865.

109 Nakamura H, Kuriyama K, Sadamori N, Mine M, Itoyama T, Sasagawa I et al. (1997) Morphological subtyping of acute myeloid leukemia with maturation (AML-M2): homogeneous pink-colored cytoplasm of mature neutrophils is characteristic of AML-M2 with t(8;21). *Leukemia*, **11**, 651–655.

110 Domingo-Claros A, Alonso E, Aventin A, Petit J, Crespo N, Ponce C and Grañena A (1996) Oligoblastic leukaemia with (8;21) translocation and haemophagocytic syndrome and granulocyte cannibalism. *Leuk Res*, **20**, 517–521.

111 Swirsky DM and Richards SY (2001) Laboratory diagnosis of acute myeloid leukaemia. *Best Practice Res Clin Haematol*, **14**, 1–17.

112 Kaneko Y, Kimpara H, Kawai S and Fujimoto T (1983) 8;21 chromosome translocation in eosinophilic leukaemia. *Br J Haematol*, **9**, 181–183.

113 Jacobsen RJ, Temple MJ and Sacher RA (1984) Acute myeloblastic leukaemia and t(8;21) translocation. *Br J Haematol*, **57**, 539–540.

114 Lorsbach RB, McNall R and Mathew S (2001) Marked bone marrow basophilia in a child with acute myeloid leukemia with a cryptic t(8;21)(q22;q22) chromosomal translocation. *Leukemia*, **15**, 1799–1801.

115 Xue Y, Yu F, Kou Z, Guo Y, Xie X and Lin B (1994) Translocation (8;21) in oligoblastic leukemia: is this a true myelodysplastic syndrome? *Leuk Res*, **18**, 761–765.

116 Brunning RD, Matutes E, Flandrin G, Vardiman J, Bennett J, Head D and Harris NL (2001) Acute myeloid leukaemia with recurrent cytogenetic abnormalities. In Jaffe ES, Harris NL, Stein H and Vardiman JW (Eds), *World Health Organization Classification of Tumours: Pathology and Genetics of Tumours of Haematopoietic and Lymphoid Tissues*, IARC Press, Lyon, pp. 81–87.

117 Hayhoe FGJ and Quaglino D (1988) *Haematological Cytochemistry*. Second edition. Churchill Livingstone, Edinburgh.

118 Kamada N, Dohy H, Okada K, Oguma N, Kuramoto A, Tanaka K and Uchino H (1981) *In vivo* and *in vitro* activity of neutrophil alkaline phosphatase in acute myelocytic leukaemia with 8;21 translocation. *Blood*, **58**, 1213–1217.

119 Bloomfield CD, Lawrence D, Byrd JC, Carroll A, Pettenati MJ, Trantravahi R *et al.* (1998) Frequency of prolonged remission duration after high-dose cytarabine intensification in acute myeloid leukemia varies by cytogenetic subtype. *Cancer Res*, **58**, 4173–4179.

120 Mrózek K, Heinonen K and Bloomfield CD (2001) Clinical importance of cytogenetics in acute myeloid leukaemia. *Bailliere's Clin Haematol*, **14**, 19–47.

121 Richards SJ, Rawstron AC, Evans PAS, Short M, Dickinson H, Follows G *et al.* (2002) Rapid identification of the prognostic cytogenetic abnormalities t(8;21), t(15;17) and inv16 in acute myeloid leukaemia using 4-colour flow cytometry. *Br J Hamatol*, **117**, Suppl.1, 56–57.

122 Khoury H, Dalal BI, Barnett MJ, Nevill TJ, Horsman DE, Shepherd JD *et al.* (2001) Correlation between karyotype and quantitative immunophenotype in acute myelogenous leukemia with t(8;21). *Am J Clin Pathol*, **116**, 598–599.

123 Hurwitz C A, Raimondi S C, Head D, Krance R, Mirro J, Kalwinsky D K *et al.* (1990) Distinctive immunophenotypic features of t(8;21)(q22;q22) acute myeloblastic leukemia in children. *Blood*, **80**, 3182–3188.

124 Porwit-Macdonald A, Janossy G, Ivory K, Swirsky D, Peters R, Wheatley K *et al.* (1996) Leukemia-associated changes identified by quantitative flow cytometry. IV. CD34 overexpression in acute myelogenous leukemia M2 with t(8;21). *Blood*, **87**, 1162–1169.

125 Baer MR, Stewart CC, Lawrence D, Arthur DC, Byrd JC, Davey FR *et al.* (1997) Expression of the neural cell adhesion molecule CD56 is associated with short remission duration and survival in acute myeloid leukemia with t(8;21)(q22;q22). *Blood*, **90**, 1643–1648.

126 Kita K, Nakase K, Miwa H, Masuya M, Nishii K, Morita N *et al.* (1992) Phenotypical characteristics of acute myelocytic leukemia associated with the t(8;21)(q22;q22) chromosomal abnormality: frequent expression of immature B-cell antigen CD19 together with stem cell antigen CD34. *Blood*, **80**, 470–477.

127 Rega K, Swansbury GJ, Atra AA, Korton C, Min T, Dainton MG *et al.* (2000) Disease features in acute myeloid leukemia with t(8;21)(q22;q22). Influence of age, secondary karyotype abnormalities, CD19 status, and extramedullary leukemia on survival. *Leuk Lymphoma*, **40**, 67–77.

128 Knuutila S, Teerenhovi L, Larramendy ML, Elonen E, Franssila KO, Nylund SJ *et al.* (1994) Cell lineage involvement of recurrent chromosomal abnormalities in hematologic neoplasms. *Genes Chromosomes Cancer*, **10**, 95–102.

129 Nucifora G, Birn DJ, Erickson P, Gao J, LeBeau MM, Drabkin HA and Rowley JD (1993) Detection of DNA rearrangements in AML1 and ETO loci and of an AML1/ETO fusion mRNA in patients with t(8;21) acute myeloid leukemia. *Blood*, **81**, 883–888.

130 Fischer K, Scholl C, Sàlat J, Fröhling S, Schlenk R, Bentz M *et al.* (1996) Design and validation of DNA probe sets for a comprehensive interphase cytogenetic analysis of acute myeloid leukemia. *Blood*, **88**, 3962–3971.

131 Nucifora G, Dickstein JI, Torbenson V, Roulston D, Rowley JD and Vardiman JW (1994) Correlation between cell morphology and expression of the AML1/ETO chimeric transcript in patients with acute myeloid leukemia without the t(8;21). *Leukemia*, **8**, 1533–1538.

132 Langabeer SE, Walker H, Rogers JR, Burnett AK, Wheatley K, Swirsky D and Goldstone AH on behalf of the MRC Adult Leukaemia Working Party (1997) Incidence of AML1/ETO fusion transcripts in patients entered into the MRC AML trials. *Br J Haematol*, **99**, 925–928,

133 Yin JAL (2002) Minimal residual disease in acute myeloid leukaemia. *Best Practice Res Clin Haematol*, **15**, 119–135.

134 Beghini A, Peterlongo P, Ripamonti CB, Larizza L, Cairoli R, Morra E and Mecucci C (2000) C-kit mutations in core binding factor leukemias. *Blood*, **95**, 726–727.

135 Kondoh K, Nakata Y, Furuta T, Hosoda F, Gamou T, Kurosawa Y *et al.* (2002) A pediatric case of secondary leukemia associated with t(16;21)(q24;q22) exhibiting the chimeric AML1-MTG16 gene. *Leuk Lymphoma*, **43**, 415–420.

136 Andersen MK, Larson RA, Mauritzson M, Schnittger S, Jhanwar SC and Pedersen-Bjergaard J (2002) Balanced chromosome abnormalities inv(16) and t(15;17) in therapy-related myelodysplastic syndromes and acute leukemia: report from an international workshop. *Genes Chromosomes Cancer*, **33**, 395–400.

137 Lu D-P, Qiu J-Y, Jiang B, Liu K-Y, Liu Y-R and Chan S-S (2002) Tetra-arsenic tetra-sulfide for the treatment of acute promyelocytic leukemia: a pilot report. *Blood*, **99**, 3136–3143.

138 Sanz MA, Martin G, Rayón C, Esteve J, Gonzáles M and Díaz-Mediavilla J (1999) A modified AIDA protocol with anthracycline-based consolidation results in high antileukemic efficacy and reduced toxicity in newly diagnosed PML/RARα positive acute promyelocytic leukemia, *Blood*, **94**, 3015–3021.

139 Tallman MS, Nabham C, Feusner JH and Rowe JM (2002) Acute promyelocytic leukemia: evolving therapeutic strategies. *Blood*, **99**, 759–767.

140 Burnett AK, Grimwade D, Solomon E, Wheatley K and Goldstone AH, on behalf of the MRC Adult Leukaemia Working Party (1999) Presenting white blood cell count and kinetics of molecular remission predict prognosis in acute promyelocytic leukaemia treated with all-*trans*-retinoic acid: result of the randomized MRC trial. *Blood*, **93**, 4131–4143.

141 Estey E, Giles FJ, Kantarjian H, O'Brien S, Cortes J, Freireich EJ *et al.* (1999) Molecular remission induced by liposomal-encapsulated all-trans-retinoic acid in newly diagnosed acute promyelocytic leukemia. *Blood*, **94**, 2230–2235.

142 Exner M, Thalhammer R, Kapiotis S, Mitterbauer G, Knöbl P, Haas OA *et al.* (2000) The 'typical' immunophenotype of acute promyelocytic leukemia (APL-M3): does it prove true for the M3-variant? *Cytometry*, **42**, 106–109.

143 Oelschlågel U, Nowak R, Mohr B, Thiede C and Ehninger G (2000) Letter to the Editor, *Cytometry*, **42**, 396–397.

144 Borowitz MJ, Bray R, Gascoyne R, Melnick S, Parker JW, Picker L and Stetler-Stevenson M (1997) U.S.-Canadian consensus recommendations on the immunophenotypic analysis of hematologic neoplasia by flow cytometry: data analysis and interpretation. *Cytometry*, **30**, 236–244.

145 Borowitz M and Silberman MA (1999) Interactive CD-ROM: *Cases in Flow Cytometry*, Carden Jennings Publishing, Charlottesville.

146 Bahia DMM, Chauffaille MdeLLF, Kimura EYS, Joffe R, Lima WM and Yamamoto M (2001) Acute promyelocytic leukemia (APL): CD117+CD65+ immunophenotype-based score system to predict the finding of t(15;17) translocation. *Blood*, **98**, 197b.

147 Sainty D, Liso V, Cantu-Rajnoldi A, Head D, Mozziconacci MJ, Arnoulet C *et al.* (2000) A new morphologic classification system for acute promyelocytic leukemia distinguishes cases with underlying *PLZF/RARA* gene rearrangements. *Blood*, **96**, 1287–96.

148 González M, Barragán E, Bolufer P, Chillón C, Colomer D, Borstein R *et al.* (2001) Pre-treatment characteristics and clinical outcome of acute promyelocytic leukaemia patients according to the PML-RARα isoforms: a study of the PETHEMA Group. *Br J Haematol*, **114**, 99–103.

149 O'Connor SJM, Evans PAS and Morgan AJ (1999) Diagnostic approach to acute promyelocytic leukaemia. *Leuk Lymphoma*, **33**, 53–63.

150 Krause JR, Stoic V, Kaplan SS and Penchansky L (1989) Microgranular promyelocytic leukemia: a multiparameter examination. *Am J Hematol*, **30**, 158–163.

151 Paietta E (1996) Adhesion molecules in acute myeloid leukemia. *Leuk Res*, **20**, 795–798.

152 Murray CJ, Estey E, Paietta E, Howard RS, Edenfield WJ, Pierce S *et al.* (1999) CD56 expression in APL: a possible indication of poor treatment outcome. *J Clin Oncol*, **17**, 293–297.

153 De Botton S, Chevret S, Sanz M, Dombret H, Thomas X, Guerci A *et al.* (2000) Additional chromosomal abnormalities in patients with acute promyelocytic leukaemia (APL) do not confer poor prognosis: results of APL 93 trial. *Br J Haematol*, **111**, 801–806.

154 Hiorns LR, Swansbury GJ, Mehta J, Min T, Dainton MG, Treleaven J *et al.* (1997) Additional chromosome abnormalities confer a worse prognosis in acute promyelocytic leukaemia. *Br J Haematol*, **96**, 314–321.

155 Schoch C, Haase D, Haferlach T, Freund M, Link H, Lengfelder E *et al.* (1996) Incidence and implication of additional chromosome abnormalities in acute promyelocytic leukaemia with translocation t(15;17) (q22;q21): a report on 50 patients. *Br J Haematol*, **94**, 493–500.

156 Kaleem Z, Watson MS, Zutter MM, Blinder MA and Hess JL (1999) Acute promyelocytic leukemia associated with additional chromosomal abnormalities and absence of Auer rods. *Am J Clin Pathol*, **112**, 113–118.

157 Warrell RP, De Thé H, Wang Z-Y and Degos L (1993) Acute promyelocytic leukemia. *N Engl J Med*, **329**, 177–189.

158 Falini B, Flenghi L, Fagioli M, Lo Coco F, Cordone I, Diverio D *et al.* (1997) Immunocytochemical diagnosis of acute promyelocytic leukemia (M3) with the monoclonal antibody PG-M3 (anti-PML). *Blood*, **90**, 4046–4053.

159 O'Connor SJM, Forsyth PD, Dalal S, Evans PA, Short MA, Shiach C *et al.* (1997) The rapid diagnosis of acute promyelocytic leukaemia using PML (5E10) monoclonal antibody. *Br J Haematol*, **99**, 596–604.

160 Grimwade D, Biondi A, Mozziconacci MJ, Hagemeijer A, Berger R, Neat M *et al.* (2000) Characterization of acute myeloid leukemia cases lacking the classic t(15;17): results of the European Working Party, Groupe Francais de Cytogenetique Hematologique, Group de Francais d'Hematologie Cellulaire, UK Cancer Cytogenetics group, and BIOMED 1 European Community-Concerted Action 'Molecular Cytogenetic Diagnosis in Haematological Malignancies', *Blood*, **96**, 1297–1308.

161 Brunel V, Lafage-Pochitaloff M, Alcalay M, Pelicci P-G and Birg F (1996) Variant and masked translocations in acute promyelocytic leukemia. *Leuk Lymphoma*, **22**, 221–228.

162 Mozziconacci M-J, Liberatore C, Brunel V, Grignani F, Arnoulet C, Ferrucci PF *et al.* (1998) In vitro responses to all-trans-retinoic acid of acute promyelocytic leukemias with non-reciprocal *PML/RARA* and *RARA/PML* fusion genes. *Genes Chromosomes Cancer*, **22**, 141–250.

163 Pui C-H and Relling MV (2000) Topoisomerase II-inhibitor-related acute myeloid leukaemia. *Br J Haematol*, **109**, 13–23.

164 Allford S, Grimwade D, Langabeer S, Duprez E, Saurin A, Chatters S *et al.* on behalf of the Medical Research

Council (MRC) Adult Leukaemia Working Party (1999) Identification of t(15;17) in AML FAB types other than M3: evaluation of the role of molecular screening for *PML/RARa* in newly diagnosed AML. *Br J Haematol*, **105**, 198–207.

165 Mancini M, Nanni M, Cedrone M, Diverio D, Avvisati G, Riccione R *et al.* (1995) Combined cytogenetic, FISH and molecular analysis in acute promyelocytic leukaemia at diagnosis and in complete remission. *Br J Haematol*, **91**, 878–884.

166 Grimwade D, Howe K, Davies L, Langabeer S, Walker H, Smith F *et al.* (1996) Establishing the presence of the t(15;17) in suspected APL; cytogenetic, molecular and PML immunofluorescence assessment of patients entered in the UK MRC ATRA trial. *Br J Haematol*, **93**, Suppl 2, 221.

167 Grimwade D (2002) The significance of minimal residual disease in patients with t(15;17). *Best Practice Res Clin Haematol*, **15**, 137–158.

168 Licht JD, Chomienne C, Goy A, Chen A, Scott AA, Head DR *et al.* (1995) Clinical and molecular characterization of a rare syndrome of acute promyelocytic leukemia associated with translocation (11;17). *Blood*, **85**, 1083–1094.

169 Redner RL, Rush EA, Faas S, Rudert WA and Correy SJ (1996) The t(5;17) variant of acute promyelocytic leukemia expresses a nucleophosmin–retinoic acid receptor fusion. *Blood*, **87**, 882–886.

170 Culligan DJ, Stevenson D, Chee Y-L and Grimwade D (1998) Acute promyelocytic leukaemia with t(11;17)(q23;q12–21) and a good initial response to prolonged ATRA and combination chemotherapy. *Br J Haematol*, **100**, 328–330.

171 Arnould C, Philippe C, Bourdon V, Grégoire MJ, Berger R and Jonveaux P (1999) The signal transducer and activator of transcription STAT5b gene is a new partner of retinoic acid receptor alpha in acute promyelocytic-like leukaemia. *Hum Mol Genet*, **8**, 1741–1749.

172 Rego EM, He L-Z and Pandolfi PP (1999) Arsenic trioxide in combination with retinoic acid is effective in the treatment of PML-RARα/APL, but not in PLZF-RARα/APL. *Blood*, **94**, Suppl. 1, 506a.

173 Le Beau MM, Larson RA, Bitter MA, Vardiman JW, Golomb HM and Rowley JD (1983) Association of an inversion of chromosome 16 with abnormal marrow eosinophils in acute myelomonocytic leukemia. *N Engl J Med*, **309**, 630–636.

174 Langabeer SE, Walker H, Gale RE, Wheatley K, Burnett AK, Goldstone AH and Linch DC (1997) Frequency of CBFβ/MYH11 fusion transcripts in patients entered into the U.K. MRC AML trials. *Br J Haematol*, **96**, 736–739.

175 Vardiman J, Mrózek K, Anastasi J, Kolitz J, Carroll AJ and Caligiuiri M *et al.*, for the Cancer and Leukemia Group B (2000) Morphology and CBFB/MYH11 transcripts in AML (CALGB study 9621). *Lab Invest*, **80**, 165A.

176 Matsuura Y, Sato N, Kimura F, Shimomura S, Yamamoto K, Enomoto Y and Takatani O (1987) An increase in basophils in a case of acute myelomonocytic leukaemia associated with bone marrow eosinophilia and inversion of chromosome 16. *Eur J Haematol*, **39**, 457–461.

177 Tien H-F, Wang C-H, Lin M-T, Lee F-Y, Liu M-C, Chuang S-M *et al.* (1995) Correlation of cytogenetic results with immunophenotype, genotype, clinical features, and ras mutation in acute myeloid leukemia: a study of 235 Chinese patients in Taiwan. *Cancer Genet Cytogenet*, **84**, 60–68.

178 Sperling C, Büchner T, Creutzig U, Ritter J, Harbott J, Löffler H and Ludwig W-D (1995) Clinical, morphologic, cytogenetic and prognostic implications of CD34 expression in childhood and adult *de novo* AML. *Leuk Lymphoma*, **17**, 417–426.

179 Osato M, Asou N, Okubo T, Nishimura S, Yamasaki H, Era T *et al.* (1997) Myelomonoblastic leukaemia cells carrying the PEBP2β/MY11 fusion gene are CD34+,c-KIT+ immature cells. *Br J Haematol*, **97**, 656–658.

180 Khoury H, Dalai BI, Nevill TJ, Horsman DE, Shepherd JD, Hogge DE *et al.* (2001) Quantitative immunophenotype (QUIP) pattern of CD34high, CD13high and CD33low identifies patients with acute myelogenous leukemia (AML) with inv(16). *Blood*, **98**, 109a.

181 Wong KF and Kwong YL (1999) Trisomy 22 in acute myeloid leukemia: a marker for myeloid leukemia with monocytic features and cytogenetically cryptic inversion 16. *Cancer Genet Cytogenet*, **109**, 131–133.

182 Arthur DC and Bloomfield CD (1983) Partial deletion of the long arm of chromosome 16 and bone marrow eosinophilia in acute nonlymphocytic leukemia: a new association. *Blood*, **61**, 994–998.

183 Ohyashiki K, Ohyashiki JH, Kondo M, Ito H and Toyama K (1988) Chromosome change at 16q22 in nonlymphocytic leukemia: clinical implications on leukemia patients with inv(16) vs. del(16). *Leukemia*, **2**, 35–40.

184 Liu P, Tarle SA, Hajra A, Claxton DF, Marlton P, Freedman M *et al.* (1993) Fusion between a transcription factor CBFβ/PEBP2β and a myosin heavy chain in acute myeloid leukemia. *Science*, **261**, 1041–1044.

185 Kolomietz E, Al-Maghrabi J, Brennan S, Karaskova J, Minkin S, Lipton J and Squire JA (2001) Primary chromosomal rearrangements of leukemia are frequently accompanied by extensive submicroscopic deletions and may lead to altered prognosis. *Blood*, **97**, 3581–3588.

186 Buonamici S, Ottaviani E, Testoni N, Montefusco V, Visani G, Bonifazi F *et al.* (2002) Real-time quantitation of minimal residual disease in inv(16)-positive acute myeloid leukemia may indicate risk for clinical relapse and may identify patients in a curable state. *Blood*, **99**, 443–449.

187 Berger R, Bernheim A, Sigaux F, Daniel M-T, Valensi F and Flandrin G (1982) Acute monocytic leukemia; chromosome studies. *Leuk Res*, **6**, 17–26.

188 Pui C-H, Raimondi SC, Srivastava DK, Tong X, Behm FG, Razzlouk B *et al.* (2000) Prognostic factors in infants with acute myeloid leukemia, *Leukemia*, **15**, 684–687.

189 Johansson B, Moorman AV, Hass OA, Watmore AE, Cheung KL, Swanton S and Secker-Walker L, on behalf of the European 11q23 Workshop participants (1998) Hematologic malignancies with t(4;11)(q21;q23)—a cytogenetic, morphologic, immunophenotypic, and clinical study of 183 cases. *Leukemia*, **12**, 779–778.

190 Martineau M, Berger R, Lillington DM and Secker-Walker L, on behalf of the European 11q23 Workshop participants (1998) The t(6;11)(q27;q23) translocation in acute leukemia: a laboratory and clinical study of 30 cases. *Leukemia*, **12**, 788–791.

191 Swansbury GJ, Slater R, Bain BJ, Moorman AV and Secker-Walker L, on behalf of the European 11q23 Workshop participants (1998) Hematological malignancies with t(9;11)(p21~22;q23)—a laboratory and clinical study of 125 cases. *Leukemia*, **12**, 792–800.

192 Lillington DM, Young B, Martineau M, Berger R, Moorman AV and Secker-Walker L, on behalf of the European 11q23 Workshop participants (1998) The t(10;11)(p12;q23) translocations in acute leukemia: a cytogenetic and clinical study of 20 patients. *Leukemia*, **12**, 801–804.

193 Moorman AV, Hagemeijer A, Charrin C, Rieder H and Secker-Walker L, on behalf of the European 11q23 Workshop participants (1998) The translocations t(11;19)(q23;p13.1) and t(11;19)(q23;p13.3): a cytogenetic and clinical profile of 53 cases. *Leukemia*, **12**, 805–810.

194 Harbott J, Mancini M, Verellen-Dumoulin C, Moorman AV and Secker-Walker L, on behalf of the European 11q23 Workshop participants (1998) Hematological malignancies with del(11q23): cytogenetic and clinical aspects. *Leukemia*, **12**, 823–827.

195 Drexler HG, Borkhardt A and Jansen JWG (1995) Detection of chromosomal translocations in leukemia-lymphoma cells by polymerase chain reaction. *Leuk Lymphoma*, **19**, 359–380.

196 Pegram LD, Megonigal MD, Lange BJ, Nowell PC, Rowley JD, Rappaport EF and Felix CA (2000) t(3;11) translocation in treatment-related acute myeloid leukemia fuses *MLL* with the GMPS (guanosine 5′ monophosphate synthetase) gene. *Blood*, **96**, 4260–4362.

197 Daheron L, Veinstein A, Brizard F, Drabkin H, Lacotte L, Guilhot F *et al.* (2001) Human LPP gene is fused to MLL in a secondary acute leukemia with a t(3;11)(q28;q23), *Genes Chromosomes Cancer*, **31**, 382–389.

198 Aventïn A, La Starza R, Martinez C, Wlodarska I, Boogaerts M, Van den Berghe H and Mecucci C (1999) Involvement of *MLL* gene in a t(10;11)(q22;q23) and a t(8;11)(q24;q23) identified by fluorescence in situ hybridization. *Cancer Genet Cytogenet*, **108**, 48–52.

199 Fuchs U, Rehkamp G, Haas OA, Slany R, Konig M, Bojesen S *et al.* (2001) The human formin-binding protein 17 (FBP17) interacts with sorting nexin, SNX2,

200 Alexander BM, Engstrom LD, Motto DG, Roulston D and Wechsler DS (2001) A novel inversion of chromosome 11 in infant acute myeloid leukaemia fuses *MLL* to Calm. A clathrin assembly protein gene. *Blood*, **98**, 576a.

201 Kuwada N, Kimura F, Matsumura T, Yamashita T, Nakamura Y, Wakimoto N *et al.* (2001) t(11;14)(q23;q24) generates an MLL-human gephyrin fusion gene along with a de facto truncated MLL in acute monoblastic leukemia. *Cancer Res*, **61**, 2665–2669.

202 Hayette S, Tigaud I, Vanier A, Martel S, Corbo L, Charrin C *et al.* (2000) AF15q14, a novel partner gene fused to the MLL gene in an acute myeloid leukaemia with a t(11;15)(q23;q14), *Oncogene*, **19**, 4446–4450.

203 Megonigal MD, Cheung NK, Rappaport EF, Nowell PC, Wilson RB, Jones DH *et al.* (2000) Detection of leukemia-associated MLL-GAS7 translocation early during chemotherapy with DNA topoisomerase II-inhibitors. *Proc Natl Acad Sci USA*, **97**, 2814–2819.

204 Ida K, Kitabayashi I, Taki T, Taniwaki M, Noro K, Yamamoto M *et al.* (1997) Adenoviral E1A-associated protein p300 is involved in acute myeloid leukemia with t(11;22)(q23;q13). *Blood*, **90**, 4699–4704.

205 Borkhardt A, Teigler-Schlegel A, Fuchs U, Keller C, Konig M, Harbott J and Haas OA (2001) An ins(X;11)(q24;q23) fuses the MLL and the Septin 6/KIAA0128 gene in an infant with AML-M2. *Genes Chromosomes Cancer*, **32**, 82–88.

206 Kwong YL and Wong KF (1997) Acute myeloid leukaemia with trisomy 11; a molecular cytogenetic study. *Cancer Genet Cytogenet*, **99**, 19–23.

207 Reinhardt D and Creutzig U (2002) Isolated myelosarcoma in children—update and review. *Leuk Lymphoma*, **43**, 565–574.

208 Mrózek K, Heinonen K, Lawrence D, Carroll AJ, Koduru PRK, Rao KW *et al.* (1997) Adult patients with *de novo* acute myeloid leukemia with t(9;11)(p22;q23) have a superior outcome to patients with other translocations involving band 11q23: a Cancer and Leukemia Group B study. *Blood*, **90**, 4531–4538.

209 Bloomfield CD, Archer KJ, Mrózek K, Lillington DM, Kaneko Y, Head DR *et al.* (2002) 11q23 balanced chromosome aberrations in treatment-related myelodysplastic syndromes and acute leukemia: report from an international workshop. *Genes, Chromosomes Cancer*, **33**, 362–378.

210 Smith FO, Rauch C, Williams DE, March CJ, Arthur D, Hilden J *et al.* (1996) The human homologue of rat NG2, a chondroitin sulfate proteoglycan, is not expressed on the cell surface of normal hematopoietic cells but is expressed by acute myeloid leukemia blasts from poor-prognosis patients with abnormalities of chromosome band 11q23. *Blood*, **87**, 1123–1133.

211 Wutcher C, Schnittger S, Schoch C, Harbott J, Martin M, Sperling C *et al.* (1998) Detection of acute leukemia cells with 11q23 rearrangements by flow cytometry:

sensitivity and specificity of monoclonal antibody 7.1. *Blood*, **92**, Suppl. 1, 228a.

212 Johansson B, Mertens F and Mitelman F (1994) Secondary chromosomal abnormalities in acute leukemias. *Leukemia*, **8**, 953–962.

213 Cimino G, Moir DT, Canaani O, Williams K, Crist WM, Katzao S *et al.* (1991) Cloning of the *ALL-1* locus involved in leukemias with the t(4;11)(q21;q23), t(9;11)(p22;q23) and t(11;19)(q23;p13) chromosome translocations. *Cancer Res*, **51**, 6712–6714.

214 Bresters D, Reus ACW, Veerman AJP, van Wering ER, van der Does-van den Berg A and Kaspers GJL (2002) Congenital leukaemia: the Dutch experience and review of the literature. *Br J Haematol*, **117**, 513–524.

215 Abou SMH, Jadayel DM, Min T, Swansbury GJ, Dainton MG, Jafer O *et al.* (2002) Incidence of *MLL* rearrangement in acute myeloid leukemia, and a *CALM-AF10* fusion in M4 type acute myeloblastic leukemia. *Leuk Lymphoma*, **43**, 89–95.

216 Lillington DM, Young BD, Berger R, Martineau M, Moorman AV and Secker-Walker LM (1998) The t(10;11)(p12;q23) translocation in acute leukaemia: a cytogenetic and clinical study of 20 patients. European 11q23 Workshop Participants. *Leukemia*, **12**, 801–804.

217 Sandberg AA, Hecht B KMc-C and Hecht F (1985) Nomenclature: the Philadelphia chromosome or Ph without superscript. *Cancer Genet Cytogenet*, **14**, 1.

218 Cascavilla N, Melillo L, d'Arena G, Greco MM, Carella AM, Sajeva MR *et al.* (2000) Minimally differentiated acute myeloid leukemia (AML M0): clinicobiological findings in 29 cases. *Leuk Lymphoma*, **37**, 105–113.

219 Black A-MW, Carroll AJ, Hagemeijer A, Michaux L, van Lom K, Olney HJ and Baer MR (2002) Rare recurring balanced chromosome abnormalities in therapy-related myelodysplastic syndromes and acute leukemia: report from an International Workshop. *Genes Chromosomes Cancer*, **33**, 401–412.

220 Peterson LC, Bloomfield CD and Brunning RD (1976) Blast crisis as an initial or terminal manifestation of chronic myeloid leukemia: a study of 28 patients. *Am J Med*, **60**, 209–220.

221 Sasaki M, Kondo K and Tomiyasu T (1983) Cytogenetic characterization of 10 cases of Ph[1]-positive acute myelogenous leukemia. *Cancer Genet Cytogenet*, **9**, 119–128.

222 Pedersen-Bjergaard J, Brondum-Nielsen K, Karle H and Johansson B (1997) Chemotherapy-related— and late occurring—Philadelphia chromosome in AML, ALL and CML. Similar events related to treatment with DNA topoisomerase II-inhibitors? *Leukemia*, **11**, 1571–1574.

223 Pearson MG, Vardiman JW, Le Beau MM, Rowley JD, Schwartz S, Kerman SL *et al.* (1985) Increased numbers of marrow basophils may be associated with a t(6;9) in ANLL. *Am J Hematol*, **18**, 393–403.

224 Heim S, Kristoffersson U, Mandahl N, Mitelman F, Bekassy AN, Garwicz S and Wiebe T (1986) High resolution banding analysis of the reciprocal transloca-

tion t(6;9) in acute nonlymphocytic leukemia. *Cancer Genet Cytogenet*, **22**, 195–201.

225 Horsman DE and Kalousek DK (1987) Acute myelomonocytic leukemia (AML-M4) and translocation t(6;9)(p23;q34): two additional patients with prominent myelodysplasia. *Cancer Genet Cytogenet*, **26**, 77–82.

226 Von Lindern M, Fornerod M, van Baal S, Jaegle M, de Wit T, Buijs A and Grosveld G (1992) The translocation (6;9), associated with a specific subtype of acute myeloid leukemia, results in the fusion of two genes, *dek* and *can*, and the expression of a chimeric, leukemia-specific *dek-can* mRNA. *Mol Cell Biol*, **12**, 1687–1697.

227 Kraemer D, Wozniak RW, Blobel G and Radu A (1994) The human CAN protein, a putative oncogene product associated with myeloid leukemogenesis, is a nuclear pore complex protein that faces the cytoplasm. *Proc Natl Acad Sci USA*, **91**, 1519–1523.

228 Fu KF, Grosveld G and Markovitz DM (1997) DEK, an autoantigen involved in chromosomal translocation in acute myelogenous leukemia, binds to the HIV-2 enhancer. *Proc Natl Acad Sci USA*, **94**, 1811–1815.

229 Secker-Walker LM, Mehta A and Bain B on behalf of the UKCCG (1995) Abnormalities of 3q21 and 3q26 in myeloid malignancy: a United Kingdom Cancer Cytogenetic Group study. *Br J Haematol*, **91**, 490–501.

230 Lavabre-Bertrand T, Bourquard P, Chiesa J, Berthéas MF, Lefort G *et al.* (2001) Diabetes insipidus revealing acute myelogenous leukaemia with a high platelet count, monosomy 7 and abnormalities of chromosome 3: a new entity? *Eur J Haematol*, **66**, 66–69.

231 Jenkins RB, Tefferi A, Solberg LA and Dewald GW (1989) Acute leukemia with abnormal thrombopoiesis and inversions of chromosome 3. *Cancer Genet Cytogenet*, **39**, 167–179.

232 Wieser R (2002) Rearrangements of the chromosome band 3q21 in myeloid leukemia. *Leuk Lymphoma*, **43**, 59–65.

233 Bloomfield CD, Garson DM, Volin L, Knuutila S and de la Chapelle A (1985) t(1;3)(p36;q21) in acute nonlymphocytic leukemia: a new cytogenetic–clinicopathologic association. *Blood*, **66**, 1409–1413.

234 Raimondi SC, Dubé ID, Valentine MD, Mirro J, Watt HJ, Larson RA *et al.* (1989) Clinicopathologic manifestations of the t(3;5) in patients with acute nonlymphocytic leukemia. *Leukemia*, **3**, 42–47.

235 Hoyle CF, Sherrington P and Hayhoe FGJ (1988) Translocation (3;6)(q21;p21) in acute myeloid leukemia with abnormal thrombopoiesis and basophilia. *Cancer Genet Cytogenet*, **30**, 261–267.

236 Raynaud SD, Baens M, Grosgeorge J, Rodgers K, Reid CDL, Dainton M *et al.* (1996) Fluorescence *in situ* hybridization analysis of t(3;12)(q26;p13): a recurring chromosomal abnormality involving the *TEL* gene (*ETV6*) in myelodysplastic syndromes. *Blood*, **88**, 682–689.

237 Pedersen-Bjergaard J, Johansson B and Philip P (1994) Translocation (3;21)(q26;q22) in therapy-

related myelodysplasia following drugs targeting DNA-topoisomerase II combined with alkylating agents, and in myeloproliferative disorders undergoing spontaneous leukaemic transformation. *Cancer Genetic Cytogenet*, **76**, 50–55.

238 Nucifora G, Begy CR, Kobayashi H, Roulston D, Claxton D, Pedersen-Bjergaard J *et al.* (1994) Consistent intergenic splicing and production of multiple transcripts and AML1 at 21q22 and three unrelated genes at 3q26 in (3;21)(q26;q22) translocation. *Proc Natl Acad Sci USA*, **91**, 4004–4009.

239 Suzukawa K, Parganas E, Gajjar A, Abe T, Takahashi S, Tani K *et al.* (1994) Identification of the break point cluster region 3′ of the ribophorin I gene at 3q21 associated with the transcriptional activation of the *EVI1* gene in acute myelogenous leukemia with inv(3)(q21q26). *Blood*, **84**, 2681–2688.

240 Ogawa S, Kurokawa M, Tanaka T, Mitani K, Inazawa J, Hangaishi A *et al.* (1996) Structurally altered Evi-1 protein generated in the 3q21q26 syndrome. *Oncogene*, **13**, 183–191.

241 Russell M, List A, Greenberg P, Woodward S, Glinsmann B, Parganas E *et al.* (1994) Expression of EVI1 in myelodysplastic syndromes and other hematologic malignancies without 3q26 translocations. *Blood*, **84**, 1243–1248.

242 Hanslip JI, Swansbury GJ, Pinkerton R and Catovsky D (1992) The translocation t(8;16)(p11;q13) defines an AML subtype with distinct cytology and clinical features. *Leuk Lymphoma*, **6**, 479–486.

243 Stark B, Resnitzky P, Jeison M, Luria D, Blau O, Avigad S *et al.* (1995) A distinct subtype of M4/M5 acute myeloblastic leukemia (AML) associated with t(8;16)(p11:p13), in a patient with the variant t(8:19) (p11:q13)—case report and review of the literature. *Leuk Res*, **19**, 367–379.

244 Velloso ERP, Mecucci C, Michaux L, van Orshoven A, Stul M, Boogaerts M *et al.* (1996) Translocation t(8;16)(p11;p13) in acute non-lymphocytic leukemia: report on two new cases and review of the literature. *Leuk Lymphoma*, **21**, 137–142.

245 Thandla S and Aplan PD (1997) Molecular biology of acute lymphocytic leukemia. *Semin Oncol*, **24**, 45–56.

246 Aguiar RCT, Chase A, Coulthard S, Macdonald D, Swirsky D, Goldman JM and Cross NCP (1997) Molecular investigation of chromosome band 8p11 in two distinct leukaemia syndromes. *Br J Haematol*, **96**, Suppl 1, 5.

247 Coulthard S, Chase A, Orchard K, Watmore A, Vora A, Goldman JM and Swirsky DM (1998) Two cases of inv(8)(p11q13) in AML with erythrophagocytosis: a new cytogenetic variant. *Br J Haematol*, **100**, 561–563.

248 Bernstein J, Dastague N, Haas OAS, Harbott J, Heerema NA, Huret JL *et al.* (2000) Nineteen cases of the t(1;22)(p13;q13) acute megakaryoblastic leukemia in infants/children and a review of 39 cases: report of the t(1;22) study group. *Leukemia*, **14**, 216–217.

249 Duchayne E, Fenneteau O, Pages M-P, Sainty D, Arnoulet C, Dastugue N *et al.* (2001) *Blood*, **99**, 581a.

250 Ng KC, Tan AM, Chong YY, Lau LC and Lu J (2002) Congenital acute megakaryoblastic leukaemia (M7) with chromosomal t(1;22)(p13;q13) translocation in a set of identical twins. *J Pediat Hematol Oncol*, **21**, 428–430.

251 Carroll A, Civin C, Schneider N, Dahl G, Pappo A, Bowman P *et al.* (1991) The t(1;22)(p13;q13) is nonrandom and restricted to infants with acute megakaryoblastic leukaemia: A Pediatric Oncology Group study. *Blood*, **78**, 748–752.

252 Lu G, Altman AJ and Benn PA (1993) Review of the cytogenetic changes in acute megakaryoblastic leukemia: one disease or several? *Cancer Genet Cytogenet*, **67**, 81–89.

253 Hitzler JK, Li Y, Ma G, Ma Z, Fernandez CV, Lee C *et al.* (2001) Variant *RBM15-MKL1* and *MKL1-RBM15* fusion transcripts in an infant with recurrent acute megakaryoblastic leukaemia and t(1;22) after allogeneic bone marrow transplantation. *Blood*, **98**, 563a.

254 Mercher T, Coniat MB, Monni R, Mauchauffe M, Khac FN, Gressin L *et al.* (2001) Involvement of a human gene related to the Drosophila spen gene in the recurrent t(1;22) translocation of acute megakaryocytic leukemia. *Proc Natl Acad Sci USA*, **98**, 5776–5779.

255 Imashuku S, Hibi S, Sako M, Lin YW, Ikuta K, Nakata Y *et al.* (2000) Hemophagocytosis by leukaemic blasts in 7 acute myeloid leukemia cases with t(16;21)(p11;p22). *Cancer*, **88**, 1970–1975.

256 Streubel B, Sauerland C, Heil G, Freund M, Bartels H, Lengfelder E *et al.* (1998) Correlation of cytogenetic, molecular genetic, and clinical findings in 59 patients with ANLL or MDS and abnormalities of the short arm of chromosome 12. *Br J Haematol*, **100**, 521–533.

257 Suenega M, Sanada I, Tsukamoto A, Sato M, Kawano F, Shido T *et al.* (1993) Trisomy 4 in a case of acute myelogenous leukemia accompanied by subcutaneous soft tissue tumors. *Cancer Genet Cytogenet*, **71**, 71–75.

258 Hoyle C, Sherrington PD and Hayhoe FGJ (1987) Cytological features of 9q– deletions in AML. *Blood*, **60**, 277–278.

259 Lunde JH and Allen EF (1994) Interstitial 9q– deletion in a case of acute myeloid leukemia arising from a granulocytic sarcoma. *Cancer Genet Cytogenet*, **78**, 239–241.

260 Mehta AB, Bain BJ, Fitchett M, Shah S and Secker-Walker LM (1997) Trisomy 13 and myeloid malignancy: characteristic blast cell morphology. A United Kingdom Cancer Cytogenetics Group Survey. *Br J Haematol*, **101**, 745–752.

261 Nichols CR, Roth BJ, Heerema N, Giep J and Tricot G (1990) Malignant hematologic neoplasia associated with primary mediastinal germ-cell tumors. *N Engl J Med*, **322**, 1425–1429.

262 Ladanyi M, Samaniego F, Reuter VE, Motzer RJ, Jhanwar SC, Bosl GJ and Chaganti RSK (1990) Cytogenetic and immunohistochemical evidence for

the germ cell origin of a subset of acute leukemias associated with mediastinal germ cell tumors. *J Natl Cancer Inst*, **82**, 221–227.

263 Vlasveld LT, Splinter TAW, Hagemeijer A, van Lom K and Löwenberg B (1994) Acute myeloid leukaemia with +i(12p) shortly after treatment of mediastinal germ cell tumour. *Br J Haematol*, **88**, 196–198.

264 Mascarello JT, Cajulis TR, Billman GF and Spruce WE (1993) Ovarian germ cell tumour evolving to myelodysplasia. *Genes Chromosomes Cancer*, **7**, 227–230.

265 Woodruff K, Wang N, May W, Adrone E, Denny C and Feig SA (1995) The clonal nature of mediastinal germ cell tumors and acute myelogenous leukemia. *Cancer Genet Cytogenet*, **79**, 25–31.

266 Mochizuki N, Shimizu S, Nagasawa T, Tanaka H, Taniwaki M, Yokota J and Morishita K (2000) A novel gene, MEL1, mapped to 1p36.3 is highly homologous to the MDS1/EVI1 gene and is transcriptionally activated in t(1;3)(p36;q21)-positive leukemia cells. *Blood*, **96**, 3209–3214.

267 Nakamura T, Yamazaki Y, Hatano Y and Miura I (1999) NUP98 is fused to PMX1 homeobox gene in human acute myelogenous leukemia with chromosome translocation t(1;11)(q23;p15), *Blood*, **94**, 741–747.

268 Salomon-Nguyen F, Della-Valle V, Mauchauffe M, Busson-Le Coniat M, Ghysdael J *et al.* (2000) The t(1;12)(q21;p13) translocation of human acute myeloblastic leukemia results in a TEL-ARNT fusion, *Proc Natl Acad Sci USA*, **97**, 6757–6762.

269 Hromas R, Shopnick, Jumean HG, Bowers C, Varell-Garcia M and Richkind K (2000) A novel syndrome of radiation-associated acute myeloid leukemia (AML) involving AML1 gene translocations. *Blood*, **95**, 4011–4013.

270 Odero MD, Carlson K, Calasanz MJ, Lahortiga I, Chinwalla V and Rowley JD (2001) Identification of new translocations involving ETV6 in hematologic malignancies by fluorescence in situ hybridization and spectral karyotyping. *Genes Chromosomes Cancer*, **31**, 134–142.

271 Jaju RJ, Fidler C, Haas OA, Strickson J, Watkins F, Clark K *et al.* (2001) A novel gene, *NSD1*, is fused to *NUP98* in the t(5;11)(q35;p15.5) in *de novo* childhood AML. *Br J Haematol*, **113**, Suppl. 1, 60.

272 Yagasaki F, Jinnai I, Yoshida S, Yokoyama Y, Matsuda A, Kusumoto S *et al.* (1999) Fusion of TEL/ETV6 to a novel ACS2 in myelodysplastic syndrome and acute myelogenous leukemia with t(5;12)(q31;p13) *Genes, Chromosomes Cancer*, **26**, 192–202.

273 Huang S-Y, Tang J-L, Liang Y-J, Wang C-H, Chen Y-C and Tien H-F′ (1997) Clinical, haematological and molecular studies in patients with chromosome translocation t(7;11): a study of four Chinese patients in Taiwan. *Br J Haematol*, **96**, 682–687.

274 Taketani T, Taki T, Ono R, Kobayashi Y, Ida K and Hayashi T (2002) The chromosome translocation t(7;11)(p15;p15) in acute myeloid leukemia results in fusion of the *NUP98* gene with a *HOXA* cluster gene,

HOXA13, but not *HOXA9*. *Genes Chromsomes Cancer*, **34**, 437–443.

275 Beverloo HB, Panagopoulos I, Isaksson M, van Wering E, van Drunen E, de Klein A *et al.* (2001) Fusion of homeobox gene HLXB9 and the ETV6 gene in an infant acute myeloid leukemias with the t(7;12)(q36;p13), *Cancer Res*, **61**, 5374–5377.

276 Rosati R, La Starza R, Veronese A, Aventin A, Schwienbacher C, Vallespi T *et al.* (2002) *NUP98* is fused to the *NSD3* gene in acute myeloid leukemia associated with t(8;11)(p11.2;p15). *Blood*, **99**, 3857–3860.

277 Chaffanet M, Gressin L, Preudhomme C, Soenen-Cornu V, Birnbaum D and Pebusque MJ (2000) *MOZ* is fused to *p300* in an acute monocytic leukemia with t(8;22). *Genes Chromosomes Cancer*, **28**, 138–144.

278 Ahuja HG, Hong J, Aplan PD, Tcheurekdjian L, Forman SJ and Slovak ML (2000) t(9;11)(p22;p15) in acute myeloid leukemia results in a fusion between NUP98 and the gene encoding transcriptional coactivators p52 and p75-lens epithelium-derived growth factor (LEDGF), *Cancer Res*, **60**, 6227–6229.

279 O'Brien SG, Vieira SAD, Connors S, Bown N, Chang J, Capdeville R and Melo JV (2002) Transient response to imatinib mesylate (STI571) in a patient with the *ETV6-ABL* t(9;12) translocation, *Blood*, **99**, 3465–3467.

280 Kobayashi H, Hosoda F, Maseki N, Sakurai M, Imashuku S, Ohki M and Kaneko Y (1997) Hematologic malignancies with the t(10;11)(p13;q21) have the same molecular events and a variety of morphologic and immunologic phenotypes. *Genes Chromosomes Cancer*, **21**, 253–259.

281 Panagopoulos I, Fioretos T, Isaksson M, Samuelsson U, Billstrom R, Strombeck B *et al* (2001) Fusion of the MORF and CBP genes in acute myeloid leukemia with the t(10;16)(q22;p13). *Hum Mol Genet*, **10**, 395–404.

282 Chase A, Reiter A, Burci L, Cazzaniga G, Biondi A, Pickard J *et al.* (1999) Fusion of ETV6 to the caudal-related homeobox gene CDX2 in acute myeloid leukemia with the t(12;13)(p13;q12), *Blood*, **93**, 1025–1031.

283 Liu Q, Schwaller J, Kutok J, Cain D, Aster JC, Williams IR and Gilliland DG (2000) Signal transduction and transforming properties of the TEL-TRKC fusions associated with t(12;15)(p13;q25) in congenital fibrosarcoma and acute myelogenous leukemia, *EMBO J*, **19**, 1827–1838.

284 Wlodarska I, Mecucci C, Baens M, Marynen P and van den Berghe H (1996) *ETV6* gene rearrangements in hematopoietic malignant disorders. *Leuk Lymphoma*, **23**, 287–295.

285 Ichikawa H, Shimizu K, Hayashi Y and Ohki M (1994) An RNA-binding protein gene, *TLS/FUS*, is fused to *ERG* in human myeloid leukemia with t(16;21) chromosomal translocation. *Cancer Res*, **54**, 2865–2868.

286 Dastague N, Duchayne E, Kuhein E, Rubie H, Mur C, Aurich J, Robert A and Sie P (1997) Acute basophilic

leukaemia and translocation t(X;6)(p11;q23). *Br J Haematol*, **98**, 170–176.

287 Secker-Walker LM, Moorman AV, Bain BJ and Mehta AB on behalf of the EU Concerted Action 11q23 Workshop (1998) Secondary acute leukaemia and myelodysplastic syndrome with 11q23 abnormalities. *Leukemia*, **12**, 840–844.

288 Andersen MK, Christiansen DH, Jensen BA, Ernst P, Hauge G and Pedersen-Bjergaard J (2001) Therapy-related acute lymphoblastic leukaemia with *MLL* rearrangements following DNA topoisomerase II-inhibitors, an increasing problem: report on two new cases and review of the literature since 1992. *Br J Haematol*, **114**, 539–543.

289 Silva MLM, Land MGP, Maradei S, Otero L, Veith M, Brito G *et al.* (2002) Translocation (11;11)(p13~15;q23) in a child with therapy-related acute myeloid leukemia following chemotherapy with DNA-topoisomerase II-inhibitors for Langerhans cell histiocytosis. *Cancer Genet Cytogenet*, **135**, 101–102.

290 Sato Y, Izumi T, Kanamori H, Davis EM, Miura Y, Larson RA *et al.* (2002) t(1;3)(p36;p21) is a recurring therapy-related translocation. *Genes Chromosomes Cancer*, **34**, 186–192.

291 Carbonell F, Swansbury J, Min T, Matutes E, Farahat N, Buccheri V *et al.* (1996) Cytogenetic findings in acute biphenotypic leukaemia. *Leukemia*, **10**, 1283–1287.

292 Kocova M, Kowalczyk JR and Sandberg AA (1985) Translocation 4;11 acute leukemia: three case reports and review of the literature. *Cancer Genet Cytogenet*, **16**, 21–32.

293 Bernard OA and Berger R (1995) Molecular basis of 11q23 rearrangements in hematopoietic malignant proliferations. *Genes Chromosomes Cancer*, **13**, 75–85.

294 Harrison CJ (2001) Acute lymphoblastic leukaemia. *Bailliére's Clin Haematol*, **14**, 593–607.

295 Hunger P, Boomer T, McGavran L, Meltesen L, Olsen S and Varella-Garcia M (2000) Detection of *E2A* trans-locations in leukemia. *Blood*, **96**, 463a.

296 Raimondi SC, Shurtleff SA, Downing JR, Rubnitz J, Mathew S, Hancock M *et al.* (1997) 12p abnormalities and the *TEL* gene (*ETV6*) in childhood acute lymphoblastic leukaemia. *Blood*, **90**, 4559–4566.

297 Raimondi SC, Pui CH, Hancock ML, Behm FB, Filatov L and Rivera GK (1993) Heterogeneity of hyperdiploid (51–67) childhood acute lymphoblastic leukemia. *Leukemia*, **10**, 213–224.

298 Chessels JM, Swansbury GJ, Reeves B, Bailey CC and Richards SM (1997) Cytogenetics and prognosis in childhood lymphoblastic leukaemia: results in MRC UKALL X. *Br J Haematol*, **99**, 93–100.

299 The Groupe Francais de Cytogénétique Hématologique (1996) Cytogenetic abnormalities in adult acute lymphoblastic leukemia: correlations with hematologic findings and outcome. A collaborative study of the Groupe Francais de Cytogénétique Hématologique. *Blood*, **87**, 3135–3142.

300 Secker-Walker-L, Prentice HG, Durrant J, Richards S, Hall E and Harrison C (1997) Cytogenetics adds independent prognostic information in adults with acute lymphoblastic leukaemia. *Br J Haematol*, **96**, 601–610.

301 Andreasson P, Höglund M, Békássy AN, Garwicz S, Heldrup J, Mitelman F and Johansson B (2000) Cytogenetic and FISH studies of a single center consecutive series of 152 childhood acute lymphoblastic leukaemias. *Eur J Haematol*, **65**, 40–51.

302 Forestier E, Johansson B, Borgström G, Kerndrup G, Johannsson J, Heim S, the NOPHO Leukemia Cytogenetic Study Group (2000) Cytogenetic findings in a population-based series of 787 childhood acute lymphoblastic leukemias from the Nordic countries. *Eur J Haematol*, **64**, 194–200.

303 Taub JW, Konrad MA, Ge Y, Naber JM, Scott JS, Matherly LH and Ravindranath Y (2002) High frequency of leukemic clones in newborn screening blood samples of children with B-precursor acute lymphoblastic leukemia. *Blood*, **99**, 2992–2996.

304 Campana D and Behm FG, Immunophenotyping, In Whittaker JA and Holmes JA, *Leukaemia and Related Disorders*, Blackwell Science, Oxford, 1998, pp. 71–86.

305 Moorman AV, Clark R, Farrell DM, Hawkins JM, Martineau M and Secker-Walker L (1996) Detecting hidden hyperdiploidy in ALL. *Br J Haematol*, **93**, Suppl 2, 331.

306 Gaynon PS, Trigg ME, Heerema NA Sensel MG, Sather HN, Hammond GD and Bleyer WA (2000) Children's Cancer Group trial in childhood acute lymphoblastic leukemia: 1983–1995. *Leukemia*, **14**, 2223–2233.

307 Maloney KW, Shuster JJ, Murphy S, Pullen J and Camitta BA (2000) Long-term results of treatment studies for childhood acute lymphoblastic leukemia, Pediatric Oncology Study Group studies from 1986–1994. *Leukemia*, **14**, 2276–2285.

308 Romana SP, Poirel H, Leconiat M, Flexor M-A, Mauchauffé M, Jonveaux P *et al.* (1995) High frequency of t(12;21) in childhood B-lineage acute lymphoblastic leukaemia. *Blood*, **86**, 4263–4269.

309 Raynaud S, Cavé H, Baens M, Bastard C, Cacheux V, Grosgeorge J *et al.* (1996) The 12;21 translocation involving TEL and deletion of the other TEL allele: two frequently associated alterations found in childhood lymphoblastic leukaemia. *Blood*, **87**, 2891–2899.

310 Kobayashi H, Satake N, Maseki N, Sakashita A and Kaneko Y (1996) The der(21)t(12;21) chromosome is always formed in a 12;21 translocation associated with childhood acute lymphoblastic leukaemia. *Br J Haematol*, **94**, 105–111.

311 Borkhardt A, Cazzaniga G, Viehmann S, Valsecchi MG, Ludwig WD, Burci L *et al.* for the 'Associazione Italiana Ematologia Oncologia Pediatrica' and the Berlin–Frankfurt–Münster' Study Group' (1997) Incidence and clinical relevance of TEL/AML1 fusion genes in children with acute lymphoblastic leukemia enrolled in the German and Italian Multicenter Therapy Trials. *Blood*, **90**, 571–577.

312 Aguiar RCT, Goldman JM and Cross NCP (1996) TEL-AML1 fusion in primary and secondary acute leukaemias of adults. *Br J Haematol*, **93**, Suppl 1, 62.

313 McLean TW, Ringold S, Neuberg D, Stegmaier K, Tantravahi R, Ritz J *et al.* (1996) TEL/AML-1 dimerizes and is associated with a favorable outcome in childhood acute lymphoblastic leukemia. *Blood*, **88**, 4252–4258.

314 Greaves M (2002) Childhood leukaemia. *BMJ*, **324**, 283–287.

315 Codrington R, O'Connor HE, Jalali GR, Carrara P, Papaioannou M, Hart SM *et al.* (2000) Analysis of *ETV6/AML1* abnormalities in acute lymphoblastic leukaemia: incidence, alternative spliced forms and minimal residual disease value. *Br J Haematol*, **111**, 1073–1079.

316 de Haas V, Oosten L, Dee R, Verhagen OJHM, Kroes W, van den Berg H and van der Schoot CE (2000) Minimal residual disease studies are beneficial in the follow-up of *TEL/AML1* patients with B-precursor acute lympho-blastic leukaemia. *Br J Haematol*, **111**, 1080–1086.

317 Hann IA, Vora A, Harrison G, Harrison C, Eden O, Hill F *et al.* on behalf of the UK Medical Research Council's Working Party on Childhood Leukaemia (2001) Determinants of outcome after intensified therapy of childhood lymphoblastic leukaemia; results from Medical Research Council United Kingdom acute lymphoblastic leukaemia XI protocol. *Br J Haematol*, **113**, 103–114.

318 Silverman LB, Gelber RD, Dalton VK, Asselin BL, Barr RD, Clavell LA *et al.* (2001) Improved outcome for children with acute lymphoblastic leukemia: results of Dana-Farber Consortium protocol 91-01, *Blood*, **97**, 1211–1218.

319 Baruchel A, Cayuela JM, Ballerini P, Landman-Parker J, Cezard V, Firat H *et al.* (1997) The majority of myeloid-antigen-positive (My+) childhood B-cell precursor acute lymphoblastic leukaemias express TEL-AML1 fusion transcripts. *Br J Haematol*, **99**, 101–106.

320 Alessandri AJ, Reid GSD, Bader SA, Massing BG, Sorensen PHB and Schultz KR (2002) ETV6 (TEL)-AML1 pre-B acute lymphoblastic leukaemia cells are associated with a distinct antigen-presenting phenotype. *Br J Haematol*, **116**, 266–272.

321 Riesch M, Niggli FK, Leibundgut K, Caflisch U and Betts DR (2001) Loss of X chromosome in childhood acute lymphoblastic leukemia. *Cancer Genet Cytogenet*, **125**, 27–29.

322 Rambaldi A, Attuati V, Bassan R, Neonato MG, Viero P, Battista R *et al.* (1996) Molecular diagnosis and clinical relevance of t(9;22), t(4;11) and t(1;19) chromosome abnormalities in a consecutive group of 141 adult patients with acute lymphoblastic leukemia. *Leuk Lymphoma*, **21**, 457–466.

323 Hunger SP (1996) Chromosomal translocations involving the E2A gene in acute lymphoblastic leukemia: clinical features and molecular pathogenesis. *Blood*, **87**, 1211–1224.

324 Lessard M, Fenneteau O, Sainty D, Valensi F, MacIntyre E and Flandrin G (1993) Translocation t(1;19) in acute lymphoblastic leukemia patients with cytological presentation simulating L3-ALL (Burkitt-like). *Leuk Lymphoma*, **11**, 149–152.

325 Uckun FM, Sensel MG, Sather HN, Gaynon PS, Arthur DC, Lange BJ *et al.* (1998) Clinical significance of translocation t(1;19) in childhood acute lymphoblastic leukemia in the context of contemporary therapies: a report of the Children's Cancer Group. *J Clin Oncol*, **16**, 527–535.

326 Khalidi H, O'Donnell MR, Slovak ML and Arber DA (1999) Adult precursor-B acute lymphoblastic leukemia with translocations involving chromosome band 19p13 is associated with poor prognosis. *Cancer Genet Cytogenet*, **109**, 58–65.

327 Hunger SP, Galili N, Carroll AJ, Crist WM, Link M and Cleary ML (1991) the t(1;19)(q23;p13) results in consistent fusion of *E2A* and *PBX1* coding sequences in acute lymphoblastic leukemias. *Blood*, **77**, 687–693.

328 Secker-Walker LM, Berger R, Fenaux P, Lay JL, Nelken B, Garson M *et al.* (1992) Prognostic significance of the balanced t(1;19) and unbalanced der(19)t(1;19) translocation in acute lymphoblastic leukaemia. *Leukemia*, **6**, 363–369.

329 Forestier E, Johansson B, Gustafsson G, Kerndrup G, Johannsson J and Heim S for the Nordic Society for Paediatric Haematology and Oncology (NOPHO) Leukaemia Cytogenetic Study Group (2000) Prognostic impact of karyotypic findings in childhood acute lymphoblastic leukaemia: a Nordic series comparing two treatment periods. *Br J Haematol*, **110**, 147–153.

330 Sang B-C, Si L, Dias P, Liu L, Wei J, Wang Z-X, Monell CR, Behm F and Gruenwald S (1997) Monoclonal antibodies specific to the acute lymphoblastic leukemia t(1;19)-associated E2A/pbx1 chimeric protein: characterization and diagnostic utility. *Blood*, **89**, 2909–2914.

331 Faderl S, Kantarjian HM, Thomas DA, Cortes J, Giles F, Pierce S *et al.* (2000) Outcome of Philadelphia chromosome-positive adult acute lymphoblastic leukaemia. *Leuk Lymphoma*, **36**, 263–273.

332 Gleissner B, Gökbuget N, Bartram CR, Janssen B, Rieder H, Janssen JWG *et al.* (2002) Leading prognostic significance of the BCR-ABL translocation in adult acute B-lineage lymphoblastic leukemia: a prospective study of the German Multicenter Trial group and confirmed polymerase chain reaction analysis. *Blood*, **99**, 1536–1543.

333 Preti HA, O'Brien S, Giralt S, Beran M, Pierce S and Kantarjian HM (1994) Philadelphia-chromosome-positive adult acute lymphocytic leukemia: characteristics, treatment results, and prognosis in 41 patients. *Am J Med*, **97**, 60–65.

334 Kobayashi S, Maruta A, Yamamoto T, Fujisawa S, Fukawa H, Kanamori H *et al.* (2000) Significance of micromegakaryocytes in Philadelphia chromosome-

positive acute lymphoblastic leukemia. *Leukemia*, **14**, 1327–1329.

335 Rieder H, Ludwig W-D, Gassman W, Maurer J, Janssen JWG, Gökbuget N et al. (1996) Prognostic significance of additional chromosome abnormalities in adult patients with Philadelphia chromosome positive acute lymphoblastic leukaemia. *Br J Haematol*, **95**, 678–691.

336 Tabernero MD, Bortoluci AM, Alaejos I, Lopez-Berges MC, Rasillo A, Garcia-Sanz R et al. (2001) Adult precursor B-ALL with BCR/ABL gene rearrangements displays a unique immunophenotype based on the pattern of CD10, CD34, CD13 and CD38 expression. *Leukemia*, **15**, 406–414.

337 Reid AG, Huntly BJP, Campbell L, Telford N, Bown N et al. (2001) Extensive deletion at the t(9;22) breakpoint occurs in a minority of patients with Philadelphia-positive acute lymphoblastic leukaemia. *Blood*, **98**, 316a.

338 Cazzaniga G, Rossi V and Biondi A (2002) Monitoring minimal residual disease using chromosomal translocations in childhood ALL. *Best Practice Res Clin Haematol*, **15**, 21–35.

339 Pui C-H, Frankel LS, Carroll AJ, Raimondi SC, Shuster JJ, Head DR et al. (1991) Clinical characteristics and treatment outcome of childhood acute lymphoblastic leukemia with the t(4;11)(q21;q23): a collaborative study of 40 cases. *Blood*, **77**, 440–447.

340 Greaves M (1999) Molecular genetics, natural history and demise of childhood leukaemia. *Eur J Cancer*, **35**, 1941–1953.

341 Behm FG, Smith FO, Raimondi SC, Pui C-H and Bernstein ID (1996) Human homologue of the rat chondroitin sulfate proteoglycan, NG2, detected by monoclonal antibody 7.1, identifies childhood acute lymphoblastic leukaemia with t(4;11)(q21;q23) or t(11;19)(q23;p13) and MLL gene rearrangements. *Blood*, **87**, 1134–1139.

342 Baskaran K, Erfurth F, Taborn G, Copeland NG, Gilbert DJ, Jenkins NA et al. (1997) Cloning and developmental expression of the murine homolog of the acute leukemia proto-oncogene AF-4. *Oncogene*, **15**, 1967–1978.

343 Peham M, Panzer S, Fasching K, Haas OA, Fischer S, Marschalek R et al. (2002) Low frequency of clonotypic Ig and T-cell receptor gene rearrangements in t(4;11) infant acute lymphoblastic leukaemia and its implication for the detection of minimal residual disease. *Br J Haematol*, **117**, 315–321.

344 Behm FG, Raimondi SC, Frestedt JL, Liu Q, Crist WM, Downing JR et al. (1996b) Rearrangement of the MLL gene confers a poor prognosis in childhood acute lymphoblastic leukaemia, regardless of presenting age. *Blood*, **87**, 2870–2877.

345 Khoury H, Dalal BI, Barnett MJ, Nevill TJ, Horsman DE, Shepherd JD et al. (2001) Distinctive immunophenotypic features in acute myelogenous leukemia with 11q23 abnormalities. *Blood*, **98**, 189b.

346 Stamatoullas A, Buchonnet G, Lepretre S, Lenain P, Lenormand B, Duval C et al. (2000) De novo acute B cell leukemia/lymphoma with t(14;18). *Leukemia*, 14, 1960–1966.

347 Harrison C (2001) The detection and significance of chromosomal abnormalities in childhood acute lymphoblastic leukaemia. *Blood Rev*, **15**, 49–59.

348 Heerema NA, Nachman JB, Sather HN, Sensel MG, Lee MK, Hutchinson R et al. (1999) Hypodiploidy with less than 45 chromosomes confers adverse risk in childhood acute lymphoblastic leukemia: a report from the Childrens Cancer group. *Blood*, **94**, 4036–4046.

349 Bernard OA, Busson-LeConiat M, Ballerini P, Mauchauffe M, Della Valle V, Monni R et al. (2001) A new recurrent and specific cryptic translocation, t(5;14)(q35;q32), is associated with expression of the Hox11L2 gene in T acute lymphoblastic leukemia. *Leukemia*, **15**, 1495–1504.

350 Delabesse E, Bernard M, Landman-Parker J, Davi F, Leboeuf D, Varet B et al. (1997) Simultaneous *SIL-TAL1* RT-PCR detection of all *tal*^d deletions and identification of novel tal^d variants. *Br J Haematol*, **99**, 901–907.

351 Brunning RD, Matutes E, Flandrin G, Vardiman J, Bennett J, Head D and Harris NL (2001) Acute myeloid leukaemia, not otherwise categorized. In Jaffe ES, Harris NL, Stein H and Vardiman JW (Eds), *World Health Organization Classification of Tumours: Pathology and Genetics of Tumours of Haematopoietic and Lymphoid Tissues*, IARC Press, Lyon, pp. 91–105.

352 Bain BJ (2003) Di Guglielmo and his syndromes. *Br J Haematol, in press.*

353 Hasserjian RP, Howard J, Wood A, Henry K and Bain B (2001) Acute erythremic myelosis (true erythroleukaemia): a variant of AML FAB-M6. *J Clin Pathol*, **54**, 205–209.

354 Bain BJ, Catovsky D, O'Brien M, Prentice HG, Lawlor E, Kumaran TO et al. (1981) Megakaryoblastic leukaemia presenting as acute myelofibrosis. A study of four cases with the platelet-peroxidase reaction. *Blood*, **58**, 206–213.

355 Brunning RD, Borowitz M, Matutes E, Head D, Flandrin G, Swerdlow SH and Bennett JM (2001) Precursor B lymphoblastic leukaemia/lymphoblastic lymphoma (precursor B-cell acute lymphoblastic leukaemia). In Jaffe ES, Harris NL, Stein H and Vardiman JW (Eds), *World Health Organization Classification of Tumours: Pathology and Genetics of Tumours of Haematopoietic and Lymphoid Tissues*, IARC Press, Lyon, pp. 111–114.

356 Brunning RD, Borowitz M, Matutes E, Head D, Flandrin G, Swerdlow SH and Bennett JM (2001) Precursor T lymphoblastic leukaemia/lymphoblastic lymphoma (precursor T-cell acute lymphoblastic leukaemia). In Jaffe ES, Harris NL, Stein H and Vardiman JW (Eds), *World Health Organization Classification of Tumours: Pathology and Genetics of Tumours of Haematopoietic and Lymphoid Tissues*, IARC Press, Lyon, pp. 115–117.

CHAPTER 3

MYELODYSPLASTIC SYNDROMES

The myelodysplastic syndromes (MDS) are a related group of bone marrow disorders that were first described in the 1930s and 1940s, being referred to by terms such as 'primary refractory anaemia' and 'pre-leukaemic anaemia' [1]. They have been increasingly recognized in the last 25–30 years since the French–American–British (FAB) group suggested criteria to distinguish them from the acute leukaemias. In the initial FAB classification of the acute leukaemias they were designated the dysmyelopoietic syndromes and were divided broadly into chronic myelomonocytic leukaemia (CMML) and refractory anaemia with excess of blasts (RAEB) [2]. The latter condition included cases that would previously have been classified not only as 'primary refractory anaemia' and 'preleukaemic anaemia' but also as 'preleukaemia', 'smouldering leukaemia', 'subacute leukaemia' or 'atypical leukaemia'. The dysmyelopoietic syndromes, renamed the myelodysplastic syndromes, were further described and classified by the FAB group in 1982 [3] with the criteria for making a distinction from acute myeloid leukaemia (AML) being further refined by the FAB group in 1985 [4] and by a World Health Organization expert group in 2001 [5–11]. The term 'myelodysplastic syndrome' (or syndromes) has now been widely accepted to designate this group of disorders.

The incidence of MDS is about 6 times that of AML. It has been estimated at 0.75/1000/year in those over 60 [12].

The MDS are a closely related group of acquired bone marrow disorders characterized by ineffective and dysplastic haemopoiesis. These conditions are intrinsic to the bone marrow and are progressive. They are consequent on the proliferation of an abnormal clone of cells that replaces normal haemopoietic cells. MDS may either be apparently primary or may evolve in the course of other bone marrow diseases or be secondary to previous exposure to cytotoxic chemotherapy, irradiation or other environmental toxins. The defect may be principally manifest in one lineage (the granulocytic/monocytic lineage, the erythroid lineage or, less often, the megakaryocyte lineage) but commonly dysplasia is bilinear or trilinear. There is usually a discrepancy between a normocellular or hypercellular bone marrow and peripheral blood cytopenia, although in up to 10% of cases the bone marrow is hypocellular. (It should be mentioned that, since MDS occurs predominantly in the elderly, it is important to interpret bone marrow cellularity in relation to the age of the patient.) Although cytopenia is most characteristic, some patients have neutrophil leucocytosis, monocytosis or thrombocytosis or, rarely, eosinophilia or basophilia. Some patients with prominent proliferative as well as dysplastic features are, in the WHO classification, designated as a mixed myelodysplastic/myeloproliferative disorder, rather than as MDS.

Dysplastic haemopoiesis is not confined to MDS, being seen, for example, during administration of certain drugs or exposure to various toxic substances such as heavy metals, in human immunodeficiency virus (HIV)-infected subjects [13] and in megaloblastic anaemia secondary to vitamin B_{12} or folic acid deficiency. The diagnosis of MDS requires the recognition of features consistent with this diagnosis and the exclusion of alternative causes. Haematological abnormalities that may occur are shown in Table 3.1. The usefulness of such features in diagnosis varies. Some abnormalities, such as an acquired Pelger–Huët

Table 3.1 Haematological features that may occur in the myelodysplastic syndromes (MDS).

Peripheral blood	Bone marrow
Erythropoiesis	
Anaemia and red cell dysplasia	Hyperplasia (common)
Normocytic normochromic (common)	Hypoplasia (uncommon) including red cell aplasia
Macrocytic (common)	Macronormoblastic erythropoiesis
Microcytic (uncommon)*	Sideroblastic erythropoiesis
Megaloblastic erythropoiesis	Dysplastic erythropoiesis with features such as binuclearity, multinuclearity,
Dimorphic blood film	nuclear lobulation or fragmentation, increased Howell–Jolly bodies,
Anisocytosis, anisochromasia	internuclear bridges, gaps in nuclear membrane, pyknosis, gigantism
Poikilocytosis (which may include ovalocytes,	
elliptocytes [16], schistocytes [16, 17],	
teardrop poikilocytes, stomatocytes,	
acanthocytes [18] and target cells)	
Polychromasia (uncommon),	
Pappenheimer bodies, basophilic stippling	
Circulating nucleated red blood cells,	
which may show dyserythropoietic or	
megaloblastic features or defective	
haemoglobinization	
Decreased reticulocyte count (usually)	
Increased reticulocyte count (rarely) [19]	
Granulopoiesis	
Neutropenia (common)	Granulocytic hyperplasia
Neutrophilia (uncommon)	Granulocytic hypoplasia
Acquired Pelger–Huët anomaly	Increased blast cells, with or without Auer rods or with giant
Neutrophils with hypersegmented	(pseudo-Chèdiak–Higashi) granules
nuclei, increased nuclear projections,	Hypogranular or hypergranular promyelocytes
ring nuclei or nuclei of bizarre shape,	Hypogranular myelocytes
increased chromatin clumping,	Increased chromatin clumping in myeloid precursors
increased apoptotic forms	Increase of monocytes and promonocytes
Agranular and hypogranular neutrophils	Cytoplasmic vacuolation
Hypergranular neutrophils or giant granules	Lack of mature neutrophils
(uncommon)	Morphologically abnormal neutrophils
Persistence of cytoplasmic basophilia	Increased or dysplastic eosinophils [20] including eosinophils with
in mature neutrophils or presence	intranuclear Charcot–Leyden crystals [21] (uncommon)
of Döhle bodies	Increased basophils (uncommon)
Macropolycytes and binucleated neutrophils	Increased mast cells
Monocytosis, abnormal monocytes	Atypical mast cells [22]
Presence of promonocytes	
Blast cells, with or without Auer rods	
Eosinophilia (uncommon)	
Hypogranular eosinophils and	
eosinophils with ring-shaped nuclei or	
non-lobulated nuclei	
Basophilia (uncommon)	
Thrombopoiesis	
Thrombocytopenia (common)	Reduction of megakaryocytes
Thrombocytosis (uncommon)	Increase of megakaryocytes
Giant platelets	Mononuclear or binuclear micromegakaryocytes
Hypogranular or agranular platelets	Megakaryocytes with hypolobulated nuclei
Platelets with giant granules	Multinucleated megakaryocytes
Micromegakaryocytes	Megakaryocytes with botryoid nuclei
Cyclical thrombocytopenia (rare) [23]	Hypogranular megakaryocytes

*Microcytic anaemia in MDS may be consequent on acquired haemoglobin H disease [14] or, rarely, acquired β thalassaemia trait [15]; it can also occur in association with sideroblastic erythropoiesis, although macrocytic anaemia is much more characteristic.

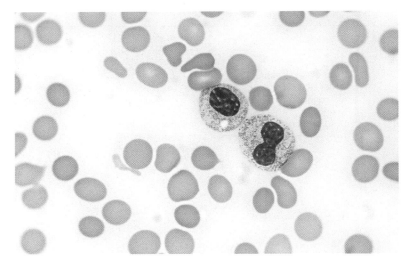

Fig. 3.1 Peripheral blood (PB) film of a patient with refractory anaemia (RA) secondary to cytotoxic chemotherapy showing the acquired Pelger–Huët anomaly; also apparent are anisocytosis, poikilocytosis and severe thrombocytopenia. The bone marrow (BM) showed trilineage myelodysplasia. May–Grünwald–Giemsa (MGG) × 870.

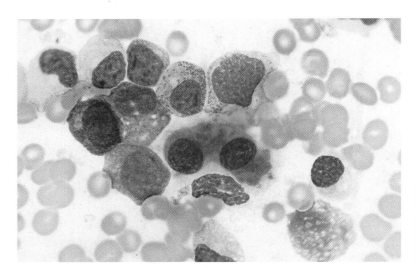

Fig. 3.2 Micromegakaryocytes in the BM of a patient with RA; there was also granulocytic hyperplasia, hypogranularity of the neutrophil series and severe erythroid hypoplasia. MGG × 870.

anomaly (Fig. 3.1) or micromegakaryocytes (Fig. 3.2), are highly characteristic and almost pathognomonic of MDS; one or other of these abnormalities occurs in a high percentage of patients [24]. Agranular neutrophils (Fig. 3.3) are also highly specific but are present in a smaller proportion of patients. Pseudo-Chédiak-Higashi granules probably have a similar degree of specificity but are rare (see Fig. 3.12). Other abnormalities such as macrocytosis, monocytosis, neutropenia, heavy granules in neutrophils or precursors (Fig 3.4) and binucleate or other apparently

tetraploid neutrophils (Fig. 3.5) are less specific and require that alternative diagnoses be excluded. In some patients the features at presentation may not be sufficient to make a firm diagnosis but on continued follow-up the diagnosis becomes certain as disease progression occurs.

The diagnosis of MDS may be aided by ferrokinetic studies to demonstrate ineffective erythropoiesis, studies with monoclonal antibodies to demonstrate aberrant antigen expression, cytochemistry (see page 164), bone marrow histology (see page 165), bone

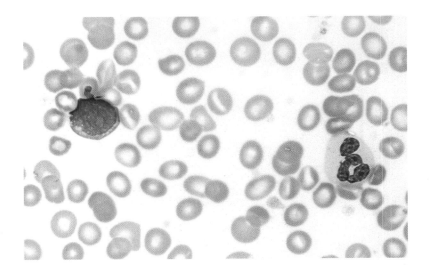

Fig. 3.3 Agranular neutrophil in the PB of a patient with refractory anaemia with excess of blasts (RAEB). A myeloblast is present, some red cells are stomatocytic and platelet numbers are markedly reduced. MGG × 870.

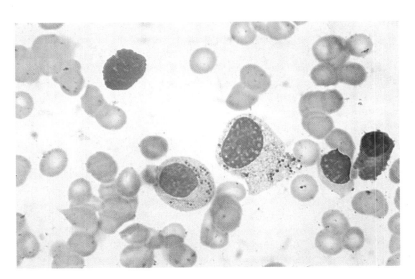

Fig. 3.4 Granulocyte precursors with abnormally heavy granules from a patient with MDS. MGG × 870 (courtesy of Dr D. Swirsky, Leeds).

marrow culture (see page 168) and cytogenetic or molecular genetic analysis to demonstrate acquired clonal abnormalities (see page 168).

MDS needs to be distinguished from the myelo-proliferative disorders (MPD), among which are included polycythaemia vera (also known as poly-cythaemia rubra vera), essential thrombocythaemia, idiopathic myelofibrosis and various chronic myeloid leukaemias. In MPD, haemopoiesis is generally effective and excessive with erythrocytosis, thrombo-cytosis, neutrophilia and basophilia being common whereas in MDS haemopoiesis is generally ineffec-tive with increased cell death in the marrow leading to various cytopenias. There is, however, some over-lap between the two groups of diseases. Chronic myelomonocytic leukaemia, which was classified by the FAB group as one of the myelodysplastic syn-dromes, shares many features with other members of the myelodysplastic group but it resembles other chronic myeloid leukaemias in that production of monocytes and, usually, neutrophils is effective and hepatomegaly and splenomegaly are common. For

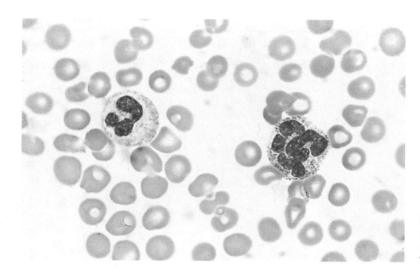

Fig. 3.5 PB film showing a normal neutrophil and a macropolycyte, probably a tetraploid cell, in a patient with MDS. MGG × 870.

this reason the WHO group preferred to classify it as a myelodysplastic/myeloproliferative disorder (MDS/MPD) [25] (see page 180). The childhood syndrome associated with monosomy 7 [26] is usually regarded as a myeloproliferative disorder but has some features of myelodysplasia and the WHO group has similarly assigned it to the MDS/MPD group of disorders. Some patients with refractory anaemia (RA) or refractory anaemia with ring sideroblasts (RARS) have effective production of platelets so that thrombocytosis rather than thrombocytopenia is seen. Although most patients with the 5q– syndrome [27–29] (see page 162) are anaemic and are regarded as having myelodysplasia, a minority initially present as essential thrombocythaemia without anaemia. Both MDS and MPD can terminate in acute leukaemia. Myelodysplasia may supervene in patients with myeloproliferative disorders and the likelihood of acute leukaemia is then greatly increased. Myelodysplastic features such as hypogranular and hypolobulated granulocytes often develop during the course of myelofibrosis. Sideroblastic erythropoiesis, the acquired Pelger–Huët anomaly and very small, presumably diploid, megakaryocytes may appear during transformation of chronic granulocytic leukaemia and may herald blast crisis. Similarly, in some patients with polycythaemia rubra vera a myelodysplastic phase may precede the development of acute leukaemia. The relationship between the MDS and the MPD, according to the WHO classification, is shown diagrammatically in Fig. 3.6.

It is likely that the great majority of cases of MDS arise through a mutation in a multipotent stem cell capable of giving rise to cells of all myeloid lineages. Less often the mutation occurs in a pluripotent stem cell capable of giving rise to lymphoid and myeloid cells. These generalizations are suggested by studies of glucose-6-phosphate dehydrogenase (G6PD) alloenzymes [30], by cytogenetic analysis [31] and by investigation of *RAS* oncogene mutations and of active and inactive alleles of X chromosome genes [32]. Lineages that appear morphologically normal may be part of the abnormal clone and in some cases the T lymphocytes [31] or both T and B lymphocytes [30, 32] are also clonal; lymphocytopenia is common in MDS. The myelodysplastic clone is unstable and with the passage of time clonal evolution occurs, often associated with the acquisition of new karyotypic abnormalities and showing itself in progressive marrow failure, an increase in the number of blast cells or the development of overt acute leukaemia, which is usually myeloid but occasionally lymphoblastic. In rare cases, cytogenetic analysis has proven that the lymphoblasts arise from the myelodysplastic clone [33].

The FAB classification of MDS is based on morphology of the blood and bone marrow supplemented by a cytochemical stain for iron. It is summarized in Table 3.2. In applying the classification (Fig. 3.7) the most important features are the numbers of blast cells and the presence of Auer rods. When the peripheral blood blast cells reach 5% or the bone

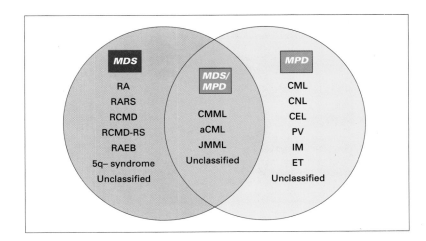

Fig. 3.6 The relationship between the myelodysplastic syndromes and the myeloproliferative disorders in the WHO classification.

Table 3.2 The French–American–British (FAB) classification of the myelodysplastic syndromes [3, 4].

Category	Peripheral blood			Bone marrow
Refractory anaemia (RA) or refractory cytopenia*	Anaemia,* blasts ≤1%, monocytes ≤1 × 10⁹/l	AND		Blasts <5%, ringed sideroblasts ≤15% of erythroblasts
Refractory anaemia with ringed sideroblasts (RARS)	Anaemia, blasts ≤1%, monocytes ≤1 × 10⁹/l	AND		Blasts <5%, ringed sideroblasts >15% of erythroblasts
Refractory anaemia with excess of blasts (RAEB)	Anaemia, blasts >1%, monocytes ≤1 × 10⁹/l blasts <5%	OR AND		Blasts ≥5% BUT Blasts ≤20%
Chronic myelomonocytic leukaemia (CMML)	Monocytes >1 × 10⁹/l, granulocytes often increased, blasts <5%			Blasts up to 20%, promonocytes often increased
Refractory anaemia with excess of blasts in transformation (RAEB-T)	Blasts ≥5%	OR	Auer rods in blasts, in blood or bone marrow OR	Blasts >20%s BUT Blasts <30%

*Or in the case of refractory cytopenia either neutropenia or thrombocytopenia.

marrow blast cells exceed 20% or Auer rods are present the case is classified as refractory anaemia with excess of blasts in transformation (RAEB-T), irrespective of other features. In classifying the remaining cases the number of monocytes is assessed. If the peripheral blood monocyte count exceeds $1 \times 10^9/l$ the case is classified as CMML regardless of other features such as the sideroblast percentage. Following allocation to the RAEB-T and CMML categories, remaining cases are classified on the basis of the numbers of blasts and numbers of ring sideroblasts. If the peripheral blood blasts exceed 1%, or the bone marrow blasts reach 5%, the case is categorized as refractory anaemia with excess of blasts (RAEB). If blasts have not reached these levels but bone marrow sideroblasts exceed 15% of erythroblasts the case is

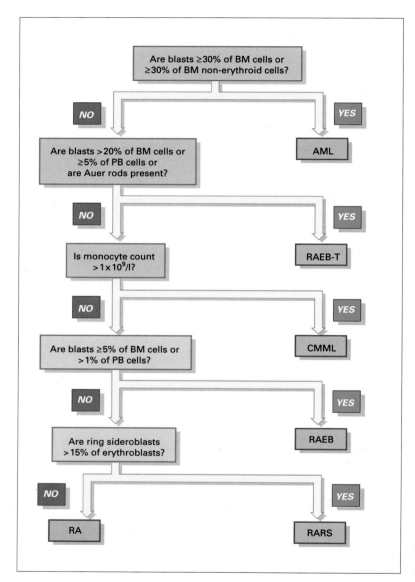

Fig. 3.7 A method of applying the French–American–British (FAB) classification of MDS [3, 4].

classified as RARS. If there is neither an excess of blasts nor more than 15% ring sideroblasts the case is classified as RA. It will be noted that the monocyte count may exceed $1 \times 10^9/l$ in both CMML and RAEB-T and the sideroblast count may exceed 15% in all categories except RA. The FAB classification of MDS is often applied incorrectly and it is sometimes stated that there is overlap between the categories. If the criteria are applied correctly as summarized here there is no ambiguity or overlap in the classification.

The FAB classification, which was widely accepted, was crucial in defining the myelodysplastic syndromes, led to their increasing recognition and, by providing a common language through which haematologists could communicate, led to improved diagnosis and management. This classification also provided a framework for research into the cytogenetic and molecular genetic abnormalities underlying these disorders. However, with the passage of the years, certain problems emerged in the use of this classification.

1 Prognostic differences were found between RA with and without evident myelodysplastic features in other lineages [34].

2 Prognostic differences were found between RARS with and without evident myelodysplastic features in other lineages. The former group have been found to have a higher incidence of clonal cytogenetic abnormality, a greater risk of leukaemic transformation and a shorter survival [35, 36].

3 Patients categorized as RAEB were found to differ in prognosis, according to the degree of elevation of the blast count.

4 Patients categorized as RAEB-T on the basis of the presence of Auer rods, but with bone marrow blasts being less than 20%, were found to have a better prognosis than those categorized as RAEB-T on the basis of the blast count in the peripheral blood or bone marrow [37]. In addition, among patients with increased blast cells those who also have Auer rods were found to have a better prognosis than those who did not [37]. The high complete remission rate of patients with RAEB-T and Auer rods [37, 38] gives support for the view that the presence of Auer rods is indicative of a condition closely related to acute leukaemia and suggests that such patients differ from others categorized as MDS who may have a lower remission rate.

5 Patients with RAEB-T with more than 20% bone marrow blasts were increasingly regarded as having, and were treated as, AML. RAEB-T is probably a heterogeneous group including patients with *de novo* RAEB-T with Auer rods or with one of two specific chromosomal rearrangements, t(8;21)(q22;q22) and inv(16)(p13q22). Such patients have a remission rate similar to that observed in AML and a bone marrow blast percentage of less than 30% is not an indication to delay treatment. The same is not necessarily true of other patients who have neither of these specific cytogenetic abnormalities nor Auer rods; they are often older, are more likely to have multilineage dysplasia and may have RAEB-T that has evolved from other categories of MDS.

6 There was some controversy as to whether CMML, particularly when the white cell count (WBC) was high, was properly classified as MDS rather than as MPD. As interpreted by haematologists seeking to apply the FAB classification, this appears to be a heterogeneous group. Reported median survivals have varied greatly (see Table 3.5, page 172). It has been suggested that the number of monocytes should be ignored and cases of CMML should be reassigned to other categories [39]. If an MDS category designated CMML is accepted then there are obvious problems in making a distinction from atypical chronic myeloid leukaemia (aCML). Both conditions may have monocytosis and dysplastic features although cases categorized as aCML more often have increased numbers of eosinophils and basophils. Both may have disease characteristics commonly associated with 'leukaemia' such as a high WBC, marked splenomegaly and infiltrative lesions. Both may represent the evolution of other categories of MDS. The FAB group made a distinction between CMML and aCML based principally on the proportion of immature granulocytes in the peripheral blood [40]. It is likely that only a much fuller understanding of the molecular basis of this group of diseases will permit the establishment of a satisfactory classification.

7 Some cases were unclassifiable.

8 The FAB classification ignores other information of prognostic value, particularly the presence of cytogenetic abnormalities. The Third MIC Cooperative Study Group proposed that cytogenetic information should be assessed within the framework of the FAB morphological classification [41]. It is also useful to consider other prognostic features and assign a prognostic score to each patient (see below).

Many of these criticisms were considered by working parties convened by the World Health Organization (WHO) in the middle and late 1990s and from their deliberations the WHO classification emerged [42]. Two fundamental changes were, firstly, an alteration of the bone marrow blast percentage which served as a criterion for separating MDS from AML and, secondly, the recognition that there are a group of disorders with features of both MDS and a MPD. These overlap syndromes were designated 'myelodysplastic/myeloproliferative disorders' (MDS/MPD). The FAB classification of the MDS will be discussed first, and is followed by a discussion of the WHO classification of MDS. The conditions that the WHO expert groups regarded as MDS/MPD, which include both CMML and aCML, will be considered in Chapter 4.

The FAB classification of the myelodysplastic syndromes

Refractory anaemia (FAB classification)

Thirty to forty per cent of cases of MDS are classified as RA (see Figs 3.1, 3.2 and 3.5). Commonly either the patient presents with symptoms of anaemia or the diagnosis is an incidental one. A small minority of patients have hepatomegaly or splenomegaly.

The patient is anaemic and there is an absolute reticulocytopenia. Red cells are commonly macrocytic but sometimes normocytic. Some anisocytosis and poikilocytosis (Fig. 3.8) may be present together with some basophilic stippling. In macrocytic cases, the degree of anisocytosis is less than that which is seen in megaloblastic anaemia and oval macrocytes are not usual.

In some cases morphological and quantitative abnormalities are confined to the red cell series but other patients are neutropenic or thrombocytopenic or show pseudo-Pelger–Huët (see Fig. 3.1) or hypogranular neutrophils or large or agranular platelets. Prognosis is worse in those patients who have severe trilineage myelodysplasia than in other patients with RA [34]. Thrombocytosis is occasionally seen, particularly in patients with the 5q– chromosomal anomaly. Occasional blasts may be present but they do not exceed 1% and monocytes do not exceed 1×10^9/l.

In the majority of patients the bone marrow is hypercellular; in a minority it is normocellular or hypocellular. Erythropoiesis is dysplastic and either normoblastic, macronormoblastic or megaloblastic. Rarely there is a virtually complete red cell aplasia (see Fig. 3.2). Such cases have, in the past, sometimes been misdiagnosed as pure red cell aplasia; their recognition as part of the spectrum of MDS is important. Ring sideroblasts may be present but do not exceed 15%. Iron stores are often increased. Some cases show dysplastic granulopoiesis and thrombopoiesis (see Fig. 3.2). Bone marrow blasts are fewer than 5%.

A significant proportion of patients with RA have deletion of the long arm of chromosome 5, designated del(5q) or 5q–, as the sole cytogenetic abnormality and have characteristics that have been designated the 5q– syndrome [27]. The WHO classification has accepted the 5q– syndrome as a distinct entity [11] (see page 162).

Other refractory cytopenias (FAB classification)

Some patients with MDS are cytopenic but not anaemic and do not fit into any of the other categories of MDS. They are grouped with the RAs and are designated refractory cytopenia. Both refractory neutropenia and refractory thrombocytopenia occur. Refractory thrombocytopenia may constitute 3–4% of patients with MDS. The peripheral blood may show

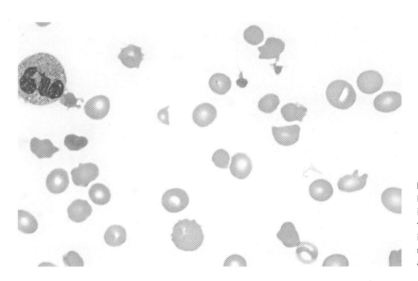

Fig. 3.8 PB film of a patient with RA showing marked poikilocytosis including the presence of several fragments and one stomatocyte. There is also anisocytosis with the presence of several macrocytes. Platelet numbers are greatly reduced. MGG × 870.

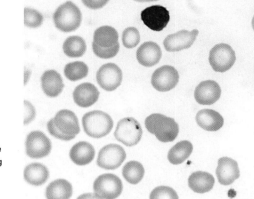

Fig. 3.9 PB film of a patient with refractory anaemia with ring sideroblasts (RARS). The film is dimorphic and one red cell contains Pappenheimer bodies. Poikilocytes including an acanthocyte are present. Pappenheimer bodies are basophilic iron-containing granules, which can be distinguished from basophilic stippling by being larger, more peripherally situated and less numerous within a cell. MGG × 870.

large or hypogranular platelets while the bone marrow shows an increase of megakaryoblasts and the presence of micromegakaryocytes. In some cases platelet lifespan is somewhat reduced but thrombocytopenia is consequent mainly on ineffective production of platelets. Thrombocytopenia may be cyclical [23].

Refractory anaemia with ring sideroblasts (FAB classification)

Refractory anaemia with ring sideroblasts (RARS), also designated primary acquired sideroblastic anaemia, constitutes 15–25% of MDS. Usually either the patient presents with symptoms of anaemia or the diagnosis is made incidentally. The serum iron is usually high with increased transferrin saturation and a high serum ferritin concentration.

The patient is anaemic with the red cells commonly being macrocytic but sometimes normocytic or microcytic. The mean cell volume (MCV) is usually normal or high but occasionally reduced. The blood film (Figs 3.9–3.10) is often dimorphic with a predominant population of normochromic macrocytes and a minor population of hypochromic microcytes. Basophilic stippling may be present. A careful search usually reveals the presence of Pappenheimer bodies (Fig. 3.9). A small number of circulating nucleated red blood cells (NRBC) can often be found and it may be noted that they show defective haemoglobinization and sometimes basophilic cytoplasmic granules adjacent to the nucleus. An iron stain will confirm the nature of Pappenheimer bodies and thus positively identify siderocytes and ring sideroblasts. Neutropenia, thrombocytopenia or dysplastic changes in neutrophils or platelets may be present but often these lineages are morphologically and quantitatively normal. A minority of patients with sideroblastic anaemia have thrombocytosis. Occasionally blast cells may be present in the peripheral blood but they are less than 1%. The monocyte count does not exceed 1×10^9/l. In some [35, 36] but not all [43] series of patients the presence of obvious involvement of other lineages has been associated with a worse prognosis than involvement apparently confined to the erythroid lineage.

The bone marrow is generally hypercellular with erythroid hyperplasia and dyserythropoiesis. Erythropoiesis may be normoblastic, macronormoblastic or megaloblastic with an appreciable percentage of erythroblasts showing either ragged, scanty cytoplasm or more ample cytoplasm that is defectively haemoglobinized and contains granules (Fig. 3.11a). On an iron stain, ring sideroblasts are readily identified (Fig. 3.11b) and constitute more than 15% of erythroblasts. Ring sideroblasts have been variously defined as erythroblasts with at least five [44] or at least 10 [45] siderotic granules surrounding a third or more of the circumference of the nucleus. There is also an increase of other abnormal sideroblasts in which the iron-containing granules are increased in size and number but are not disposed in a ring. In RARS, siderotic granules are often present

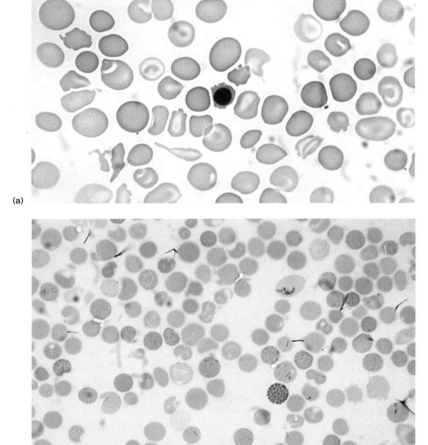

(a)

(b)

Fig. 3.10 PB film of a patient with RARS with acquired haemoglobin H disease. (a) MGG-stained film showing anisocytosis, poikilocytosis (including target cells), one hypochromic cell and a nucleated red blood cell (NRBC). (b) Haemoglobin H preparation showing a typical 'golf-ball' cell with haemoglobin H inclusions. MGG × 870 (courtesy of Dr Jane Mercieca, St Helier).

in early erythroid cells from basophilic erythroblasts onwards whereas in secondary sideroblastic anaemia the changes may be confined to late erythroblasts. Ultrastructural examination shows that in ring sideroblasts the iron is deposited in mitochondria whereas in most other abnormal sideroblasts and in the sideroblasts of normal bone marrow the iron is in cytoplasmic micelles. Iron stores are commonly increased. This may be a feature of other categories of MDS in advance of any transfusion therapy but it is most common in sideroblastic anaemia. If a patient with sideroblastic anaemia develops coincidental severe iron deficiency the percentage of ring sideroblasts falls in most but not all cases and rarely ring sideroblasts totally disappear only to reappear when iron stores are replenished. A silver stain has been found to be more sensitive than a Perls' stain in the detection of ring sideroblasts, particularly in patients with low or absent iron stores [46]. Patients with sideroblastic anaemia may have dysgranulopoiesis or dysthrombopoiesis but often these cell lines are morphologically normal. Bone marrow blasts are fewer than 5%.

One patient has been described with acquired erythropoietic porphyria associated with (probably radiation-induced) RARS [47].

It should be mentioned that the FAB group actually suggested that ring sideroblasts should be counted as a percentage of all nucleated bone marrow cells rather than as a percentage of erythroblasts [4]; counting

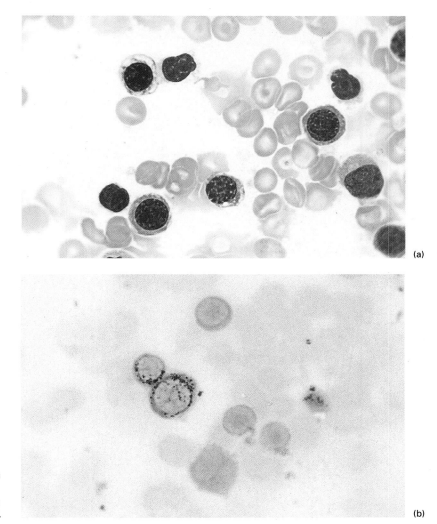

(a)

(b)

Fig. 3.11 BM films of a patient with RARS. (a) Erythroid hyperplasia with only slight dyserythropoiesis. One erythroblast shows defective haemoglobinization and has basophilic granules within its cytoplasm. MGG × 870. (b) Perls' reaction for iron showing two ring sideroblasts. Perls' stain × 870.

ring sideroblasts as a percentage of erythroblasts now appears to be accepted [44] and I have described the classification on this basis.

Refractory anaemia with excess of blasts (FAB classification)

Refractory anaemia with excess of blasts (RAEB) constitutes 15–25% of MDS. Patients usually present with symptoms of anaemia or with infection or bruising.

Patients with RAEB may show the red cell features of either RA or RARS. Neutropenia, thrombocytopenia and dysplastic changes in neutrophils and platelets

are more common than in these two conditions. Peripheral blood blast cells are usually present (see Fig. 3.3) but are fewer than 5% of white cells. The monocyte count does not exceed $1 \times 10^9/l$.

The bone marrow blasts are usually increased to at least 5% but do not exceed 20%; in those cases without 5% of blasts in the bone marrow the peripheral blood blasts must be greater than 1% for the criteria of RAEB to be met. Blasts are often small with scanty cytoplasm and appear undifferentiated on a May–Grünwald–Giemsa (MGG) stain. Bilineage or trilineage myelodysplasia (Figs 3.12 & 3.13) is more common in RAEB than in RA or RARS. Ring

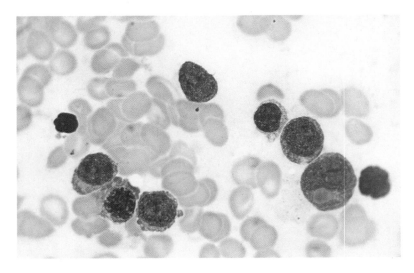

Fig. 3.12 BM film of a patient with RAEB showing increased, relatively small blasts and a myeloid precursor with a pseudo-Chédiak–Higashi granule. MGG × 870.

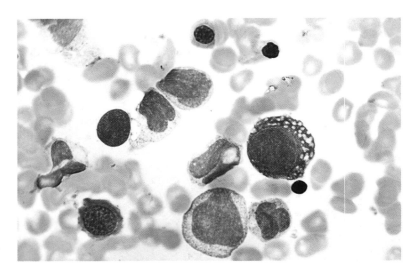

Fig. 3.13 BM film of a patient with RAEB showing a blast and a heavily vacuolated red cell precursor. MGG × 870.

sideroblasts may be present and may exceed 15% of erythroblasts.

The FAB designation 'refractory anaemia with excess of blasts' is preferred to the earlier designation 'refractory anaemia with excess of myeloblasts' since the blasts present are not invariably myeloblasts.

Chronic myelomonocytic leukaemia (FAB classification)

Chronic myelomonocytic leukaemia (CMML), as defined by the FAB group, constitutes about 15% of

MDS; for CMML as defined by the WHO group see page 195. Patients usually present with symptoms of anaemia, with the clinical picture of leukaemia or with both. Anaemia is less common than in RA or RARS whereas hepatomegaly and splenomegaly are much more common than in other types of myelodysplasia. A minority of patients have pleural, pericardial or peritoneal effusions, synovitis, lymphadenopathy or skin infiltration [12, 48]. Rarely gum hypertrophy occurs [12]. Serum lysozyme is usually increased and urinary lysozyme is sometimes increased. Rare cases of renal failure may be related

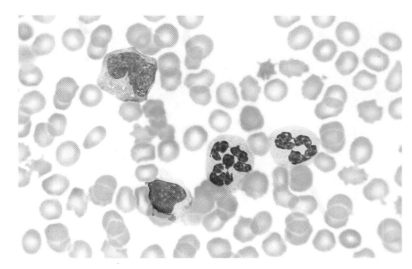

Fig. 3.14 PB film of a patient with chronic myelomonocytic leukaemia (CMML) showing a monocyte, a lymphocyte and two neutrophils, one of which is a macropolycyte. The red cells are poikilocytic and platelet numbers are reduced. MGG × 870.

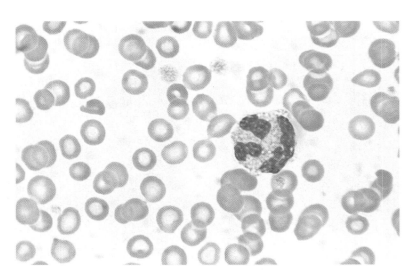

Fig. 3.15 PB film of a patient with CMML showing a binucleate macropolycyte. There is also anisocytosis, poikilocytosis, hypochromia and thrombocytopenia. MGG × 870.

to elevated urinary lysozyme [49]. Associated immunological dysfunction is common. Immunoglobulin concentrations are increased in about a third of patients and 5–10% have a monoclonal protein. Autoantibodies are present in about a half of patients; these may include cold agglutinins. The direct antiglobulin test is positive in about 10% of patients. Immunological abnormalities may occur in other categories of MDS but they appear to be most common in CMML.

The peripheral blood (Figs 3.14 & 3.15) shows a monocytosis with the monocyte count being greater than $1 \times 10^9/l$. Monocytes are sometimes morphologically abnormal with hypersegmented or bizarre-shaped nuclei or with features of immaturity such as increased cytoplasmic basophilia and prominent cytoplasmic granules. Some promonocytes may be present but monoblasts are rarely seen. The neutrophil count is usually also elevated but this is not essential for the diagnosis. Neutrophils sometimes show dysplastic features. Anaemia may be present and is usually normocytic and normochromic. Macrocytosis may also occur and in patients with sidero-blastic erythropoiesis, hypochromic microcytes and a

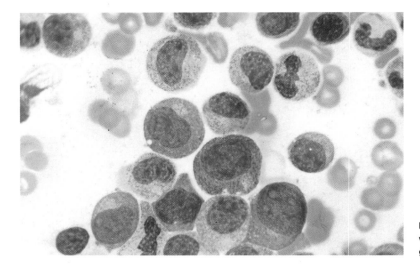

Fig. 3.16 BM film from a patient with CMML showing predominantly granulocytic hyperplasia. MGG × 870.

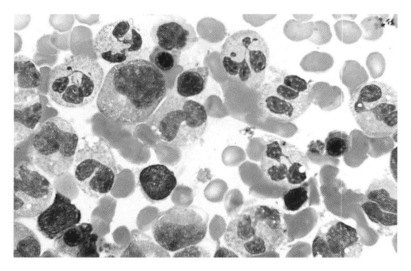

Fig. 3.17 BM film of a patient with CMML showing granulocytic dysplasia. The neutrophils are hypogranular and in addition there is a defect of nuclear lobulation with unusually long filaments separating lobes, an appearance showing some similarities to the inherited condition known as myelokathexis. MGG × 870 (courtesy of Dr A. Copplestone, Plymouth).

dimorphic blood film are present. Occasional patients with a positive direct antiglobulin test have haemolysis with spherocytes on the blood film. Those with an increase of immunoglobulins, either polyclonal or monoclonal, usually have increased rouleaux formation and an elevated erythrocyte sedimentation rate. The platelet count may be normal or low and dysplastic features may be present. Peripheral blood blasts are fewer than 5%.

The bone marrow (Figs 3.16 & 3.17) is hypercellular. Promonocytes are prominent with relatively few mature monocytes. In some cases there is marked granulocytic hyperplasia with monocyte precursors being inconspicuous. However, it should be noted that it can be difficult to distinguish promonocytes and promyelocytes on a Romanowsky-stained film; esterase cytochemistry is useful in making this distinction. Blasts vary from low levels to 20%. Ring sideroblasts may be present and may exceed 15% of the erythroblasts. Dysplastic features may be observed in all lineages but in some patients with CMML, dysplasia in erythroid and megakaryocyte lineages is minimal. Various haematological features have been found to be of prognostic significance, including, in one series of 213 patients, high WBC, monocyte count and lymphocyte count, low haemoglobin concentration (Hb), low platelet count, circulating granulocyte precursors and a higher bone marrow blast percentage [50]; in multivariate analysis, the independent prognostic features were an Hb below 12 g/dl, circulating granulocyte precursors, a lymphocyte count of more than $2.5 \times 10^9/l$ and bone marrow blast cells above 10% [50].

CMML requires separation not only from other MDS but also from other chronic myeloid leukaemias. There is no difficulty in distinguishing it from Ph-positive chronic granulocytic leukaemia since this condition shows few dysplastic features prior to transformation and has a very characteristic peripheral blood film (see page 192). The distinction from atypical (Ph-negative) chronic myeloid leukaemia (aCML) is more difficult. The most useful distinguishing feature is the presence of appreciable numbers of myelocytes and usually promyelocytes and blasts in the peripheral blood in aCML. A cut-off point of 15% of immature granulocytes has been suggested for making the distinction but in the great majority of cases of CMML there are fewer than 5% [51]. The FAB group have suggested a cut-off point of 10% [19]. Eosinophilia and basophilia are sometimes present in aCML but are very unusual in CMML, with the exception of secondary cases, which sometimes show basophilia, and cases associated with t(5;12)(q33;p13), which are likely to show eosinophilia (see page 195). The FAB group also found the percentage of bone marrow erythroblasts to be lower in aCML, averaging 6% in comparison with 18% in CMML [40]. The degree of dysplasia is not useful in making the distinction since cases of aCML shows dysplastic features even more frequently than cases of CMML [40]. The FAB group have also suggested that cases of CMML with a WBC of greater than $13 \times 10^9/l$ are more likely to behave clinically as a MPD and might be classified with other chronic myeloid leukaemias while those with a WBC of $13 \times 10^9/l$ or less are appropriately regarded as MDS [40]. One comparison of these two groups of patients found splenomegaly to be more common in those with a WBC of at least $13 \times 10^9/l$ but there was no significant difference in the prevalence of cytogenetic abnormalities, the likelihood of leukaemic transformation or length of survival [52]. Another comparison found some haematological differences but no statistically significant differences in the frequency of hepatosplenomegaly,

abnormal karyotype, leukaemic transformation or survival [53].

aCML appears to have a worse prognosis than CMML and making a distinction between these two conditions is probably valid. However, it should be noted that RA and RAEB can evolve not only into CMML but also into aCML [54]; whether aCML and CMML are part of the spectrum of a single disease or represent two or more distinct diseases will only be established when more is known of the underlying molecular mechanisms of leukaemogenesis. This dilemma has not been solved by the WHO classification.

Refractory anaemia with excess of blasts in transformation (FAB classification)

Cases of refractory anaemia with excess of blasts in transformation (RAEB-T) constitute 5–10% of patients with MDS. This category encompasses transformation both of RAEB and CMML since all cases that meet the criteria for numbers of blasts, Auer rods or both are assigned to this category. Patients usually present with symptoms of anaemia or with infection or haemorrhage. Hepatomegaly and splenomegaly may be present.

The peripheral blood may show 5% or more blasts, blasts containing Auer rods or both. Any of the other features described in the other MDS may be present with anaemia, neutropenia, thrombocytopenia and dysplastic neutrophils and platelets being usual. Some patients have monocytosis.

The bone marrow blasts are usually above 20% but do not exceed 30%. To meet the criteria for RAEB-T, either peripheral blood or bone marrow blasts must be increased or Auer rods must be present (see Table 3.2). Trilineage myelodysplasia is usual.

The WHO classification of the myelodysplastic syndromes

The following cases, some or all of which were included in the FAB classification of MDS, are excluded from the WHO classification:
1 Cases with bone marrow blasts of 20% or more;
2 Cases with t(8;21)(q22;q22), t(15;17)(q22;q21), inv(16)(p13q22) or t(16;16)(p13;q22), even when the bone marrow blast cells are less than 20%;
3 Cases meeting the WHO criteria for CMML;
4 Cases with a platelet count above $600 \times 10^9/l$.

Table 3.3 The WHO classification of myelodysplastic syndromes (MDS) [5–11].

Disease	Peripheral blood findings	Bone marrow findings
Refractory anaemia (RA)	Anaemia, blasts rarely seen and always less than 1%	Dysplasia confined to erythroid lineage, <5% blasts, <15% ringed sideroblasts
Refractory anaemia with ringed sideroblasts (RARS)	Anaemia, no blasts	Dysplasia confined to erythroid lineage, <5% blasts, ≥15% ringed sideroblasts
Refractory cytopenia with multilineage dysplasia (RCMD)*	Cytopenias (bicytopenia or pancytopenia), no or rare blasts, no Auer rods, $<1 \times 10^9$/l monocytes	Dysplasia in ≥10% of the cells of two or more myeloid cell lineages, <5% blasts, <15% ringed sideroblasts, no Auer rods
Refractory cytopenia with multilineage dysplasia and ringed sideroblasts (RCMD-RS)*	Cytopenias (bicytopenia or pancytopenia), no or rare blasts, no Auer rods, $<1 \times 10^9$/l monocytes	Dysplasia in ≥10% of the cells of two or more myeloid cell lineages, <5% blasts, ≥15% ringed sideroblasts, no Auer rods
Refractory anaemia with excess blasts-1 (RAEB-1)*	Cytopenias, <5% blasts, no Auer rods, $<1 \times 10^9$/l monocytes	Unilineage or multilineage dysplasia, 5–9% blasts, no Auer rods
Refractory anaemia with excess blasts-2 (RAEB-2)*	Cytopenias, 5–19% blasts, Auer rods sometimes present, $<1 \times 10^9$/l monocytes	Unilineage or multilineage dysplasia, 10–19% blasts, Auer rods sometimes present
Myelodysplastic syndrome-unclassified (MDS-U)*	Cytopenias, no or rare blasts, no Auer rods	Unilineage dysplasia, <5% blasts. No Auer rods
MDS associated with isolated del(5q)	Anaemia, platelet count usual normal or elevated, <5% blasts	Megakaryocytes in normal or increased numbers but with hypolobated nuclei, <5% blasts, no Auer rods, 5q– as sole cytogenetic abnormality

*If cases are therapy-related, this should be specified and it should be further specified whether cases are alkylating agent–related (the majority) or topoisomerase II-interactive-drug-related (a small minority); therapy-related cases are categorized with therapy-related AML.

Other cases continued to be classified as MDS but may be assigned to a different category. Table 3.3 summarizes the criteria for the WHO categories of MDS [5–11] and Fig. 3.18 shows diagrammatically how cases are assigned to categories.

Refractory anaemia (WHO classification)

As defined in the WHO classification [5, 6] (Table 3.3), refractory anaemia (RA) comprises 5–10% of MDS [55]. Significant dysplasia is confined to the erythroid lineage, i.e. other lineages show no more than 10% of cells with dysplastic features.

There is anaemia. The peripheral blood film may show mild to marked anisocytosis and poikilocytosis. Cells are usually normochromic and either normocytic or macrocytic but occasional cases have a population of hypochromic cells. Blast cells are uncommon and are, by definition, always less than 1%.

The bone marrow is usually hypercellular but may be normocellular or hypocellular. Erythroid dysplasia varies from slight to moderate. By definition, ring sideroblasts are less than 15% of erythroblasts and blasts are less than 5%. Up to a quarter of patients have a clonal cytogenetic abnormality, usually del(20q), trisomy 8 or abnormalities of 5, 7 or both [6]. However, cases with an isolated 5q– are excluded from the RA category.

RA shows a low rate of evolution to AML. In one series only 6% of patients developed AML and the median survival was 66 months [55].

Refractory anaemia with ringed sideroblasts (WHO classification)

Refractory anaemia with ringed (or ring) sideroblasts (RARS), as defined in the WHO classification [5, 7] (Table 3.3), has ringed sideroblasts constituting 15%

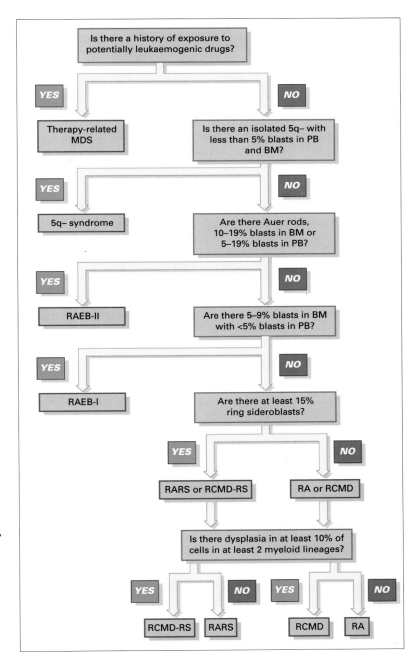

Fig. 3.18 A method of applying the WHO classification of the myelodysplastic syndromes. Abbreviations: BM, bone marrow; MDS, myelodysplastic syndrome; PB, peripheral blood; RA, refractory anaemia; RCMD, refractory cytopenia with multilineage dysplasia; RCMD-RS refractory cytopenia with multilineage dysplasia and ring sideroblasts; RAEB, refractory anaemia with excess of blasts; RARS, refractory anaemia with ring sideroblasts.

or more of bone marrow erythroid cells. Ringed sideroblasts are defined as erythroblasts with at least a third of the nucleus encircled by 10 or more siderotic granules, demonstrated with an iron stain. Such cases comprise about 11% of cases of MDS [55]. Significant dysplasia is confined to the erythroid lineage, i.e. other lineages show no more than 10% of cells with dysplastic features.

There is anaemia. The peripheral blood film shows normochromic cells, which may be normocytic but are often macrocytic. There is a population of hypochromic microcytes, giving a dimorphic appearance. Pappenheimer bodies may be present. The platelet count may be increased but does not exceed $600 \times 10^9/l$.

The bone marrow shows erythroid hyperplasia. There may be other dyserythropoietic features, in addition to the ring sideroblasts. Iron-laden macrophages may be prominent. Clonal cytogenetic abnormalities are present in less than 10% of cases [7]. Cases with an isolated 5q– are excluded from the RARS category.

RARS shows a very low rate of evolution to AML. In one series 1.4% of patients developed AML and the median survival was 69 months [55].

Refractory cytopenia with multilineage dysplasia (WHO classification)

Refractory cytopenia with multilineage dysplasia without significant numbers of ring sideroblasts (RCMD) [5, 8] comprises about a quarter of cases of MDS [55]. There is bicytopenia or pancytopenia with dysplastic features in 10% or more of cells in at least two lineages.

There is anaemia and neutropenia, thrombocytopenia or both. In addition to red cell abnormalities, neutrophils and platelets may show dysplastic features. Peripheral blood blasts are less than 1% and monocytes are less than $1 \times 10^9/l$.

The bone marrow is usually hypercellular with bilineage or trilineage dysplasia. Blasts are less than 5% and ring sideroblasts are less than 15%. Clonal cytogenetic abnormalities are present in around a half of patients and may be complex.

In one series of patients, median survival was 33 months with 10% transformation to AML [55].

Refractory cytopenia with multilineage dysplasia and ringed sideroblasts (WHO classification)

Refractory cytopenia with multilineage dysplasia and ring sideroblasts (RCMD-RS) [5, 8] comprises about 15% of cases of MDS [55]. With the exception of the sideroblastic erythropoiesis (by definition, at least 15% of erythroblasts are ring sideroblasts) the haematological features are similar to those of RCMD.

In one series of patients, the median survival was 32 months with 13% transformation to AML [55].

Refractory anaemia with excess of blasts-1 (WHO classification)

The WHO classification divides refractory anaemia with excess of blasts (RAEB) into two categories, RAEB-1 and RAEB-2, on the basis of blast numbers [5, 9]. RAEB-1 has 5–19% bone marrow blasts and less than 5% circulating blasts. Auer rods are absent. Trilineage dysplasia is usual. RAEB-1 comprises around a fifth of cases of MDS [55]. Clonal cytogenetic abnormalities, including trisomy 8, abnormalities of chromosomes 5 and 7 and complex karyotypes are present in around 50% of patients. Transformation to AML occurs in about a fifth of patients, the others dying of the effects of bone marrow failure. The median survival is around 18 months [55].

Refractory anaemia with excess of blasts-2 (WHO classification)

Cases of MDS are categorized as RAEB-2 if the bone marrow blasts are 10–19%, if the peripheral blood blasts are 5–19% (regardless of bone marrow blast count) or if Auer rods are present [5, 9]. In one series such cases comprised 18.5% of cases of MDS [55]. Clinical features are similar to those in RAEB-1. Clonal cytogenetic abnormalities are also similar. In one series of patients, somewhat more than a third suffered transformation to AML [55]. The median survival of 10 months was significantly worse than the median survival of RAEB-1 [55].

Myelodysplastic syndrome associated with isolated del(5q) chromosome ('5q– syndrome') (WHO classification)

Deletion of part of the long arm of chromosome 5 (5q–) was the second recurrent cytogenetic abnormality for which an association with a specific human neoplasm was recognized. The clinical and haematological features are sufficiently consistent that the WHO classification recognizes this as an entity. As defined in the WHO classification [5, 10] this is MDS associated with an isolated 5q– with peripheral blood and bone marrow blasts being less than 5%. In the FAB classification, patients with the 5q– anomaly fell into the RA, RARS or RAEB categories, the latter group being excluded from the equivalent WHO category.

Patients are mainly women, usually middle-aged or elderly. The peripheral blood usually shows a

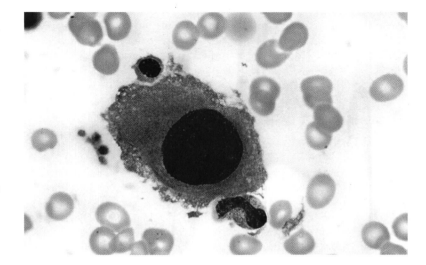

Fig. 3.19 BM film from a patient with the 5q– syndrome showing a megakaryocyte of normal size but with a hypolobated nucleus. This type of dysplastic megakaryocyte rather than a micromegakaryocyte (see Fig. 3.2) is characteristic of this syndrome. MGG × 870.

macrocytic anaemia, sometimes with thrombocytosis. The WBC may be reduced.

The bone marrow is usually hypercellular as a result of erythroid hyperplasia. Erythropoiesis is dysplastic and may be sideroblastic. Megakaryocytes are present in normal numbers or are increased and are cytologically abnormal. They have non-lobed or bilobed nuclei but are mainly more than 30–40 μm in diameter (Fig. 3.19) [28]; they thus differ from the mononuclear and binuclear micromegakaryocytes (see Fig. 3.1) associated with other forms of MDS, which are no larger than other haemopoietic cells.

The 5q– syndrome is associated with a variety of deletions, among which del(5)(q13q33) is prominent.

In one series of patients classified largely according to the WHO criteria, the 5q– syndrome comprised around 2% of patients [55]. The rate of leukaemic transformation was 3% and the median survival was 116 months. In this series a small number of patients with more than 5% bone marrow blasts had a strikingly worse prognosis [55]; such patients were excluded from the WHO classification as finally published.

FISH studies show that, although morphological abnormalities may be confined to the erythroid or erythroid and megakaryocyte lineages this is a trilineage disorder [29].

Myelodysplastic syndrome, unclassifiable (WHO classification)

The WHO group recognized that there were some cases of MDS that did not fit the categories described above but who nevertheless did have MDS [11]. Such patients include those with thrombocytopenia or neutropenia with unilineage dysplasia who would have been included in the FAB category of 'refractory cytopenia'. There are small numbers of patients with macrocytosis [56] or sideroblastic erythropoiesis [57] who have clonal haemopoiesis but are not anaemic and do not meet the other criteria for inclusion in the WHO categories of MDS. Such cases of 'refractory macrocytosis' and 'refractory sideroblastic erythropoiesis' should be assigned to the MDS, unclassifiable category.

Other categories or features of the myelodysplastic syndromes

Hypocellular MDS

The FAB group initially described MDS as having a hypercellular or normocellular bone marrow. Subsequently it became apparent that some cases, approximately 10% in all, had a hypocellular bone marrow. CMML is quite uncommon among hypocellular MDS but otherwise cases may fall into any FAB category. Their prognosis does not differ from MDS in general [58], and although it is necessary to recognize these cases as MDS it does not appear to be important to assign them to a separate category. The differential diagnosis of hypocellular MDS includes hypocellular AML and aplastic anaemia. It is not yet clear whether cases with a severely hypocellular bone marrow and a clonal cytogenetic abnormality but without morphological dysplasia should be classified as MDS or as aplastic anaemia. Although such cases clearly have a neoplastic clone of cells in the bone marrow the clinical course may be that of aplastic anaemia [59].

MDS with myelofibrosis

Some patients with MDS have considerable reticulin deposition. It is important to distinguish these cases from M7 AML with myelofibrosis. M7 AML has more than 30% (or by WHO criteria, more than 20%) blasts whereas MDS with myelofibrosis has fewer. Patients with MDS and myelofibrosis have a high incidence of complex chromosomal abnormalities and a poor prognosis [60]. As long as a bone marrow aspirate adequate for diagnostic purposes is obtained they can be assigned to FAB categories. However, in view of the worse prognosis the presence of reticulin fibrosis should be noted and a separate categorization could be justified.

Therapy-related MDS

Therapy-related MDS has distinctive haematological and cytogenetic features. This entity is not specifically mentioned in the FAB classification whereas, in the WHO classification, it is classified with therapy-related AML. Marked trilineage dysplasia is common, even in cases that in the FAB classification would be categorized as RA. Eosinophilia and basophilia are more common than in *de novo* cases. Hypocellularity and reticulin fibrosis are common. Cytogenetic abnormalities are more often present than in *de novo* MDS and often include particularly adverse abnormalities such as abnormalities of both chromosome 5 and 7 and complex karyotypic abnormalities. Therapy-related MDS has a very poor prognosis both with regard to leukaemic transformation and to survival. It should be recognized as a separate category.

Cytochemical reactions in MDS

The only cytochemical reactions essential in the diagnosis and classification of MDS are a Perls' stain for iron, which is necessary for assessing the presence and number of ring sideroblasts, and a Sudan black B (SBB) or myeloperoxidase (MPO) stain to ensure that all cases with Auer rods are recognized and classified

as RAEB-T (FAB classification) or RAEB-2 (WHO classification). These and other cytochemical reactions may provide evidence of dysplastic maturation and can thus be useful both in confirming the diagnosis and in assessing the number of lineages involved. In CMML, staining for non-specific esterase (NSE) activity may be necessary to identify the monocytic component in the bone marrow [2].

Cytochemical stains for MPO, SBB and naphthol AS-D chloroacetate esterase (chloroacetate esterase, CAE) may show mature neutrophils with negative reactions [61] and, similarly, mature monocytes may be deficient in NSE activity. Particularly in CMML, individual cells may show reactivity for both CAE and NSE, activities that are normally characteristic of granulocytic and monocytic lineages, respectively. The neutrophil alkaline phosphatase score is reduced in a third to a half of patients and in a minority is elevated.

When patients with MDS have an increase of bone marrow blasts the cells show the cytochemical reactions expected of myeloblasts, monoblasts or megakaryoblasts. Relatively undifferentiated myeloblasts are the form most commonly present so that positive reactions for SBB, MPO and CAE may be weak and confined to a minority of cells. In some cases the blasts do not give positive reactions with any cytochemical markers of myeloid cells. Such cells are generally very immature myeloblasts, confirmed by immunophenotyping, but in a minority of cases the cells appear to be lymphoblasts.

Erythroblasts may be periodic acid–Schiff (PAS) stain positive with the positive reaction being confined to proerythroblasts or being present in early, intermediate and late erythroblasts [62]. Although PAS positivity is seen in some reactive conditions its presence in patients with MDS or leukaemia is likely to indicate that the lineage is part of the abnormal clone. Erythroblasts may also show aberrant strong paranuclear positivity for acid phosphatase and NSE; such reactions are not confined to MDS and AML but may be seen in megaloblastic anaemia [61]. In MDS, the percentage of haemoglobin F and the percentage of cells containing haemoglobin F may both be increased. A cytochemical stain such as the Kleihauer reaction will identify the increased percentage of cells containing haemoglobin F. Such an increase is not confined to MDS. A minority of cases of MDS have acquired haemoglobin H disease [14]; they can be identified by haemoglobin electrophoresis or with a

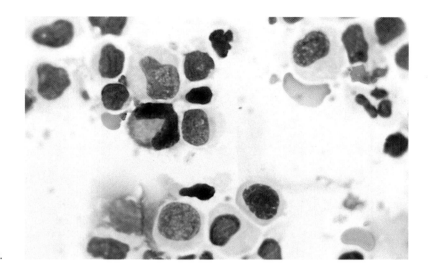

Fig. 3.20 Immunocytochemistry of a bone marrow film from a patient with refractory anaemia with excess of blasts in transformation (RAEB-T) showing several platelets and a micromegakaryocyte, which have given positive reactions with a monoclonal antibody directed at platelet glycoprotein Ib (CD42b). Alkaline phosphatase-anti-alkaline phosphatase (APAAP) technique × 870.

cytochemical stain using new methylene blue or brilliant cresyl blue.

Immunophenotyping in MDS

Immunological markers have generally been considered to have only a limited place in the diagnosis of MDS. They have a role in identifying micro-megakaryocytes (Fig. 3.20) and in demonstrating or confirming the nature of blasts, particularly when myeloblasts are very immature and lack characteristic cytochemical reactions, when megakaryoblasts are present or, uncommonly, when there is a lymphoblastic or biphenotypic/bilineage transformation of MDS. If an extensive panel of reagents is used, in conjunction with assessment of light-scattering characteristics of cells, immunophenotyping can be more informative and can give strong support for a diagnosis of MDS in patients lacking convincing morphological evidence of this diagnosis [63]. Abnormalities demonstrated in the granulocytic lineage may include detection of hypogranular neutrophils (reduced sideways light scatter) or a discrete population of blasts (comparison of CD45 expression and sideways light scatter) and detection of abnormal antigen expression—reduced expression of CD16 or CD11b or expression of non-myeloid antigens [63]. Abnormalities detected in erythroid cells are reduced CD71 expression and asynchronous expression of CD71 or glycophorin A in comparison with CD45 [63].

There appears to be little relationship between immunophenotype and FAB or WHO categories of MDS.

Bone marrow trephine biopsy

Bone marrow aspiration and trephine biopsy are complementary investigations. A biopsy often gives extra information not provided by an aspirate [64–68]. Cellularity can be more reliably assessed and increased reticulin is apparent. Cellularity is most often increased but may be normal or decreased. Abnormal distribution of cells is often detectable. Erythroid islands may be absent or very large (Fig. 3.21). They may show an excess of proerythroblasts or have all precursors at the same stage of development [64]. Late in the disease course there may be marked reduction of erythropoiesis. Granulocytic precursors may be clustered centrally rather than showing their normal paratrabecular distribution (Figs 3.22 & 3.23). This phenomenon has been designated 'abnormal localization of immature precursors' (ALIP) [64]. ALIPs can be diagnostically important if they are detected in RA since their presence confirms MDS rather than a secondary anaemia. Abnormal megakaryocytes (mononuclear, binuclear and multinucleated forms) are readily assessed on a biopsy (Fig. 3.24). Megakaryocytes may be clustered or found in a paratrabecular position (Fig. 3.25). Dysgranulopoiesis and dyserythropoiesis may be detectable but they are more readily apparent in a bone marrow

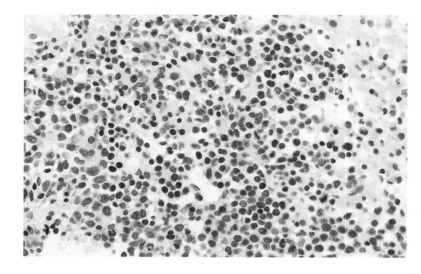

Fig. 3.21 Histological section of a trephine biopsy from a patient with RAEB showing a large ill-formed erythroid island. Haematoxylin and eosin (H & E) × 348.

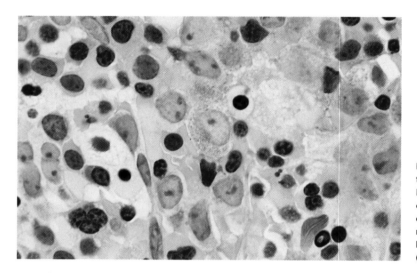

Fig. 3.22 Histological section of a trephine biopsy from a patient with RAEB-T showing erythroblasts, some of which are dysplastic, and a collection of blasts and promyelocytes that are not adjacent to bone—abnormal localization of immature precursors (ALIP). H & E × 870.

film. Apoptosis is increased [69]. Biopsies may show non-specific abnormalities such as increased macrophages, prominent mast cells, lymphoid follicles and plasma cell aggregates. Ring sideroblasts are detectable only in plastic-embedded specimens. Sections of paraffin-embedded trephine biopsies not only do not permit the detection of ring sideroblasts but also do not permit a reliable assessment of iron overload since iron may be leached out during decalcification.

Immunohistochemistry is an important supplement to histology. Use of anti-glycophorin antibodies highlights the presence of clusters of immature erythroid cells and helps to distinguish them from ALIPs. Polyclonal antibodies directed at von Willebrand's factor or monoclonal antibodies recognizing epitopes on platelet antigens, such as CD42a, CD42b or CD61, highlight megakaryocytes and facilitate the recognition of small mononuclear megakaryocytes. Positive staining with antibodies to granulocyte antigens can confirm the presence of ALIPs (see Fig. 3.23). Reactions with some antibodies give prognostic information [70]; increased numbers of CD34-positive cells and positive reactions for the p53 protein (a protein encoded by a cancer-suppressor gene, *TP53*) are

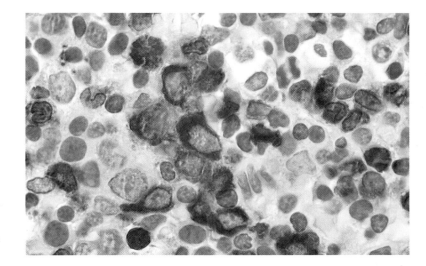

Fig. 3.23 Histological section of a trephine biopsy from a patient with RARS showing an ALIP demonstrated by immunocytochemistry with a monoclonal antibody to myeloperoxidase. Immunoperoxidase technique × 870.

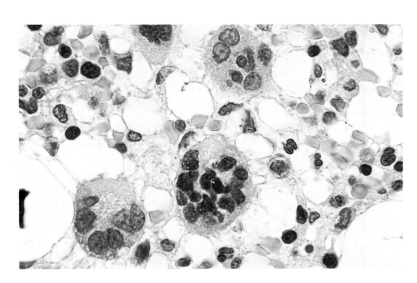

Fig. 3.24 Histological section of a trephine biopsy from a patient with RAEB showing dysplastic megakaryocytes and general disorganization of BM architecture. H & E × 870.

mainly seen in RAEB and RAEB-T and are indicative of a worse prognosis; p53 positivity is indicative of the fact that the product of the mutated gene has a longer half life than the normal protein.

The experience of different groups differs as to whether FAB subtypes of MDS constitute recognizable histological entities. Tricot *et al.* [64] could not recognize entities that corresponded to the FAB categories. Delacrétaz *et al.* [66], however, reached concordant diagnoses in 24 of 28 cases examined independently. Both groups found ALIPs in more than half the biopsies but Tricot *et al.* [65] found them

in all subtypes of MDS (although preferentially in RAEB and RAEB-T) whereas Delacrétaz *et al.* [66] found ALIP to be very uncommon in the cases that did not have an excess of blasts in the aspirate.

A biopsy is particularly useful in assessing cases with a normocellular or hypocellular bone marrow and cases with increased reticulin, in which a poor aspirate that is unlikely to be representative is obtained. It is thus particularly likely to be useful in secondary MDS in which both reduced cellularity and increased reticulin are much more common than in primary MDS. A biopsy is helpful in distinguishing

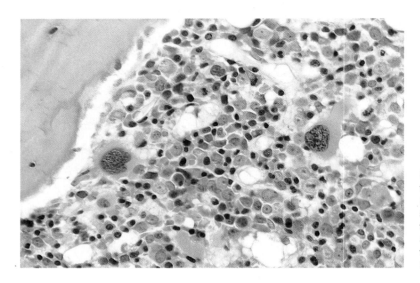

Fig. 3.25 Histological section of a trephine biopsy from a patient with myelodysplastic syndrome (MDS) showing abnormal megakaryocyte topography; a megakaryocyte is abnormally sited, adjacent to the bony trabecula. H & E × 348 (courtesy of Dr S. Davis).

hypocellular MDS, which may have increased reticulin and foci of blasts, from aplastic anaemia, which does not show these features.

Bone marrow culture

There is some correlation between the FAB categories and the results of bone marrow culture. A normal growth pattern of granulocyte–macrophage colony-forming units (CFU-GM) is most often seen in FAB RA and RARS categories whereas an abnormal pattern is usual in CMML, RAEB and RAEB-T. In one study a marked abnormality of colony growth was observed in RARS with obvious dysplasia of other lineages but not in RARS with dysplasia apparently limited to the erythroid lineage [71]. The abnormal pattern may be either reduced colonies, increased colonies and/or clusters (the commonest pattern in CMML) or reduced colonies and increased clusters (in some but not all studies predictive of transformation to acute leukaemia). Growth of BFU-E (erythroid burst-forming units), CFU-E (erythroid colony-forming units) and CFU-Meg (megakaryocyte colony-forming units) is often reduced or absent but shows no correlation with FAB subtype.

Automated blood cell counters and the myelodysplastic syndromes

Automated blood cell counters using peroxidase cytochemistry (the Bayer H.1 series and Advia 120

instruments) can give diagnostically useful information in patients with MDS [72] (Fig. 3.26). Peroxidase deficiency of neutrophils can be detected by an abnormal position of the neutrophil cluster; less often peroxidase-deficient neutrophils are present as a distinct population. In other cases the peroxidase activity of dysplastic neutrophils is increased. The presence of blasts in RAEB and RAEB-T can be suspected because of the presence of large peroxidase-negative cells or because of the presence of cells that have nuclei with abnormal light-scattering qualities. Red cell histograms and scattergrams may show increased heterogeneity of red cell size and haemoglobinization, macrocytosis, microcytosis (rarely) or, when there is sideroblastic erythropoiesis, a bimodal distribution of red cell size or haemoglobin concentration. The platelet histogram may show the presence of giant platelets.

Other automated instruments that size cells by electrical conductivity or light scatter give similar but not identical information about red cell and platelet size distribution but give more limited information about white cell characteristics.

All automated instruments are able to detect the presence of blast cells in the majority of cases in which they are detected by microscopy.

Cytogenetic and molecular genetics abnormalities in MDS

Various clonal cytogenetic abnormalities have been

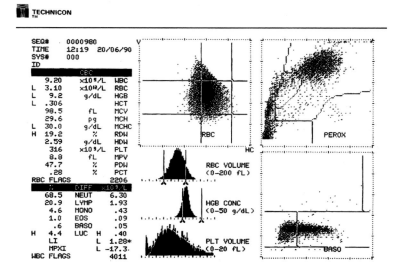

Fig. 3.26 Histograms and scatterplot produced by a Bayer H.1 automated counter in a case of RARS showing both macrocytes and hypochromic cells.

described in association with MDS (Table 3.4) [41, 73–82] among which the commonest anomalies are del(5q) (usually referred to as 5q–), monosomy 5, del(7q) (also referred to as 7q–), monosomy 7 (Fig. 3.27) and trisomy 8. Some abnormalities are particularly characteristic of secondary MDS (Table 3.4). MDS is commonly associated with loss of chromosomal material, either through monosomy, deletion or unbalanced translocation. Balanced translocations are less common.

There is no close relationship between specific cytogenetic abnormalities and FAB categories, although some trends are apparent. The frequency with which cytogenetic abnormalities are observed increases from 30 to 50% in RA, RARS and CMML to about 60% in RAEB and almost 70% in RAEB-T [78]. Single abnormalities are most likely to be found in RA, RARS and CMML whereas RAEB-T shows the highest rate of occurrence of complex rearrangements (whether this is defined as a minimum of two, three or four abnormalities in a karyotype). The commonest abnormalities, –5, 5q–, –7, 7q– and +8, are seen in all FAB categories but 5q– as a single defect is preferentially associated with good prognosis subtypes and with the features of the 5q– syndrome (see above). Other abnormalities associated with RA are +8, 20q–, –7, i(17q) and 17p–. The uncommon chromosomal rearrangement, idic(X)(q13), is associated with RARS [76]. In some series of patients rearrangements of chromosome 11 have been asso-

ciated preferentially with RARS and rearrangements of chromosome 12 with CMML. However in a large series of patients with CMML abnormalities of chromosome 12 were not common [50].

The WHO classification recognizes the 5q– syndrome as an entity (see above). Otherwise the relationship of the WHO categories to cytogenetic abnormalities is similar to that described for the FAB categories, with clonal abnormalities and, in particular, complex karyotypic abnormalities being more common in the categories of MDS with a worse prognosis. Not surprisingly, adverse cytogenetic abnormalities appear to be more common in the WHO RCMD and RCMD-RS categories of MDS than in RA and RARS [83].

Certain abnormalities are associated with particular clinical or morphological features but not with specific FAB or WHO categories. Monosomy 7 is seen in all FAB categories but in children is associated with a specific syndrome (categorized in the WHO classification as one of the MDS/MPD group of disorders) and in adults is commonly associated with pancytopenia, a hypocellular bone marrow, trilineage myelodysplasia and a relatively poor prognosis. Hypocellular MDS (see above) has shown an association with trisomy 6, trisomy 8, 7q– and 5q–. 11q– has been associated with increased ring sideroblasts whether or not the patient falls into the FAB RARS category.

Abnormalities of 3q21 and 3q26 are associated with thrombocytosis and with increased and abnormal

Table 3.4 Cytogenetic abnormalities associated with the myelodysplastic syndromes (MDS). (Derived from references 41, 74, 75, 77–79, 81, 82 and other sources.)

	Loss of chromosomal material	Gain of chromosomal material	Chromosomal rearrangement
Common:	−5* 5q− −7* 7q−* 9q− 20q−* −Y*†	+8	

Less common:	1p−
	 11q−
	 12p−*
	 13q−
	 17p−*
	 −17*
	 −20
	 21q−
	 −22
			11q23 rearrangements including:
			   t(2;11)(p21;q23)
			   t(9;11)(p21;q23)*
			   t(11;16)(q23;p13.3)*
			   del(11)(q23)
			 12p11–13 rearrangements including:
			   t(5;12)(q33;p13)‡
			   t(10;12)(q24;p13)‡
			 i(17q)
			 21q22 rearrangements including:
			   t(3;21)(q26;q22)*

Uncommon or rare rearrangements:	3p−*
	 6p−*
	 −8
	 −14
	 14q−
	 −15
	 16q−
	 17q−*
	 18q−
	 −18*
	 −19
	 −21
		+4
		 +6
		 +11
		 +13
		 +14
		 +16
		 +19
		 +21
			Xp11* and Xp13* including:
			   idic(X)(13)
			 3q21 and/or 3q26 rearrangements
			   t(1;3)(p26;q21)*
			   inv(3)(q21q26)*
			   t(3;3)(q21;q26)*
			   del(3)(q21)
			   ins(3)(q26;q21q26)
			   t(3;4)(q26;q21)
			   t(3;5)(q21;q31)*
			   t(3;8)(q26;q24)
			   t(3;12)(q26;p13)
			   t(3;19)(q21;p13)
			   t(3;5)(q25;q34)
			   t(6;9)(p23;q34.5)
			 11q23 rearrangements less often associated with MDS including:
			   t(1;11)(p32;q23)*
			   t(3;11)(p21;q23)
			   t(11;17)(q23;q25)
			   t(11;19)(q23;q13.1)*
			   t(11;21)(q24;q11.2)
			 Rearrangements of 17q21*
			 Rearrangements of 19p13* or 19q13*
			 i(21q)
			 Ring chromosomes
			 Double minute chromosomes

Chromosomal rearrangements that are usually unbalanced:
  der(Y)t(Y;1)(q12;q21)¶
  der(1)t(1;7)(q10;p10)*¶§
  der(1)t(1;13)(q11;q10)¶
  der(1)t(1;15)(q12;p11)¶
  der(16)t(1;16)(q11;q11)*¶
  −5,−7,+der(5)t(5;7)(q11;p11)*
  −17,t(5;17)(p11;p11)**
  −17,t(7;17)(p11;p11)**

*Commoner among cases of secondary MDS.

†−Y is usually an age-related change rather than being indicative of clonal haemopoiesis [73].

‡These chromosomal abnormalities are likely to be associated with haematological features leading to their being classified, In the WHO classification as an MPD/MDS.

§This translocation has also been described as dic(1;7)(p11;q11) and as t(1;7)(cen;cen).

¶These translocations result in trisomy for all or part of 1q.

**These translocations result in deletion of 17p.

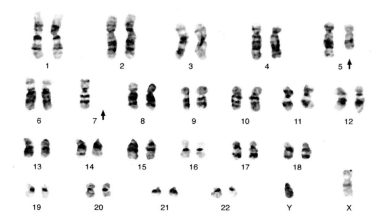

Fig. 3.27 Karyogram from a male patient with MDS showing a partial deletion of the long arm of chromosome 5 and monosomy 7. The karyogram is 45,XY,del(5)(q21q33),–7 (courtesy of Professor Lorna Secker-Walker).

megakaryocytes; the megakaryocytes are more pleomorphic than those of the 5q– syndrome with micromegakaryocytes, large non-lobulated megakaryocytes and multinucleated and other dysplastic forms being seen.

Deletion of the short arm of chromosome 17 has been found to be associated with MDS with distinctive haematological features and this has sometimes been referred to as the 17p– syndrome. Cases are usually FAB categories RA, RAEB, RAEB-T or CMML. A significant proportion are therapy-related. There is characteristic dysgranulopoiesis with an acquired Pelger–Huët anomaly of neutrophils and eosinophils, small vacuolated neutrophils and myeloperoxidase deficiency [84, 85]. There is usually trilineage myelodysplasia and although the blast count is often less than 5% at presentation there is rapid progression to AML [86]. There may be myeloproliferative as well as myelodysplastic features with most patients having leucocytosis and monocytosis and some having thrombocytosis [86]. Immature granulocytes may be increased in the peripheral blood, some patients have eosinophilia and a smaller number have basophilia [86]. A trephine biopsy shows increased reticulin fibrosis [86]. 17p– can be detected by interphase FISH as well as by classical cytogenetic analysis. Similar morphological abnormalities occur in other diseases with loss of 17p including AML and MPD in evolution. The 17p– syndrome can result not only from simple deletion of the short arm of 17 but also from monosomy 17, i(17q) and unbalanced translocations with loss of 17p such as –17,t(5;17)(p11;p11) and –17,t(7;17)(p11;p11). The relevant abnormality is often part of a complex

cytogenetic abnormality. The 17p– syndrome is related to loss of the *TP53* tumour-suppressor gene. The other *TP53* allele is often mutated. Prognosis of this syndrome is poor.

The molecular basis of MDS has been defined in only a small proportion of subtypes. Patients with translocations that are also seen in AML have the same molecular genetic changes as are seen in patients with overt leukaemia. This is true of t(6;9), abnormalities of 3q21 and 3q26 and translocations with 11q23 and 21q22 breakpoints. In patients with loss of all or part of a chromosome, e.g. –5, 5q–, –7, 7q– and 20q–, it is likely that deletion of a tumour-suppressing gene is critical in development of MDS. Such deletion, of the *TP53* gene, has been demonstrated for MDS associated with 17p–. Mutations in *RAS* and, to a lesser extent *FMS* and *TP53*, are common in MDS and are indicative of a worse prognosis [87]. In one series of patients with CMML, 25 of 65 patients were found to have a *RAS* mutation [50].

MDS may be associated with mutations of mitochondrial as well as nuclear DNA [88, 89]. For example, mutations of cytochrome c oxidase I and II and cytochrome b have been described in at least 36 patients and other patients have had mutations in mitochondrial genes encoding transfer RNA (mtRNA) [89, 90]. Mitochondrial mutations are likely to precede clonal expansion rather than be the event leading to it [89]. They may be the cause of sideroblastic erythropoiesis. One reported patient with RARS who had a cytochrome c oxidase mutation developed 5q– during the course of the disease, illustrating further clonal evolution [83].

Table 3.5 Median survival in months in the FAB categories of myelodysplasia.

Number of cases	RA	RARS	CMML	RAEB	RAEB-T	Reference
101	20	14	4	13	2.5	[91]
141	32	76	22	10.5	5	[92]
109	64	71	8	7	5	[93]
237	50	>60	>60	9	6	[94]
107	23	31	9.4	8	4	[95]
569	26.5	42	12	8.5	5	[60]
109	91	142	47	19	5	[96]
838	65	58	20	16	10	[97]
226	24	36	12	12.5	12	[98]
816	48	80	28	18	6	[81]
1600	37	50	19	12	5	[55]
213			12			[50]

This table includes only data from series containing more than 100 patients and in which the FAB criteria have been applied with minor or no modifications. Figures have been rounded to the nearest month. See Table 3.2 for abbreviation definitions.

Table 3.6 The percentage of patients transforming to acute leukaemia in the FAB categories of myelodysplasia.

Number of cases	Length of follow-up	RA	RARS	CMML	RAEB	RAEB-T	Reference
101	'Long term'	16	7	0	38	47	[91]
141	4 months to 16 years	11	5	13	28	55	[92]
109	4–9 years	15	0	32	27	50	[93]
256	5 years	26	16	17	66	60	[94]
569	2–12 years	16	4	49	42	58	[60]
838	3–9 years	27	21	47	76	80	[97]
1600	Long term	10	8	13	28	45	[55]
213	Long term			19			[50]

This figure contains only data from series containing more than 100 patients in which the FAB criteria have been applied with minor or no modifications. See Table 3.2 for abbreviation definitions.

Evolution of MDS

Patients with MDS may die of marrow failure as a direct consequence of MDS or may die following transformation to acute leukaemia. The likelihood of either outcome and the rapidity with which it occurs varies between the different FAB and WHO categories so that both the percentage of patients developing acute leukaemia and the prognosis as reflected in the median survival differ significantly between FAB categories (Tables 3.5 & 3.6). Myelodysplastic syndromes may also evolve into other MDS. Change is usually into a worse prognostic category and very rarely into one more favourable. Thus, RA and RARS may evolve into either CMML or RAEB, which in turn may both evolve into RAEB-T. Variation in the number of monocytes can alter the classification,

mainly between CMML and RAEB and rarely ring sideroblasts disappear so that RARS converts to RA. When acute leukaemia supervenes it may develop within a brief period or there may be a stepwise evolution over many weeks or months. The acute leukaemia that occurs in MDS is almost always AML but rare cases of acute lymphoblastic leukaemia (ALL) and of bilineage/biphenotypic leukaemia have been reported; this occurrence is consistent with the evidence suggesting that in at least some cases the cell giving rise to the MDS clone is a pluripotent stem cell capable of both myeloid and lymphoid differentiation. However, it should be noted that in the great majority of cases of apparent lymphoid or biphenotypic transformation it has not been demonstrated that the acute leukaemia has arisen in the MDS clone. Since MDS is predominantly a disease of the

Table 3.7 Factors that have been reported to have prognostic significance in the myelodysplastic syndromes (MDS)*. (Derived from references 48, 55, 60, 67, 81, 92, 99–107 and other sources.)

	Better prognosis	Intermediate prognosis	Worse prognosis
Clinical features	Younger Female *De novo* MDS		Older (e.g. >60 years) Male Secondary MDS or t-MDS Splenomegaly (in CMML)*
FAB category	RA or RARS		RAEB or RAEB-T
WHO category	RA, RARS or 5q– syndrome	RCMD or RCMD-RS	RAEB-1 or RAEB-2 (RAEB-2 worse than RAEB-1)
Peripheral blood features			Anaemia (Hb ≤9 or ≤10 g/dl) Neutropenia (neutrophil count <0.5, 0.5–1.0, 1–3 or ≤ 2.5 cf. >2.5 × 10^9/l) Thrombocytopenia (platelet count <20, 20–50, 50–100, 100–150 or >150 × 10^9/l) Presence of blast cells Dyserythropoiesis Dysgranulopoiesis Dysthrombopoiesis Neutrophilia (in CMML)* Monocytosis (in CMML)*† Presence of CD34-positive cells
Biochemistry			Elevated LDH
Bone marrow aspirate			Increased blast cells (<5%, 5–10%, 10–20%, 20–30%) Increased percentage of CD34-positive cells Dyserythropoiesis Dysgranulopoiesis Dysthrombopoiesis Reduced megakaryocytes
Bone marrow trephine biopsy	Increased mast cells		Abnormal localization of immature precursors (ALIP) Increased CD34-positive cells Presence of fibrosis Megakaryocyte atypia Reduced erythropoiesis Increased haemosiderin
Bone marrow culture	Normal numbers of CFU-GM		Reduced CFU-GM; increased colonies and/or clusters
Cell kinetics			Low labelling index
Ferrokinetics	Near normal iron utilization at 14 days		Low iron utilization at 14 days, increased ineffective erythropoiesis
Karyotype	Normal karyotype	Some normal and some abnormal metaphases	All abnormal metaphases
	5q–, 20q– or –Y as sole abnormality	Trisomy 8 and any other abnormality not associated with good prognosis or poor prognosis	Abnormality of chromosome 7 or both 5 and 7; complex, karyotype, e.g. at least 3 abnormalities in the karyotype

*Referring mainly to the FAB classification; t-MDS, therapy-related MDS
†In some but not all series.
CFU-GM, colony-forming units—granulocyte, macrophage. See Table 3.2 for other abbreviation definitions.

elderly a significant proportion of patients with MDS die of other diseases. The likelihood of this outcome is of course greatest in those in the best prognostic categories, RA and RARS. Occasional patients with MDS, particularly with RA and RARS, die of iron overload.

Prognosis of MDS

A number of factors can be correlated with prognosis of MDS (Table 3.7). The FAB classification divides patients into two broad prognostic groups, RA plus RARS and RAEB plus RAEB-T. There is no consistent or statistically significant difference between median survivals in RA and RARS, although leukaemic transformation is less common in RARS [100] (see Tables 3.5 & 3.6). The prognosis of RAEB-T is somewhat worse than that of RAEB and in large series of patients the difference in survival becomes significant [100]. The prognosis of CMML has been very variable between different series of patients (see Table 3.5). The considerable variation in prognosis within the CMML group is likely to relate to how many patients with a high white cell count (in some series indicative of worse prognosis) are included and to the wide range of bone marrow blast counts within this group (0–20%), prognostic differences having been found between patients with MDS with fewer than 5% blasts, 5–10% blasts and 10–20% blasts [81] and in CMML between cases with fewer than 5% blasts and those with 5–20% blasts [102] and between those with fewer than 10% and more than 10% blasts [50]. The WHO classification can be used to divide MDS into three prognostic groups (see Table 3.7).

Because of the considerable heterogeneity within FAB categories, efforts have been made to use other criteria to give a clearer idea of prognosis in the individual patient. The Third MIC Cooperative Study Group proposed consideration of cytogenetic information [41] and this approach has since been validated by the demonstration that specific karyotypic abnormalities have independent prognostic significance [75, 81, 96, 106, 108]. In general, cases with a normal karyotype have been found to have a better prognosis than those with a clonal cytogenetic abnormality and in some series of patients those with a mixture of normal and abnormal metaphases had a better prognosis than those with only abnormal metaphases. In general, the best prognosis is associated with a normal karyotype, isolated 5q–, isolated 20q– and isolated –Y. An intermediate prognosis is found in association with trisomy 8 and miscellaneous single and some double defects. The worst prognosis is associated with abnormalities of chromosome 7, complex karyotypes (e.g. defined as three or more unrelated abnormalities) and certain specific translocations; (1;3)(p36;q21), t(6;9)(p21–22;q34), rearrangements with an 11q23 breakpoint, 3q21q26 abnormalities and perhaps also t(1;7)(p11;q11) have been associated with a high probability of transformation to AML and poor prognosis. Rearrangements of 11q23 are specifically associated with evolution to AML of M4 and M5 categories [82] and in the WHO classification these patients are classified as AML rather than MDS, regardless of the blast percentage.

Karyotypic abnormalities have been incorporated, together with other variables shown to indicate prog-

Table 3.8 The International Prognostic Scoring System for MDS [81].

Score	0	0.5	1.0	1.5	2
Prognostic variables					
% blasts	<5	5–10	–	11–20	20–30*
Karyotype†	Good	Intermediate	Poor	–	–
Cytopenias‡	0–1	2–3			

*Cases with 20–30% blasts are classified as AML not MDS in the WHO classification.

†Good prognosis karyotype—normal, –Y, del(5q), del(20q). Poor prognosis karyotype—complex (≥3 abnormalities) or chromosome 7 abnormalities. Intermediate prognosis karyotype—other abnormalities.

‡Cytopenias—Hb <10 g/dl, neutrophil count <1.5 × 10^9/l, platelet count <100 × 10^9/l.

Individual scores are summed and cases are then assigned to four risk groups, indicative of an increasingly bad prognosis. A score of 0 is indicative of low risk; a score of 1 is indicative of intermediate risk-1; a score of 1.5–2.0 is indicative of intermediate risk-2; a score of ≥2.5 is indicative of high risk.

nosis, into a number of scoring systems. These include the Lille scoring system [103, 108], the Lausanne–Bournemouth system [96] and the International Prognostic Scoring System [81]. Of these, the International Prognostic Scoring System (Table 3.8) is the most widely accepted.

References

1 Doll DC and List AF (1992) Myelodysplastic syndromes: introduction. *Semin Oncol*, **19**, 1–3.

2 Bennett JM, Catovsky D, Daniel MT, Flandrin G, Galton DAG, Gralnick HR and Sultan C (1976) Proposals for the classification of the acute leukaemias (FAB cooperative group). *Br J Haematol*, **33**, 451–458.

3 Bennett JM, Catovsky D, Daniel MT, Flandrin G, Galton DAG, Gralnick HR and Sultan C (1982) Proposals for the classification of the myelodysplastic syndromes. *Br J Haematol*, **51**, 189–199.

4 Bennett JM, Catovsky D, Daniel MT, Flandrin G, Galton DAG, Gralnick HR and Sultan C (1985) Proposed revised criteria for the classification of acute myeloid leukemia. *Ann Intern Med*, **103**, 626–629.

5 Brunning RD, Bennett JM, Flandrin G, Matutes E, Head D, Vardiman JW and Harris NL (2001) Myelodysplastic syndromes: introduction. In Jaffe ES, Harris NL, Stein H and Vardiman JW (Eds), *World Health Organization Classification of Tumours: Pathology and Genetics of Tumours of Haematopoietic and Lymphoid Tissues*, IARC Press, Lyon, pp. 63–67.

6 Brunning RD, Bennett JM, Flandrin G, Matutes E, Head D, Vardiman JW and Harris NL (2001) Refractory anaemia. In Jaffe ES, Harris NL, Stein H and Vardiman JW (Eds), *World Health Organization Classification of Tumours: Pathology and Genetics of Tumours of Haematopoietic and Lymphoid Tissues*, IARC Press, Lyon, p. 68.

7 Brunning RD, Bennett JM, Flandrin G, Matutes E, Head D, Vardiman JW and Harris NL (2001) Refractory anaemia with ringed sideroblasts. In Jaffe ES, Harris NL, Stein H and Vardiman JW (Eds), *World Health Organization Classification of Tumours: Pathology and Genetics of Tumours of Haematopoietic and Lymphoid Tissues*, IARC Press, Lyon, p. 69.

8 Brunning RD, Bennett JM, Flandrin G, Matutes E, Head D, Vardiman JW and Harris NL (2001) Refractory cytopenia with multilineage dysplasia. In Jaffe ES, Harris NL, Stein H and Vardiman JW (Eds), *World Health Organization Classification of Tumours: Pathology and Genetics of Tumours of Haematopoietic and Lymphoid Tissues*, IARC Press, Lyon, p. 70.

9 Brunning RD, Bennett JM, Flandrin G, Matutes E, Head D, Vardiman JW and Harris NL (2001) Refractory anaemia with excess of blasts. In Jaffe ES, Harris NL, Stein H and Vardiman JW (Eds), *World Health Organization Classification of Tumours: Pathology and Genetics of*

Tumours of Haematopoietic and Lymphoid Tissues, IARC Press, Lyon, p. 71.

10 Brunning RD, Bennett JM, Flandrin G, Matutes E, Head D, Vardiman JW and Harris NL (2001) Myelodysplastic syndrome associated with isolated del(5q) chromosome abnormality ('5q– syndrome'). In Jaffe ES, Harris NL, Stein H and Vardiman JW (Eds), *World Health Organization Classification of Tumours: Pathology and Genetics of Tumours of Haematopoietic and Lymphoid Tissues*, IARC Press, Lyon, p. 73.

11 Brunning RD, Bennett JM, Flandrin G, Matutes E, Head D, Vardiman JW and Harris NL (2001) Myelodysplastic syndrome, unclassifiable. In Jaffe ES, Harris NL, Stein H and Vardiman JW (Eds), *World Health Organization Classification of Tumours: Pathology and Genetics of Tumours of Haematopoietic and Lymphoid Tissues*, IARC Press, Lyon, p. 72.

12 Hamblin TJ and Oscier DG (1987) The myelodysplastic syndrome—a practical guide. *Hematol Oncol*, **5**, 19–34.

13 Bain BJ (1997) The haematological features of HIV infection. *Br J Haematol*, **99**, 1–8.

14 Mercieca J, Bain B, Barlow G and Catovsky D (1996) Teaching cases from the Royal Marsden and St Mary's Hospitals, Case 10: microcytic anaemia and thrombocytosis. *Leuk Lymph*, **18**, 185–186.

15 Hoyle C, Kaeda J, Leslie J and Luzzatto L (1991) Case report: acquired β thalassaemia trait in MDS. *Br J Haematol*, **79**, 116–117.

16 Rummens JL, Verfaillie C, Criel A, Hidajat M, Vanhoof A, van den Berghe H and Louwagie A (1986) Elliptocytosis and schistocytes in myelodysplasia: report of two cases. *Acta Haematol*, **75**, 174–177.

17 Samson RE, Abdalla SH and Bain BJ (1998) Teaching cases from the Royal Marsden and St Mary's Hospitals Case 18. Severe anaemia and thrombocytopenia with red cell fragmentation. *Leuk Lymphoma*, in press.

18 Doll DC, List AF, Dayhoff DA, Loy TS, Ringerberg QS and Yarbro JW (1989) Acanthocytosis associated with myelodysplasia. *J Clin Oncol*, **7**, 1569–1572.

19 De Pree C, Cabrol C, Frossard JL and Beris P (1995) Pseudoreticulocytosis in a case of myelodysplastic syndrome with translocation t(1;14)(q42;q32). *Semin Hematol*, **32**, 232–236.

20 Matsushima T, Murukami H and Tsuchiya J (1994) Myelodysplastic syndrome with bone marrow eosinophilia: clinical and cytogenetic features. *Leuk Lymph*, **15**, 491–497.

21 Ma SK, Wong KF, Chan JKC and Kwong YL (1995) Refractory cytopenia with t(1;7), +8 abnormality and dysplastic eosinophils showing intranuclear Charcot–Leyden crystals: a fluorescence *in situ* hybridization study. *Br J Haematol*, **90**, 216.

22 Valent P, Spanblöchl E, Bankl H-C, Sperr WR, Marosi C, Pirc-Danoewinata H *et al.* (1994) Kit ligand/mast cell growth factor-independent differentiation of mast cells

in myelodysplasia and chronic myeloid leukemic blast crisis. *Blood*, **84**, 4322–4333.

23 Pavord S, Sivakumaran M, Furber P and Mitchell V (1996) Cyclical thrombocytopenia as a rare manifestation of myelodysplastic syndrome. *Clin Lab Haematol*, **18**, 221–223.

24 Kuriyama K, Tomonaga M, Matsuo T, Ginnai I and Ichimaru M (1986) Diagnostic significance of detecting pseudo-Pelger–Huët anomalies and micromegakaryocytes in myelodysplastic syndrome. *Br J Haematol*, **63**, 665–669.

25 Vardiman JW (2001) Myelodysplastic/myeloproliferative disease: introduction. In Jaffe ES, Harris NL, Stein H and Vardiman JW (Eds), *World Health Organization Classification of Tumours: Pathology and Genetics of Tumours of Haematopoietic and Lymphoid Tissues*, IARC Press, Lyon, pp. 47–48.

26 Evans JPM, Czepulkowski B, Gibbons B, Swansbury GJ and Chessels JM (1988) Childhood monosomy 7 revisited. *Br J Haematol*, **69**, 41–45.

27 van den Berghe H, Vermaelen K, Mecucci C, Barbieri D and Tricot G (1985) The 5q– anomaly. *Cancer Genet Cytogenet*, **17**, 189–255.

28 Thiede T, Engquist L and Billstrom R (1988) Application of megakaryocytic morphology in diagnosing 5q– syndrome. *Eur J Haematol*, **41**, 434–437.

29 Bigoni R, Cuneo A, Milani R, Cavazzini P, Bardi A, Roberti MG *et al.* (2001) Multilineage involvement in the 5q– syndrome: a fluorescent *in situ* hybridization study on bone marrow smears. *Haematologica*, **86**, 375–381.

30 Prchal JT, Throckmorton DW, Carroll AJ, Fuson EW, Gams RA and Prchal JF (1978) A common progenitor for human myeloid and lymphoid cells. *Nature*, **274**, 590–591.

31 Rashkind WH, Tirumali N, Jacobson R, Singer J and Fialkow PJ (1984) Evidence for a multistep pathogenesis of a myelodysplastic syndrome. *Blood*, **63**, 1318–1323.

32 Janssen JWG, Buschle M, Layton M, Drexler HG, Lyons J, van den Berghe H *et al.* (1989) Clonal analysis of myelodysplastic syndrome: evidence of multipotent stem cell origin. *Blood*, **73**, 248–254.

33 Ikeda T, Sato K, Yamashita T, Kanai Y, Kuwada N, Matsumura T *et al.* (2001) Burkitt's acute lymphoblastic leukaemia transformation after myelodysplastic syndrome. *Br J Haematol*, **115**, 69–71.

34 Rosati S, Mick R, Xu F, Stonys E, Le Beau MM, Larson R and Vardiman JW (1996) Refractory cytopenia with multilineage dysplasia: further characterization of an 'unclassifiable' myelodysplastic syndrome. *Leukemia*, **10**, 20–26.

35 Garand R, Gardais J, Bizet M, Bremond J-L, Accard F, Callat M-P *et al.* (1992) Heterogeneity of acquired sideroblastic anaemia (AISA). *Leuk Res*, **16**, 463–468.

36 Aul C, Hildebrandt B, Giagnounides A, Germing U and Gatterman N (1999) Clinical course and cytogenetic patterns in two types of acquired idiopathic sideroblastic

anaemia (AISA): results from a prospective follow-up study in 225 patients. *Leuk Res*, **23**, Suppl 1, 48.

37 Seymour JF and Estey EH (1993) The prognostic significance of Auer rods in myelodysplasia. *Br J Haematol*, **85**, 67–76.

38 Scoazec J-Y, Imbert M, Crofts M, Jouault H, Juneja SK, Vernant J-O and Sultan C (1985) Myelodysplastic syndrome or acute myeloid leukemia? A study of 28 cases presenting with borderline features. *Cancer*, **55**, 2390–2394.

39 Bennett JM, Cox C, Moloney WC, Rosenthal DS and Storniolo AM (1988) Chronic myelomonocytic leukemia (myelodysplasia with monocytosis). *XXII Congress of the International Society of Hematology*, Milan, Abstract Sym-M-3-6.

40 Bennett JM, Catovsky D, Daniel MT, Flandrin G, Galton DAG, Gralnick HR *et al.* (1994) The chronic myeloid leukaemias: guidelines for distinguishing granulocytic, atypical chronic myeloid, and chronic myelomonocytic leukaemia. Proposals from the French–American–British Cooperative Leukaemia Group. *Br J Haematol*, **87**, 746–754.

41 Third MIC Cooperative Study Group (1988) Recommendations for a morphologic, immunologic and cytogenetic (MIC) working classification of the primary and therapy-related myelodysplastic disorders. *Cancer Genet Cytogenet*, **32**, 1–10.

42 Jaffe ES, Harris NL, Stein H and Vardiman JW (Eds) (2001) *World Health Organization Classification of Tumours: Pathology and Genetics of Tumours of Haematopoietic and Lymphoid Tissues*, IARC Press, Lyon.

43 Sanz GF, Sanz MA, Vallespi T and del Cânizo MC (1990) Two types of acquired sideroblastic anaemia (AISA). *Br J Haematol*, **75**, 633–634.

44 Kouides PA and Bennett JM (1996) Morphology and classification of the myelodysplastic syndromes and their pathological variants. *Semin Hematol*, **33**, 95–110.

45 Cazzola M, Barosi G, Gobbi PG, Invernizzi R, Riccardi A and Ascari E (1988) Natural history of idiopathic refractory sideroblastic anemia. *Blood*, **71**, 305–312.

46 Tham KT, Cousar J and Macon WR (1990) Brief scientific reports. Silver stain for ringed sideroblasts: a sensitive method that differs from Perls' reaction in mechanism and clinical application. *Am J Clin Pathol*, **94**, 73–76.

47 Takeda Y, Sawada H, Tashima M, Okuma M and Kondo M (1996) Erythropoietic protoporphyria without cutaneous photosensitivity and with ringed sideroblasts in an atomic bomb survivor. *Lancet*, **347**, 395–396.

48 Worsley A, Oscier DG, Stevens J, Darlow S, Figes A, Mufti GJ and Hamblin TJ (1988) Prognostic features of chronic myelomonocytic leukaemia. *Br J Haematol*, **68**, 17–21.

49 Solal-Celigny P, Desaint B, Herrera A, Chastang C, Amar M, Vroclans M *et al.* (1983) Chronic myelomonocytic leukemia according to the FAB classification: analysis of 35 cases. *Blood*, **63**, 634–638.

50 Onida F, Kantarjian HM, Smith TL, Ball G, Keating MJ, Estey EH *et al.* (2002) Prognostic features and scoring systems in chronic myelomonocytic leukemia: a retrospective analysis of 213 patients. *Blood*, **99**, 840–849.

51 Krsnik I, Srivastava PC and Galton DAG (1992) Chronic myelomonocytic leukaemia and atypical chronic myeloid leukaemia. In Schmalzl F and Mufti GK (Eds), *Myelodysplastic Syndromes*, Springer-Verlag, Berlin, pp. 131–139.

52 Germing U, Gatterman N, Minning H, Heyll A and Aul C (1997) Problems in the classification of CMML. Dysplastic vs. proliferative type. *Leuk Res*, **22**, 871–878.

53 Cerve RAJ, Sanz GF, Vallespi T, del Cañizo MC, Irriguible F, López F *et al.* (1997) Does WBC really define two different subtypes of chronic myelomonocytic leukemia (CMML)? *Leuk Res*, **21**, Suppl 1, S7.

54 Oscier DG (1994) Atypical chronic myeloid leukaemia. Is it a separate entity? *Leuk Res*, **18**, Suppl, 37.

55 Germing U, Gatterman N, Strupp C, Aivado M and Aul C (2001) Validation of the WHO proposals for a new classification of primary myelodysplastic syndromes: a retrospective analysis of 1600 patients. *Leuk Res*, **24**, 983–992.

56 May SJ, Smith SA, Jacobs A, Williams A and Bailey-Wood R (1985) The myelodysplastic syndromes; analysis of laboratory characteristics in relation to the FAB classification. *Br J Haematol*, **59**, 311–319.

57 Bowen DT and Jacobs A (1989) Primary acquired sideroblastic erythropoiesis in non-anaemic and minimally anaemic subjects. *J Clin Pathol*, **42**, 56–58.

58 Ohyashiki JH, Iwabuchi A and Toyama K (1996) Clinical aspects, cytogenetics and disease evolution in myelodysplastic syndromes. *Leuk Lymphoma*, **23**, 409–415.

59 Geary CG, Marsh JCW and Gordon-Smith EC (1996) Hypoplastic myelodysplasia (MDS). *Br J Haematol*, **94**, 579–583.

60 Maschek H, Gutzmer R, Choritz H and Georgii A (1992) Life expectancy in primary myelodysplastic syndromes: a prognostic score based on histopathology from bone marrow biopsies of 569 patients. *Eur J Haematol*, **53**, 280–287.

61 Schmalzl F, Konwalinka G, Michlmayr G, Abbrederis K and Braunsteiner H (1978) Detection of cytochemical and morphological abnormalities in 'Preleukaemia'. *Acta Haematol*, **59**, 1–18.

62 Hayhoe FGJ and Quaglino D (1988) *Haematological Cytochemistry*. Second edition. Churchill Livingstone, Edinburgh.

63 Stetler-Stevenson M, Arthur DC, Jabbour N, Xie XY, Molldrem J, Barrett AJ *et al.* (2001) Diagnostic utility of flow cytometric immunophenotyping in myelodysplastic syndrome. *Blood*, **98**, 979–987.

64 Tricot G, de Wolf Peeters C, Hendrickx B and Verwilghen RL (1984) Bone marrow histology in myelodysplastic syndromes. *Br J Haematol*, **56**, 423–430.

65 Tricot G, Vlietinck R, Boogaerts MA, Hendrickx B, de Wolf Peeters C, van den Berghe H and Verwilghen RL (1985) Prognostic factors in the myelodysplastic syndrome: importance of initial data on peripheral blood counts, bone marrow cytology, trephine biopsy and chromosomal analysis. *Br J Haematol*, **60**, 19–32.

66 Delacrétaz F, Schmidt P-M, Piguet D, Bachmann F and Costa J (1987) Histopathology of myelodysplastic syndromes: the FAB classification. *Am J Clin Pathol*, **87**, 180–186.

67 Bartl R, Frisch B and Baumgart R (1992) Morphological classification of the myelodysplastic syndromes (MDS): combined utilization of bone marrow aspirates and trephine biopsies. *Leuk Res*, **16**, 15–33.

68 Bain BJ, Clark D, Lampert I and Wilkins BS (2001) *Bone Marrow Pathology*. Third edition. Blackwell Science, Oxford.

69 Clark DM and Lampert I (1990) Apoptosis is a common histopathological finding in myelodysplasia: the correlate of ineffective haematopoiesis. *Leuk Lymphoma*, **2**, 415–418.

70 Deliliers GL, Annaloro C, Soligo D and Oriani A (1998) The diagnostic and prognostic value of bone marrow immunostaining in myelodysplastic syndromes. *Leuk Lymphoma*, **28**, 231–239.

71 Gatterman N, Aul C and Schneider W (1990) Two types of acquired sideroblastic anaemia (AISA). *Br J Haematol*, **74**, 45–52.

72 d'Onofrio G and Zini G, translated by Bain BJ (1997) *Morphology of the Blood*. Heinemann, London.

73 United Kingdom Cancer Cytogenetics Study Group (1992) Loss of the Y chromosome from normal and neoplastic bone marrows. *Genes Chromosomes Cancer*, **5**, 83–88.

74 Musilova J and Michalova K (1988) Chromosome study of 85 patients with myelodysplastic syndromes. *Cancer Genet Cytogenet*, **33**, 39–50.

75 Yunis JJ, Lobell M, Arnesen MA, Oken MM, Mayer MG, Ryder RE and Brunning RD (1988) Refined chromosome study helps define prognostic subgroups in most patients with primary myelodysplastic syndromes and acute myelogenous leukaemia. *Br J Haematol*, **68**, 189–194.

76 Dierlamm J, Michaux L, Criel A, Wlodarska I, Zeller W, Louwagie A *et al.* (1995) Dicentric (X)(q13) in haematological malignancies: presentation of five new cases, application of fluorescence *in situ* hybridization (FISH) and review of the literature. *Br J Haematol*, **91**, 885–891.

77 Secker-Walker L, Mehta A and Bain B on behalf of the UKCCG (1995) Abnormalities of 3q21 and 3q26 in myeloid malignancy: a United Kingdom Cancer Cytogenetic Group Study. *Br J Haematol*, **91**, 490–502.

78 Jotterland M and Parlier V (1996) Diagnostic and prognostic significance of cytogenetics in adult

primary myelodysplastic syndromes. *Leuk Lymphoma*, **23**, 253–266.

79 Fenaux P, Morel P and Lai JL (1996) Cytogenetics of myelodysplastic syndromes. *Semin Hematol*, **33**, 127–138.

80 Mrózek K, Heinonem K, de la Chapelle A and Bloomfield CD (1997) Clinical significance of cytogenetics in acute myeloid leukemia. *Semin Oncol*, **24**, 17–31.

81 Greenberg P, Cox C, Le Beau MM, Fenaux P, Morel P, Sanz G *et al.* (1997) International Scoring System for evaluating prognosis in myelodysplastic syndromes. *Blood*, **89**, 2079–2088.

82 Bain BJ, Moorman AV, Mehta AB and Secker-Walker LM, on behalf of the European 11q23 Workshop participants. (1998) Myelodysplastic syndromes with 11q23 abnormalities. *Leukemia*, **12**, 834–839.

83 Dunkley SM, Manoharan A and Kwan YL (2002) Myelodysplastic syndromes: prognostic significance of multilineage dysplasia in patients with refractory anemia or refractory anemia with ringed sideroblasts. *Blood*, **99**, 3870–3871.

84 Lai JL, Preudhomme C, Zandecki M, Flactif M, Vanrumbeke M, Lepelley P *et al.* (1995) Myelodysplastic syndrome and acute myeloid leukemia with 17p deletion. An entity characterized by specific dysgranulopoiesis and a high incidence of P53 mutations. *Leukemia*, **9**, 370–381.

85 Jary L, Mossafa H, Fourcade C, Genet P, Pulik M and Flandrin G (1997) The 17p– syndrome: a distinct myelodysplastic syndrome entity? *Leuk Lymphoma*, **25**, 163–168.

86 McClure RF, Dewald GW, Hoyer JD and Hanson CA (1999) Isolated isochromosome 17q: a distinct type of mixed myeloproliferative disorder/myelodysplastic syndrome with an aggressive clinical course. *Br J Haematol*, **106**, 445–454.

87 Padua RA and West RR (2000) Oncogene mutation and prognosis in the myelodysplastic syndromes. *Br J Haematol*, **111**, 873–874.

88 Gatterman N, Retzlaff S, Wang Y-L, Hofhaus G, Heinisch J, Aul C and Schneider W (1997) Heteroplasmic point mutations of mitochondrial DNA affecting subunit 1 of cytochrome c oxidase in two patients with acquired idiopathic sideroblastic anemia. *Blood*, **90**, 4961–4972.

89 Gatterman N (1999) From sideroblastic anemia to the role of mitochondrial DNA mutations in myelodysplastic syndromes. *Leuk Res*, **24**, 141–151.

90 Reddy PL, Shetty VT, Dutt D, York A, Dar S, Mundle SD *et al.* (2002) Increased incidence of mitochondrial cytochrome c-oxidase gene mutations in patients with myelodysplastic syndromes. *Br J Haematol*, **116**, 564–575.

91 Vallespi T, Torrabadella M, Julio A, Irriguible D, Jaen A, Acebedo G and Triginer J (1985) Myelodysplastic syndromes: a study of 101 cases according to the FAB classification. *Br J Haematol*, **61**, 83–92.

92 Mufti GJ, Stevens JR, Oscier DG, Hamblin TJ and Machin D (1985) Myelodysplastic syndromes: a scoring system with prognostic significance. *Br J Haematol*, **59**, 425–433.

93 Foucar K, Langdon RM, Armitage JO, Olson DB and Carroll TJ (1985) Myelodysplastic syndromes. A clinical and pathological analysis of 109 cases. *Cancer*, **56**, 553–561.

94 Kerkhofs H, Hermans J, Haak HL and Leeksma CHW (1987) Utility of the FAB classification for myelodysplastic syndromes: investigation of prognostic factors in 237 cases. *Br J Haematol*, **65**, 73–81.

95 Garcia S, Sanz MA, Amigo V, Colomina P, Carrera MD, Lorenzo JI and Sanz GF (1988) Prognostic factors in chronic myelodysplastic syndromes: a multivariate analysis. *Am J Hematol*, **27**, 163–168.

96 Parlier V, van Melle G, Beris Ph, Schmidt PM, Tobler A, Haller E and Bellomo MJ (1994) Hematologic, clinical, and cytogenetic analysis in 109 patients with primary myelodysplastic syndrome: prognostic significance of morphology and chromosome findings. *Cancer Genet Cytogenet*, **78**, 219–231.

97 Oguma S, Yoshida Y, Uchino H, Maekawa T, Nomure T, Mizoguchi H and the Refractory Anaemia Study Group of the Department of Health and Welfare (1995) Clinical characteristics of Japanese patients with primary myelodysplastic syndromes: a cooperative study based on 838 cases. *Leuk Res*, **19**, 219–225.

98 Cunningham I, MacCallum SJ, Nicolls MD, Byth K, Hewson JW, Arnold B *et al.* (1995) The myelodysplastic syndromes: an analysis of prognostic factors in 226 cases from a single institution. *Br J Haematol*, **90**, 602–606.

99 Varela BL, Chuang C, Woll JE and Bennett JM (1985) Modifications in the classification of primary myelodysplastic syndromes: the addition of a scoring system. *Hematol Oncol*, **3**, 55–63.

100 Sanz GF, Sanz MA, Vallespi T, Cañizo MC, Torrabadella M, Garcia S *et al.* (1989) Two regression models and a scoring system for predicting survival and planning treatment in myelodysplastic syndromes: a multivariate analysis of prognostic factors in 370 patients. *Blood*, **74**, 395–408.

101 del Cañizo MC, Sanz G, San Miguel JF, Vallespi T, Irriguible D, Torrabadelle M and Sanz MA (1989) Chronic myelomonocytic leukemia—clinicobiological characteristics: a multivariate analysis in a series of 70 cases. *Eur J Haematol*, **42**, 466–473.

102 Storniolo AM, Moloney WC, Rosenthal DS, Cox C and Bennett JM (1990) Chronic myelomonocytic leukemia. *Leukemia*, **4**, 766–770.

103 Aul C, Gatterman N, Heyll A and Germing U (1992) Primary myelodysplastic syndromes: analysis of prognostic factors in 235 patients and proposals for an improved scoring system. *Leukemia*, **6**, 52–59.

104 Toyama K, Ohyasho K, Yoshida Y and Abe T (1993) Clinical implications of chromosomal abnormalities in 401 patients with MDS: a multicentric study in Japan. *Leukemia*, **7**, 499–508.

105 Parlier V, van Melle G, Beris P, Schmidt PM, Tobler A, Haller E and Bellomo MJ (1995) Prediction of 18 month survival in patients with primary myelodysplastic syndrome: a regression model and scoring system based on the combination of chromosome findings and the Bournemouth score. *Cancer Genet Cytogenet*, **81**, 158–165.

106 Nowell PC (1992) Chromosome abnormalities in myelodysplastic syndromes. *Semin Oncol*, **19**, 25–33.

107 Boogaerts MA, Veroef GEG and Demuynck H (1996) Treatment and prognostic factors in myelodysplastic syndromes. *Bailliére's Clin Haematol*, **9**, 161–183.

108 Morel P, Hebbar M, Laï JL, Duhamel A, Preudhomme C, Wattel E *et al.* (1993) Cytogenetic analysis has strong independent prognostic value in *de novo* myelodysplastic syndromes and can be incorporated into a new scoring system: a report of 408 cases. *Leukemia*, **7**, 1315–1323.

CHAPTER 4

CHRONIC MYELOID LEUKAEMIAS

The World Health Organization (WHO) classification assigns some chronic myeloid leukaemias to a myeloproliferative category and others, in which there are also dysplastic features, to a myeloproliferative/ myelodysplastic category [1, 2]. In addition, there are several specific types of chronic myeloid leukaemia that are mentioned in the WHO classification but are not assigned to a separate category. The WHO classification is summarized in Table 4.1. It should be noted that, in the FAB classification, chronic myelomonocytic leukaemia was regarded as a myelodysplastic syndrome whereas in the WHO classification it is regarded as one of the diseases with overlapping dysplastic and proliferative features. The term 'chronic myeloid leukaemia' is often used to refer to a specific entity associated with the Philadelphia chromosome (see below). It seems preferable that this condition be designated 'chronic granulocytic leukaemia' with the term chronic myeloid leukaemia being used as a general term to include all chronic myeloid leukaemias, a use analogous to the use of the term 'acute myeloid leukaemia'.

The classification of the chronic myeloid leukaemias is based on peripheral blood differential counts, cytological features in blood and bone marrow, cytogenetics and molecular genetics. Bone marrow findings are less useful in diagnosis than the peripheral blood features. Cytochemistry can be of some value if cytogenetic and molecular genetic analysis are not available but otherwise it is redundant. Immunophenotyping is of little value during the chronic phase of these diseases although it may give evidence of dysplastic maturation; during acute transformation it has a role in identifying the lineage of blasts.

Table 4.1 Classification of the chronic myeloid leukaemias, based on the WHO classification.

Myeloproliferative disorders
Chronic myelogenous leukaemia (also known as chronic myeloid leukaemias and chronic granulocytic leukaemia)
  Ph positive, *BCR-ABL* fusion gene
  Ph negative, *BCR-ABL* fusion gene
Chronic neutrophilic leukaemia
Chronic eosinophilic leukaemia
The 8p11 syndrome (*PDGFRB* rearranged)*
Basophilic leukaemia*
Mast cell leukaemia*

Myelodysplastic/myeloproliferative disorders
Chronic myelomonocytic leukaemia
  Chronic myelomonocytic leukaemia with eosinophilia
Myelodysplastic/myeloproliferative disorder associated with
  t(5;12)(q33;p13)*
Atypical chronic myeloid leukaemia
Juvenile myelomonocytic leukaemia

---

*Not separate categories in the WHO classification.

Chronic granulocytic leukaemia

Chronic granulocytic leukaemia (CGL) is a disease entity with specific haematological, cytogenetic and molecular genetic features. Alternative designations are chronic myelogenous leukaemia, chronic myeloid leukaemia and chronic myelocytic leukaemia. The incidence is of the order of 1.6/100 000/year with a median age of onset of 67 years [3]. The disease is bi- or triphasic with a chronic and an acute phase and, sometimes, an intervening accelerated phase.

The chronic phase of chronic granulocytic leukaemia

Clinical and haematological features

CGL is predominantly a disease of adults. The usual clinical presentation is with splenomegaly, hepatomegaly, symptoms of anaemia, and systemic symptoms such as sweating and weight loss. Occasionally this is an incidental diagnosis when a blood count is performed for another reason.

The peripheral blood usually shows anaemia and leucocytosis with a very characteristic differential count (Fig. 4.1) [4]. The two predominant cell types are the myelocyte and the mature neutrophil (Fig. 4.2). More immature granulocyte precursors are present but promyelocytes are fewer than myelocytes and blasts are fewer than promyelocytes. Almost all patients have an absolute basophilia and more than 90% have eosinophilia. The absolute monocyte count is increased but not in proportion to the increase in mature neutrophils and the percentage of monocytes is almost always less than 3%. Occasional nucleated red blood cells and occasional megakaryocyte nuclei may be present. The platelet count is most often normal or somewhat elevated but is low in about 5% of cases. Rarely the haemoglobin concentration is elevated. Dysplastic features are lacking during the chronic phase of the disease. The neutrophil alkaline phosphatase (NAP) score is low in about 95% of patients.

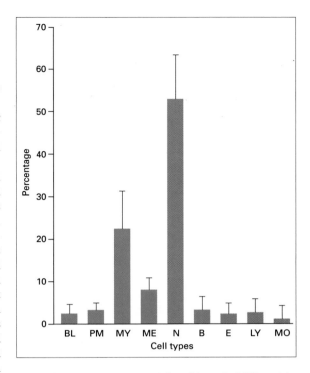

Fig. 4.1 Diagrammatic representation of the typical differential count in 50 untreated cases of chronic granulocytic leukaemia (CGL) (all demonstrated to be Ph positive) (modified from reference 4). Each differential count was of 1500 cells. BL, blasts; PM, promyelocytes; MY, myelocytes; ME, metamyelocytes; N, neutrophils; B, basophils; E, nucleated erythroid cells; LY, lymphocytes; MO, monocytes. The mean and the standard deviation are indicated.

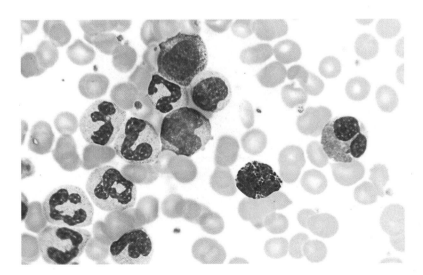

Fig. 4.2 Peripheral blood (PB) film of a patient with CGL showing two promyelocytes, a myelocyte, an eosinophil, a basophil and numerous neutrophils and band forms. May–Grünwald–Giemsa (MGG) × 870.

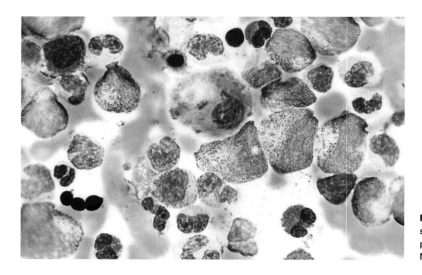

Fig. 4.3 BM film of a patient with CGL showing granulocytic hyperplasia and a phagocyte containing cellular debris. MGG × 870.

Haematological features differ somewhat between different molecular variants of CGL (see below). The features described above are those seen in the great majority of patients who have a p210 BCR-ABL protein. The rare cases with a p190 BCR-ABL protein (more characteristic of Ph-positive acute lymphoid leukaemia (ALL) than of CGL) have a more prominent relative and absolute monocytosis while those with the very rare p230 BCR-ABL protein may have a neutrophilic variant of CGL [5].

The bone marrow is intensely hypercellular with marked granulocytic hyperplasia (Fig. 4.3) and with the myeloid/erythroid (M:E) ratio being greater than 10:1. There is hyperplasia of neutrophil, eosinophil and basophil lineages. Megakaryocytes are either normal in number or increased. On average, they are smaller and their lobe count is reduced in comparison with normal megakaryocytes. The trephine biopsy shows either granulocytic or mixed granulocytic and megakaryocytic hyperplasia. Rarely the bone marrow is fibrotic at presentation.

Several staging systems have been proposed for the further categorization of patients with CGL, in order to give an indication of prognosis. The most widely used system is that of Sokal *et al.* [6]. The system of Hasford *et al.* [7] may be more appropriate for interferon-treated patients [8].

Cytogenetic and molecular genetic features

CGL was the first malignant disease for which a consistent association with an acquired non-random cytogenetic abnormality was recognized. In 1960 Nowell and Hungerford [9] reported its association with an abnormal 'minute chromosome', initially designated the Philadelphia[1] (Ph[1]) chromosome after the city of its discovery. Subsequently it was demonstrated that there was a characteristic translocation, t(9;22)(q34;q11), with the derivative chromosomes 22q− being the previously reported Philadelphia chromosome [10]. It should be noted that the favoured designation of the abnormal chromosome 22 is now Philadelphia rather than Philadelphia[1] with the abbreviation Ph rather than Ph[1]. The 9;22 translocation results in fusion of some of the sequences of the *BCR* (breakpoint cluster region) gene at 22q11 with some of the sequences of the c-*ABL* oncogene, which have been translocated from 9q34. A hybrid gene, *BCR-ABL*, is formed on chromosome 22. *BCR-ABL* encodes a constitutively activated tyrosine kinase, which is important in leukaemogenesis. There is also an *ABL-BCR* fusion gene on chromosome 9 that is not always transcribed and, since a protein product has not been identified [11], is unlikely to be relevant to leukaemogenesis. The translocation occurs in a pluripotent stem cell so that the clone of cells with this abnormality includes the granulocytic, monocytic, erythroid and megakaryocytic lineages, and also some precursors of at least B lymphocytes and possibly T lymphocytes.

The typical t(9;22) giving rise to the Ph chromosome is found in about 95% of cases of CGL. A

Table 4.2 Molecular variants of *BCR-ABL* and associated clinicopathological features.

Protein	Breakpoint	Disease association
p210$^{BCR-ABL}$	M-bcr	The great majority of cases of typical CGL. About a third of cases of Ph-positive ALL
p190$^{BCR-ABL}$	m-bcr	A minority of cases of CGL, often with monocytosis or dysplastic features. About two thirds of cases of Ph-positive ALL. Rare cases of AML
p230$^{BCR-ABL}$	μ-bcr	Neutrophilic variant of CGL, or CGL with marked thrombocytosis

ALL, acute lymphoblastic leukaemia; AML, acute myeloid leukaemia: CGL, chronic granulocytic leukaemia, Ph, Philadelphia chromosome.

minority of cases have a simple variant translocation (involving either chromosome 9 or chromosome 22 but not both) or a complex variant translocation (with involvement of chromosomes 9, 22 and a third chromosome). There are also patients with otherwise typical CGL who demonstrate neither a t(9;22) nor a variant translocation but nevertheless have a molecular rearrangement leading to formation of a *BCR-ABL* gene. The fusion gene may be at 9q34, at 22q11 or on a third chromosome [11, 12]. Cases without a Ph chromosome but with *BCR-ABL* rearrangement should be classified as Ph-negative CGL. Their clinical and haematological features, response to treatment and prognosis are identical to those of Ph-positive cases.

At a molecular level, breakpoints in the *BCR* gene vary so that at least three different *BCR-ABL* fusion genes can occur, leading to the formation of one of three abnormal proteins of different molecular weights designated p210, p190 and p230 [5]. These show different disease associations (Table 4.2). Ph-positive thrombocythaemia, which should be regarded as a variant of CGL, is associated with p210.

Fluorescence *in situ* hybridization (FISH) demonstrates that a significant minority of patients with CGL have a large deletion of chromosome 9 material adjacent to the breakpoint on the derivative chromosome 9 [13]. Most patients also have a smaller deletion of chromosome 22 material. This loss of chromosomal material is associated with a neutrophil dysplasia (chromatin clumping, Pelger–Huët anomaly and hypogranularity) [14], resistance to interferon therapy [15] and a considerably worse prognosis [13–16]. Chromosome 9 deletions appear to occur at the time of the initial translocation and are more common in patients with variant translocations [16].

The characteristic chromosomal rearrangement of CGL can be detected by conventional cytogenetics (Fig. 4.4), FISH, Southern blot analysis for rearrangement of the *BCR* gene and reverse transcriptase polymerase chain reaction (RT-PCR) for detection of *BCR-ABL* messenger RNA (mRNA). It should be noted that if Southern blot analysis is done using only a single commercially available probe, only *M-BCR* rearrangement will be detected [12]; use of a further

Fig. 4.4 Karyotype of a patient with CGL showing t(9;22)(q34;q11). The 22q– derivative chromosome is the Philadelphia chromosome (courtesy of Professor Lorna Secker-Walker, London).

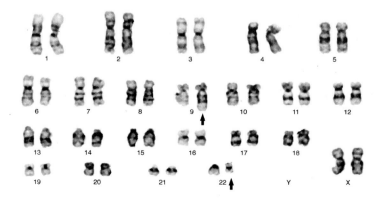

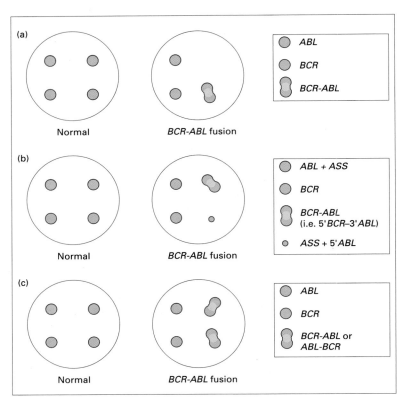

Fig. 4.5 Diagrammatic representation of three FISH strategies for detection of *BCR-ABL* fusion: (a) Dual-colour, single-fusion FISH. Normal cells have two red *ABL* signals and two green *BCR* signals. When t(9;22) is present, there is a red *ABL* signal, a green *BCR* signal and a yellow *BCR-ABL* fusion signal; (b) extra-signal, dual-colour FISH. The *ABL* probe encompasses also the upstream *ASS* (argininosuccinate synthetase) gene. A normal cell has two orange *ASS-ABL* signals and two green *BCR* signals. When t(9;22) has occurred, there are single normal red and green signals, a yellow fusion signal representing *BCR-ABL* (i.e., 5' *BCR*-3' *ABL*) and a small extra red signal representing *ASS* and 5' *ABL*; (c) dual-colour, dual-fusion FISH. Both probes are split by the t(9;22) translocation when there is a M-bcr breakpoint; normal cells have two red *ABL* signals and two green *BCR* signals whereas the translocation leads to a cell having single red *ABL* and green *BCR* signals and two yellow fusion signals representing *BCR-ABL* and *ABL-BCR*. The strategies outlined in (b) and (c) increase the specificity of the technique.

probe permits detection of *m-BCR* rearrangement also. However Southern blot analysis is now little used. FISH can be performed with a single probe for the *ABL* gene and a mixture of probes for the *BCR* gene, permitting detection of rearrangements within the major and minor breakpoint cluster regions. The use of two probes for 5' and 3' *ABL*, two probes for 5' and 3' *BCR* or two probes for each gene increases the specificity of FISH. Various FISH strategies are illustrated in Fig. 4.5. FISH permits the detection of deletions of chromosome 9 or chromosome 22 material, which are not detected by conventional cytogenetic analysis. Cases in which CGL is suspected should have conventional cytogenetic analysis performed and if a classical t(9;22) is not detected should be further studied by FISH, Southern blot analysis or RT-PCR. Such analysis is also indicated in patients with apparent essential thrombocythaemia with a high basophil count or with unusually small megakaryocytes since such patients may have a *forme fruste* of CGL.

During therapy, CGL can be monitored by conventional cytogenetic analysis, FISH or RT-PCR and its modifications [17]. Cytogenetic analysis has the advantage that the clonal evolution will be detected. However, if there is a major cytogenetic response to therapy, the technique is insensitive since conventionally only 20 metaphases are examined. FISH is a more sensitive technique as it is possible to scan many more metaphases. RT-PCR is more sensitive than FISH and can be made quantitative by use of techniques such as 'real time-PCR' (RQ-PCR). Neither FISH nor RT-PCR permits the detection of secondary cytogenetic abnormalities. It is important that the specific technique that is to be used for follow up of minimal residual disease is applied also to the diagnostic sample since deletions of chromosome 9 or 22 material will complicate interpretation.

Cytogenetic monitoring during follow-up may lead to the detection of clonal evolution within the Ph-positive clone. Less often, when therapy leads to reduction in the size of the Ph-positive clone and reappearance of Ph-negative metaphases, new clonal abnormalities may emerge from among the Ph-negative cells. This has been reported during interferon therapy but appears to be particularly common during imatinib mesylate (STI571) therapy with four instances being observed among 73 patients in two reported series [18, 19]; the abnormalities observed included those that occur in secondary leukaemias such as 5q– (2 cases) and monosomy 7 (1 case).

CGL in accelerated phase and blast transformation

After a variable period in chronic phase, usually several years, CGL undergoes further evolution. There may be an abrupt transformation to an acute leukaemia, designated blast transformation, or there may be an intervening phase of accelerated disease. The International Bone Marrow Transplant Registry has defined criteria for 'advanced disease', a similar concept to accelerated phase [20]. The WHO expert group have suggested the following criteria for accelerated phase: (i) myeloblasts constitute 10–19% of peripheral blood white cells or bone marrow nucleated cells; (ii) peripheral blood basophils are 20% or more of nucleated cells; (iii) there is persistent thrombocytopenia (platelet count $<100 \times 10^9/l$) that is not a result of treatment or persistent thrombocytosis (platelet count $>1000 \times 10^9/l$) that does not respond to treatment; (iv) there is an increasing white cell count (WBC) and increasing spleen size that does not respond to treatment; (v) cytogenetic evolution is present or (vi) there is marked granulocyte dysplasia or prominent proliferation of small dysplastic megakaryocytes in large clusters or sheets [21]. Whether cytogenetic evolution alone should be regarded as indicative of accelerated disease has been disputed, since patients classified as being in accelerated phase only for this reason appear to have a better prognosis than patients with other features of disease acceleration [3].

Blast transformation may be myeloid or lymphoid. It is important to make the distinction since there is far more chance of a useful response to therapy in a lymphoblastic transformation. Lymphoid blast crisis is more likely to emerge suddenly without a preceding accelerated phase [22]. Transformation may occur initially in the bone marrow or in extramedullary tissues. The WHO expert group have suggested the following criteria for blast transformation: (i) myeloblasts constitute at least 20% of peripheral blood white cells or bone marrow nucleated cells; (ii) there is extramedullary proliferation of blast cells

or (iii) there are large aggregates and clusters of blasts in bone marrow biopsy specimens [21].

Clinical and haematological features

During the accelerated phase of CGL there may be refractory splenomegaly with recurrence of symptoms present at presentation. The peripheral blood often shows marked basophilia, refractory leucocytosis, anaemia and either thrombocytopenia or marked thrombocytosis. Dysplastic features may appear including the acquired Pelger–Huët anomaly of neutrophils or eosinophils.

Blast transformation may be similarly associated with recurrence of fever, weight loss and sweating. In addition there may be bone pain together with lymphadenopathy or other evidence of extramedullary disease. Bruising and bleeding may occur. Increasing numbers of blast cells, out of proportion to the numbers of maturing granulocytic cells, appear in the blood and there may also be circulating micromegakaryocytes and giant dysplastic platelets (Fig. 4.6). A minority of patients have hypogranular neutrophils or the acquired Pelger–Huët anomaly [23]. Blast transformation may be myeloid, lymphoid or biphenotypic/bilineage. Myeloid transformation may be mixed or may be predominately myeloblastic, monoblastic, myelomonocytic, hypergranular promyelocytic, eosinophilic, basophilic and/or mast cell, megakaryoblastic or erythroid. In pure lymphoid blast crisis there are increasing numbers of blast cells but without the dysplastic features associated with myeloid transformation and without a striking increase in the basophil count. In lymphoid transformation the blasts usually resemble those of the FAB categories of L1 or L2 ALL but rarely they resemble the blasts of L3 ALL [24].

Since the blast cells of acute transformation often show no evidence of differentiation, immunophenotyping may be necessary to confirm their lineage. Lymphoid blast crisis is usually B lineage but occasionally T lineage. B-lineage lymphoid blast crisis may be early precursor B cell or have a common ALL or a pre-B phenotype. Biphenotypic/bilineage leukaemias are relatively much more common in CGL in transformation than in *de novo* acute leukaemias.

In the accelerated phase, the bone marrow may show dysplastic features, some increase of blast cells and a striking increase of basophils. With the onset of acute transformation, there are increasing numbers

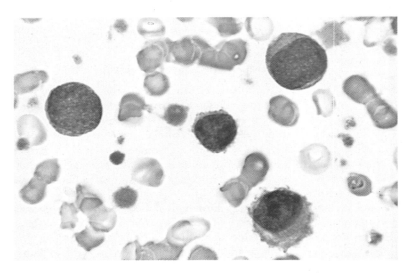

Fig. 4.6 PB film of a patient with megakaryoblastic transformation of CGL showing large platelets, several blast cells and a micromegakaryocyte. MGG × 870.

of blast cells, which rapidly replace maturing granulocytic cells. Myeloblasts are usually relatively undifferentiated with few granules. Auer rods are uncommon. Dysplastic features are usually present in various lineages. These may include numerous micromegakaryocytes and ring sideroblasts are sometimes present. The blast percentage is generally higher in lymphoid transformation [22].

In the accelerated phase the trephine biopsy shows disorganization and dysplastic features. There may be increasing numbers of blast cells, initially in a paratrabecular and periarteriolar distribution but subsequently also in the intertrabecular space. Following the onset of blast transformation, there is progressive replacement of maturing granulocytic cells by blast cells. In megakaryoblastic transformation there are often also large numbers of dysplastic megakaryocytes including micromegakaryocytes, occurring in clumps. Reticulin fibrosis is increased. Collagen fibrosis can occur, sometimes with associated osteosclerosis; this is most commonly associated with myeloid transformation, particularly megakaryocytic/megakaryoblastic transformation.

Cytogenetic and molecular genetic features

Additional cytogenetic abnormalities often develop several months before the development of blast crisis. The commonest abnormalities, in order of frequency, are +8 (34%), +Ph (31%), i(17q) (21%), +19 (13%), −Y (9% of males), +21 (7%), +17 (6%) and −7 (5%),

followed by −17, +6, +10 and +14 (all between 3 and 5%) [25]. The secondary cytogenetic abnormality usually described as i(17q) may, in fact, be idic(17p11) [25]. Secondary abnormalities are more common in myeloid transformation than lymphoid transformation. The abnormalities most often reported with lymphoid blast crisis are +Ph, del(9p)— usually as ider(9q), del(7)(q22) and −7. Abnormalities most often reported with myeloid transformation are +Ph, i(17q), +8, +19, t(3;21)(q26;q22), inv(3) (q21q26), t(3;3)(q21;q26), and del(13)(q12q14) [11, 12]. However, a recent analysis suggests that there is actually little relationship between the nature of secondary cytogenetic events and lineage at blast transformation. Johansson *et al.* [25] reviewed all published cases and concluded that i(17q) was more common in myeloid blast crisis whereas hypodiploidy and −7 were more common in lymphoid blast crisis [25]. In addition, although balanced translocations show a similar prevalence in myeloid and lymphoid blast crisis, the specific balanced translocations associated with myeloid blast crisis include those also seen in acute myeloid leukaemia (AML) and the myelodysplastic syndromes (MDS) (such as chromosomal rearrangements with a 3q21 or 3q26 breakpoint —t(3;21), t(3;3) and inv(3), t(8;21), t(15;17) and inv(16), which are not seen in lymphoid blast crisis [25]. Chromosome 3q21 and 3q26 abnormalities are often associated with large numbers of lymphocyte-sized micromegakaryocytes [26]. An isochromosome of 17q is associated with Pelger–Huët neutrophils and prominent peripheral blood basophilia, the basophil count being usually more than 10% and often more than 20% [25, 27].

Molecular genetic abnormalities sometimes present include upregulation of *MYC* and *EVI1*, mutation of *RAS* and point mutations and amplification of *BCR-ABL* [11, 28–30]. Amplification of *BCR-ABL* has been associated with refractoriness to imatinib mesylate therapy [30]. Tumour-suppressor genes may also be implicated in disease progression. *TP53* abnormalities are common and usually associated with myeloid blast crisis whereas *RB1* abnormalities are mainly associated with lymphoid and possibly megakaryoblastic blast crisis [11, 28, 29]. Homozygous deletions of *CDKN2A*, encoding p16^{INK4A}, are associated with lymphoid blast crisis [25, 31].

Chronic neutrophilic leukaemia

Chronic neutrophilic leukaemia is a rare Ph-negative condition which, as defined by the WHO group, is characterized by an increased neutrophil count with only small numbers of circulating granulocyte precursors and no dysplastic features. It appears likely that some cases result from mutation in a multipotent stem cell and others from a mutation in a committed granulocyte precursor [32].

Clinical and haematological features

Chronic neutrophilic leukaemia occurs predominantly in the middle-aged and elderly. Characteristic clinical features are anaemia, splenomegaly and sometimes hepatomegaly. The median survival is 2 to 3 years [32].

The neutrophil count is markedly increased but the peripheral blood shows few granulocyte precursors (Fig. 4.7). Toxic granulation, Döhle bodies and ring-shaped neutrophil nuclei may be present. Typical myelodysplastic features such as hypogranular neutrophils, the acquired Pelger–Huët anomaly and micromegakaryocytes are not usually seen. A variant has been described in which dysplastic features are prominent [33] but in the WHO classification such cases would not be classified as neutrophilic leukaemia. The NAP score is usually high but may be reduced. Serum vitamin B$_{12}$ concentration is increased. There may be hyperuricaemia, and gout has occurred. Serum granulocyte colony-stimulating factor (G-CSF) is reduced. Some cases have developed bone marrow fibrosis and osteosclerosis [34]; an alternative classification of such cases would be as the hypercellular phase of idiopathic myelofibrosis.

In the WHO classification, the following criteria for the diagnosis of chronic neutrophilic leukaemia are suggested: (i) peripheral blood showing white cell count (WBC) at least 25×10^9/l, neutrophils and band forms more than 80% of white cells, blast cells less than 1% and immature granulocytes (metamyelocytes to promyelocytes) less than 10% of white cells; (ii) bone marrow showing neutrophil hyperplasia with normal maturation and blast cells less than 5% of nucleated cells; (iii) hepatosplenomegaly; (iv) no identifiable cause of reactive neutrophilia, or, if a

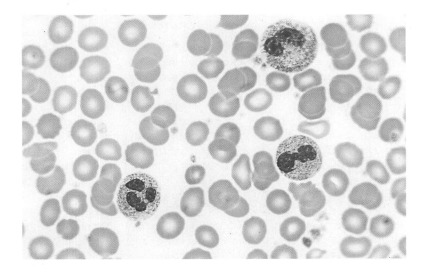

Fig. 4.7 PB film of a patient with neutrophilic leukaemia showing an increase of mature neutrophils, which show toxic granulation. MGG × 870.

potential cause is present (e.g. a non-haematological tumour), demonstration of clonality of myeloid cells; (v) no Ph chromosome or *BCR-ABL* fusion gene; (vi) no evidence of polycythaemia rubra vera, idiopathic myelofibrosis or essential thrombocythaemia and (vii) no dysplasia with the monocyte count being less than $1 \times 10^9/l$ [35]. In the WHO classification, the presence of dysplasia would lead to the case being assigned to either the category 'myelodysplastic/ myeloproliferative disease, unclassifiable' or to that of 'atypical chronic myeloid leukaemia'.

It is important to distinguish chronic neutrophilic leukaemia from the neutrophilic leukaemoid reaction that can occur in association with multiple myeloma and other plasma cell dyscrasias in which cytogenetic abnormalities are absent and myeloid cells are considered to be polyclonal [32, 36]. However the report of evolution to acute myelomonocytic leukaemia in only one and a half years in one such patient is puzzling, since the short time interval does not suggest a therapy-related leukaemia and raises the alternative possibility that the patient did actually have chronic neutrophilic leukaemia [37].

Blastic transformation of chronic neutrophilic leukaemia has occurred in a fifth of reported cases [32, 38, 39]. It may be more frequent in patients with prominent myelodysplastic features and may be preceded by the development of dysplastic features in those patients who initially lacked dysplasia [35]. In other patients, the disease terminates with a rising white cell count that is refractory to chemotherapy [40].

Cytogenetic and molecular genetic features

By definition, the Ph chromosome and *BCR-ABL* rearrangement are absent. A number of clonal cytogenetic abnormalities have been reported including trisomy 8, trisomy 9, trisomy 21, 11q– and 20q– and other rearrangements involving the long arm of chromosome 20 [32, 38, 39] but the karyotype is more often normal [32, 35]. In those with an initially normal karyotype, a clonal cytogenetic abnormality may appear during the course of the disease.

Chronic eosinophilic leukaemia

Cases of leukaemia with eosinophilic differentiation and with 20% or more blasts in the bone marrow are regarded, in the WHO classification, as acute leukaemia. Eosinophil proliferation is also sometimes associated with ALL and in these cases the eosinophilia is usually reactive. Cases of leukaemia in which eosinophils predominate or are prominent but with bone marrow blast cells being fewer than 20% are referred to as eosinophilic leukaemia or chronic eosinophilic leukaemia. There are also other chronic leukaemias with eosinophilia but with monocytosis or with an increase of immature cells of neutrophil lineage that may be more appropriately classified as, respectively, chronic myelomonocytic leukaemia with eosinophilia or atypical chronic myeloid leukaemia. In addition, a number of specific entities can be recognized, which are best defined on the basis of cytogenetic and molecular genetic criteria (see below).

Clinical and haematological features

Patients with eosinophilic leukaemia usually present with anaemia, thrombocytopenia, hepatomegaly, splenomegaly, lymphadenopathy, and signs and symptoms of damage to the heart and other tissues caused by release of eosinophil granule contents. Survival is variable but often quite short, as a consequence either of disease progression or of organ damage.

Eosinophils are increased in the blood and there may also be an increase of eosinophil precursors including blast cells (Fig. 4.8). An eosinophil count in excess of $1.5 \times 10^9/l$ is a WHO criterion for this diagnosis [41] but in many patients the count is much higher. Eosinophils often show morphological abnormalities such as vacuolation, degranulation, hypolobulation and hyperlobulation. Some patients also have neutrophilia or monocytosis.

The bone marrow shows increased eosinophils and precursors and sometimes also an increase in blast cells.

A particular problem occurs in establishing the diagnosis of eosinophilic leukaemia in patients with a marked increase of mature eosinophils but with no excess of blast cells. The differential diagnosis is between reactive eosinophilia, eosinophilic leukaemia and the idiopathic hypereosinophilic syndrome. The nature of the latter condition is not certain. Although some patients can be recognized in retrospect as having had eosinophilic leukaemia, others die as a result of eosinophil-mediated tissue damage without any incontrovertible evidence of a leukaemic process having emerged. Marked eosinophilia and the presence

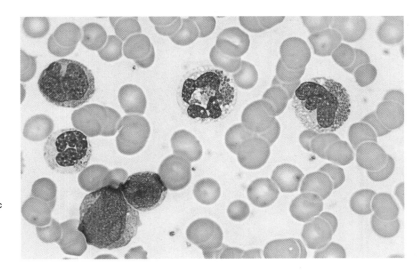

Fig. 4.8 PB film of a patient with chronic eosinophilic leukaemia with trisomy 10 showing a neutrophil, two abnormal eosinophils, a granulocyte precursor and two blast cells. MGG × 870.

of morphological abnormalities in eosinophils are of little use in confirming the diagnosis of leukaemia since they may occur also in reactive eosinophilia and in the idiopathic hypereosinophilic syndrome. The demonstration of a clonal cytogenetic abnormality (see below) can be regarded as confirmatory of leukaemia. If there is neither an increase in blast cells nor a cytogenetic abnormality the non-committal diagnosis of idiopathic hypereosinophilic syndrome is preferable.

A WHO expert group has provided guidance as to how eosinophilic leukaemia is distinguished from the various conditions with which it may be confused: (i) the presence of non-neoplastic diseases, e.g. parasitic infection or connective tissue disease, likely to cause reactive eosinophilia is excluded; (ii) the presence of haematological neoplasms likely to cause reactive eosinophilia, e.g. non-Hodgkin's lymphoma, is excluded; (iii) the presence of other haematological neoplasms in which eosinophils are part of the leukaemic clone, e.g. CGL, is excluded; (iv) the presence of a phenotypically aberrant cytokine-producing T-cell population is excluded; (v) if circulating blast cells are more than 2% or bone marrow blasts are more than 5% (but less than 20%) or if cytogenetic or other evidence of clonality is found a diagnosis of eosinophilic leukaemia is made; (vi) if no explanation of the eosinophilia is found and if the eosinophilia is persistent a diagnosis of idiopathic hypereosinophilic syndrome is made [42]. Some cases classified as idiopathic hypereosinophilic syndrome subsequently

develop a granulocytic sarcoma or transform into AML, providing evidence that the disorder was leukaemic/myeloproliferative from the outset.

Cytogenetic and molecular genetic features

A number of clonal chromosomal abnormalities have been observed in eosinophilic leukaemia, in addition to the t(5;12)(q33;p13) and t(8;13)(p11;q12) anomalies, which are described below. Those which have been observed in more than one patient include monosomy 7, trisomy 8, i(17q), trisomy 15, del(20) (q11q12), t(5;12)(q31;q13) and t(1;5)(q23;q33) [42]. The molecular basis of the leukaemia in these miscellaneous cases is not known, although it is likely that an oncogene in the 5q31–35 region is involved in a proportion of cases.

The 8p11 syndrome

A recurring cytogenetic abnormality, t(8;13) (p11–12;q12) is associated with a rare biphenotypic syndrome resulting from mutation in a pluripotent lymphoid/myeloid stem cell. Presentation may be as a myeloproliferative disorder with eosinophilia, as precursor T-cell lymphoblastic lymphoma or, rarely, as a precursor B-cell lymphoblastic leukaemia/lymphoma [42–45]. There is a slight male preponderance and a relatively young age of presentation (median age of presentation of reported patients is 32 years) [45].

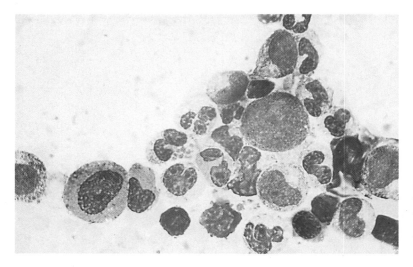

Fig. 4.9 BM film from a patient with the 8p11 syndrome who had a myeloproliferative disorder with prominent eosinophilia, subsequently transforming to AML (courtesy of Dr D. Macdonald). MGG × 870.

Clinical and haematological features

Presentation may be with simultaneous precursor T-cell lymphoblastic lymphoma and a myeloproliferative disorder with eosinophilia or, alternatively, with a myeloproliferative disorder with eosinophilia (Fig. 4.9) with subsequent development of precursor T-cell lymphoblastic lymphoma or granulocytic sarcoma/acute myeloblastic leukaemia. At least four patients have been reported who presented with or developed precursor B-cell lymphoblastic leukaemia/lymphoma, associated with bone marrow eosinophilia, in one case, preceded by T-lymphoblastic lymphoma and in another followed by acute myeloid leukaemia [46–48]. Two patients have been reported with preceding polycythaemia [46]. T lymphoblasts, B lymphoblasts and myeloid cells belong to the cytogenetically abnormal neoplastic clone. Generalized lymphadenopathy is common at presentation with the cases without lymphoma showing myeloid metaplasia of lymph nodes. The prognosis is poor although some patients have survived following bone marrow transplantation.

Cytogenetic and molecular genetic features

The majority of cases have been associated with t(8;13)(p11–12;q12) (Figs 4.10 and 4.11) but at least two other translocations with an 8p11–12 breakpoint have been recognized in association with the same syndrome [43, 45, 49]. In each instance there is formation of a fusion gene incorporating part of the *FGFR1* (**F**ibroblast **G**rowth **F**actor **R**eceptor 1) gene at 8p11 [49–53] (Table 4.3). *FGFR1* encodes a receptor tyrosine kinase for fibroblast growth factors. Partner genes of *FGFR1* have been *FOP, CEP110* and *ZNF198*. Patients with a *BCR-FGFR1* fusion gene may also represent the same syndrome; although their haematological features have been closer to those of CGL, one of the three reported patients progressed to lymphoid blast crisis at 6 months, with populations of both B-lymphoblasts and T-lymphoblasts being present [54], suggesting that these cases may represent a variant of the 8p11 syndrome. The observation of isolated cases with other cytogenetic abnormalities with disruption of the *FGFR1* gene suggests that there are further mechanisms of leukaemogenesis involving this gene.

Although at present allogeneic stem cell transplantation seems to be the treatment of choice in this syndrome, the development of specific blockers of the ATP-binding site of the FGFR1 protein means that an alternative form of therapy may become available.

Basophilic leukaemia

Cases of leukaemia showing basophilic differentiation with 30% or more of blast cells in the bone marrow are included in the FAB classification of acute leukaemia; they generally fall into the M2Baso or M4Baso categories but some are best categorized as M0Baso (see page 36). Cases of basophilic leukaemia with fewer blast cells generally have a chronic course. The majority have been demonstrated to have the Ph

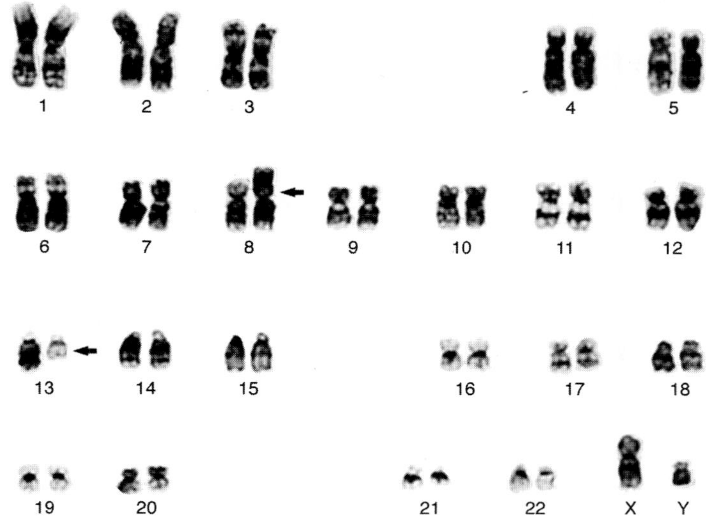

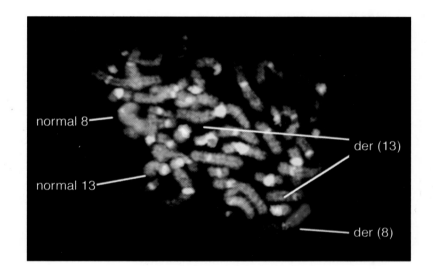

Fig. 4.10 Karyogram showing t(8;13) in a patient with the 8p11 syndrome (with thanks to Jill Elliot and the Regional Cytogenetics Service, Sheffield Childrens Hospital).

Fig. 4.11 FISH analysis from a patient with the 8p11 syndrome and t(8;13)(p11;q12) (with thanks to Dr A. Chase and the Cytogenetics Department, Hammersmith Hospital).

Table 4.3 Chromosomal rearrangements associated with the 8p11 stem cell syndrome and *FGFR1* rearrangement [49–53].

Chromosomal rearrangement	Molecular event, if known
t(6;8)(q27;p12)	*FOP-FGFR1*
t(8;9)(p12;q33)	*CEP110-FGFR1*
t(8;12)(p11;q15)*	*FGFR1* disrupted
t(8;13)(p11–12;q12)	*ZNF198-FGFR1*
t(8;17)(p12;q25)*	*FGFR1* disrupted
ins(12;8)(p11;p11p21)*	*FGFR1* disrupted
t(8;22)(p11;q11)†	*BCR-FGFR1*

*Single cases.
†Three patients.

chromosome [55] and are best regarded as a variant of CGL. Only Ph-negative cases should be categorized as basophilic leukaemia.

Clinical and haematological features

Patients with basophilic leukaemia may have signs and symptoms consequent on histamine excess [56].

Cytogenetic and molecular genetic features

By definition, cases are Ph negative and do not have *BCR-ABL* fusion.

Mast cell leukaemia/systemic mastocytosis

Mast cell leukaemia occurs either as a *de novo* leukaemia or as the terminal phase of systemic mastocytosis. Both these types of mast cell disease behave clinically as acute leukaemia and have been discussed in Chapter 1. Chronic mast cell leukaemia is part of the spectrum of systemic mastocytosis. Since there are few circulating mast cells and the clinical course is subacute or chronic it is probably better regarded as a myeloproliferative disorder rather than as a chronic leukaemia. However, for completeness, it is discussed here.

Clinical and haematological features

Chronic mast cell leukaemia is merely the more aggressive end of the spectrum of systemic mastocytosis. The usual clinical features are anaemia, hepatomegaly, splenomegaly, lymphadenopathy and symptoms of histamine excess including peptic ulceration. The peripheral blood shows only small numbers of mast cells, cases with large numbers behaving as acute leukaemia. The mast cells are often cytologically atypical (Fig. 4.12) with scanty granules and lobulated nuclei or with a higher than normal nucleocytoplasmic ratio. There may also be eosinophilia and monocytosis and eosinophils may be degranulated and vacuolated. The bone marrow is hypercellular and infiltrated by mast cells. There is often also granulocytic hyperplasia with prominent eosinophils together with increased lymphocytes. On trephine biopsy sections, there is a focal or diffuse infiltrate of mast cells, which are often spindle shaped. There may be granulocytic (neutrophilic and eosinophilic) and

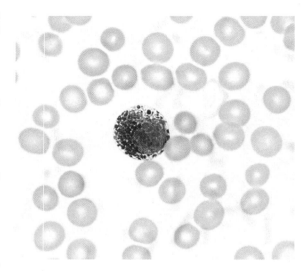

Fig. 4.12 PB film of a patient with systemic mastocytosis showing an abnormal mast cell. This cell is smaller than a normal mast cell and the cytoplasm is not so densely packed with granules. MGG × 870.

megakaryocytic hyperplasia, lymphoid infiltration, myelofibrosis and osteosclerosis. Mast cells stain metachromatically with a Giemsa stain and with toluidine blue and alcian blue; in histological sections they are more readily detected with these stains than with a haematoxylin and eosin (H & E) stain. Their presence can be confirmed by a positive chloroacetate esterase (CAE) reaction and by a positive immunocytochemical or immunohistochemical reaction for mast cell tryptase and c-KIT.

Cytogenetic and molecular genetic features

A variety of cytogenetic abnormalities have been observed. The molecular basis of the disease is almost always related to mutations in the *c-KIT* gene [57].

Atypical (Ph-negative) chronic myeloid leukaemia

Cases designated atypical chronic myeloid leukaemia (aCML) differ from CGL clinically, haematologically and cytogenetically.

Clinical and haematological features

There is a male preponderance. Most cases present

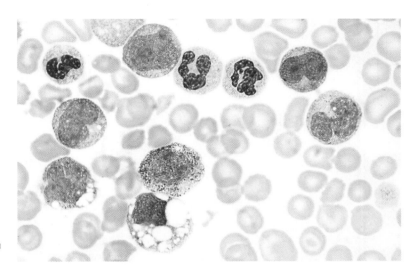

Fig. 4.13 PB film from a patient with chronic myeloid leukaemia supervening in idiopathic myelofibrosis. MGG × 870.

Table 4.4 French–American–British (FAB) criteria for the classification of certain chronic myeloid leukaemias [59].

	CGL	aCML	CMML
Basophils	>2%	<2%	<2%
Monocytes	<3%	>3–10% (usually >10%)	>3–10%
Granulocyte dysplasia	–	++	+
Immature granulocytes	>20%	10–20%	<10%
Blasts	<2%	>2%	<2%
BM erythroid cells	–	–	+

aCML, atypical chronic myeloid leukaemia; BM, bone marrow; CGL, chronic granulocytic leukaemia; CMML, chronic myelomonocytic leukaemia.

with splenomegaly, symptoms of anaemia and the haematological features of chronic myeloid leukaemia. Others initially present with MDS, mainly refractory anaemia, and subsequently develop the features of aCML [58]. Similar haematological features can also develop in the terminal phase of polycythaemia rubra vera, essential thrombocythaemia and idiopathic myelofibrosis (Fig. 4.13). Patients are on average 15–20 years older than those with CGL. The French–American–British (FAB) group [59] have suggested guidelines for distinguishing aCML from CGL and CMML (Table 4.4). However, whether aCML and CMML are two distinct conditions or merely two heterogeneous overlapping groups will only be determined when the molecular basis of each is better understood.

The peripheral blood shows leucocytosis (Fig. 4.14) with an increase of both neutrophils and their precursors but, in comparison with CGL, monocytosis is usually more prominent while eosinophilia and basophilia are less common [60]. On average, the white cell count is lower than in CGL whereas anaemia and thrombocytopenia are more common. Dysplastic features are common. Neutrophils may be hypogranular or have nuclei of abnormal shape. Some neutrophils may show the acquired Pelger–Huët anomaly. Promyelocytes, myelocytes and metamyelocytes are sometimes hypogranular. Monocytes may be immature. The neutrophil alkaline phosphatase score is commonly decreased but in a minority of patients is increased.

The bone marrow findings reflect those in the peripheral blood. There is granulocytic hyperplasia but, in contrast to CGL, the M:E ratio is usually less than 10:1. Basophil and eosinophil precursors are less often increased whereas monocyte precursors are sometimes more prominent (Fig. 4.15). Megakaryocytes are reduced in about a third of patients and may be dysplastic (Fig. 4.16). Blasts may be somewhat increased but are fewer than 30% or, in the WHO classification, blasts plus promonocytes are fewer than 20%.

aCML may terminate in blast crisis. This is usually a myeloid crisis but occasional lymphoid blast crises have been observed [61] suggesting that this condition, like CGL, may arise in a pluripotent stem cell.

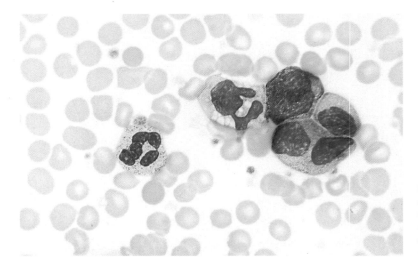

Fig. 4.14 PB film of a patient with atypical (Philadelphia-negative) chronic myeloid leukaemia (aCML) showing a neutrophil, a monocyte, a promyelocyte and two myelocytes, one of which is binucleate. MGG × 870.

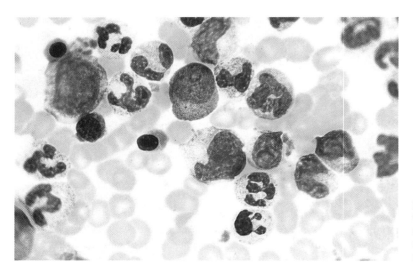

Fig. 4.15 Bone marrow (BM) film of the same patient as shown in Fig. 4.14 showing granulocytic hyperplasia with dysplastic features and several cells of monocyte lineage. MGG × 870.

Although aCML is usually readily distinguished from chronic phase CGL it can be difficult to make the distinction from CGL in early transformation when there may be both dysplastic features and an atypical differential count. Cytogenetic and molecular genetic analysis may be necessary.

Making a distinction from CMML can be more difficult. Useful features are a higher white cell count, a higher incidence of eosinophilia and basophilia and the presence of circulating granulocyte precursors, usually between 10 and 20%.

Cytogenetic and molecular genetic features

A number of clonal chromosomal abnormalities have been reported. No consistent association has been recognized although trisomy 8 is relatively common. *BCR-ABL* rearrangement has been reported in rare cases classified as aCML [62] but such cases are better regarded as true CGL with atypical features. Some patients categorized as aCML are found to have t(5;12)(q33;p13) but they are better regarded as a distinct syndrome (see below). Two patients have

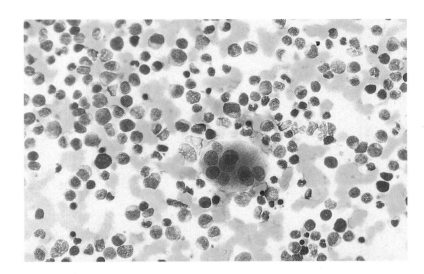

Fig. 4.16 BM film of a patient with aCML showing a multinucleated megakaryocyte. MGG × 384.

been reported with t(5;10)(q33;q21.2–22) with formation of an *H4/D10S170-PDGFRB* fusion gene and may be regarded as part of the same syndrome [49]. In the majority of patients there is neither a translocation nor a fusion gene and the leukaemogenic mechanism is unknown.

Chronic myelomonocytic leukaemia (WHO classification)

Chronic myelomonocytic leukaemia (CMML), as defined by the FAB group, has been discussed on page 156 and some of the diagnostic criteria are summarized in Fig. 3.2. In the WHO classification, CMML is defined as a myelodysplastic/myeloproliferative disorder with a monocyte count of greater than $1 \times 10^9/l$, no Ph chromosome or *BCR-ABL* fusion gene and fewer than 20% blasts plus promonocytes in the blood and marrow [63]. In addition, in cases that do not have significant dysplasia in two or more myeloid lineages there must be a clonal cytogenetic abnormality or the monocytosis must have persisted for at least three months with there being no other detectable cause of the monocytosis. CMML is further divided into CMML-1, with blasts being less than 5% in the blood and less than 10% in the bone marrow, and CMML-2, with blasts being above these levels in blood, bone marrow or both, or with Auer rods being present. The WHO classification recognizes a further subcategory of CMML with eosinophilia when the eosinophil count is greater than $1.5 \times 10^9/l$.

Some of these patients have a translocation with rearrangement of the *ETV6* gene, most often t(5;12) (q33;p13) with formation of a *PDGFRB-ETV6* fusion gene, and are better recognized as a discrete entity (see below). Uncommonly, there are other translocations involving the *PDGFRB* gene, such as t(5;7) (q33;q11.2), with formation of a *HIP1-PDGFRB* fusion gene (one patient), or t(5;17)(q33;p13) with formation of a *RAB5-PDGFRB* fusion gene (one patient) [49].

The clinical and haematological features of CMML, as defined in the WHO classification, are similar to those described for CMML as defined by the FAB group (see page 156). In the majority of patients there is neither a translocation nor a fusion gene and the leukaemogenic mechanism is unknown.

Myeloproliferative/myelodysplastic condition with t(5;12)(q31~33;p13) and related abnormalities

A recurring cytogenetic abnormality, t(5;12)(q33;p13), has been associated with a number of cases of a chronic myeloproliferative/myelodysplastic disorder, often categorized as eosinophilic leukaemia or as CMML with eosinophilia [42, 49, 51, 64]. In the WHO classification, most cases would fall into the category of CMML with eosinophilia. Patients are usually relatively young (the median age of presentation of reported patients is 42 years) and there is a remarkable male preponderance with almost all reported patients having been male [64].

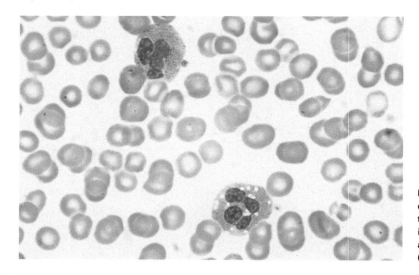

Fig. 4.17 PB film from a patient with chronic eosinophilic leukaemia with t(5;12)(q33;p13). One of the eosinophils is vacuolated but cytological abnormalities were fairly minor (courtesy of Dr Elisa Granjo, Porto).

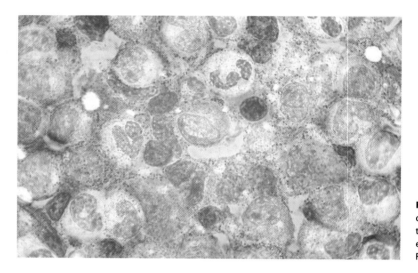

Fig. 4.18 BM film from a patient with chronic eosinophilic leukaemia with t(5;12)(q33;p13) showing marked eosinophil hyperplasia (same patient as Fig. 4.17).

Clinical and haematological features

Clinical features may include hepatomegaly and splenomegaly. The great majority of patients have had eosinophilia (Figs 4.17 and 4.18), and hypereosinophilic syndromes have occurred. Some patients have had neutrophilia, monocytosis, basophilia and anaemia and some have shown trilineage myelodysplasia. Acute transformation occurred in 16% of the reported patients [64]. The median survival of all patients is less than 2 years [64].

Cytogenetic and molecular genetic features

Cytogenetic analysis shows t(5;12)(q31–33;p12–13) (Fig. 4.19). The molecular mechanism of leukaemogenesis is fusion of the **P**latelet-**D**erived **G**rowth **F**actor **R**eceptor-**β** (*PDGFRB*) gene at 5q33 with the *ETV6* (previously known as *TEL*) gene at 12p13 [42, 65]. The 5q breakpoint appears variable because these rearrangements are often complex and FISH analysis may be misleading [64]. *PDGFRB* encodes a receptor tyrosine and the fusion gene is likely to lead

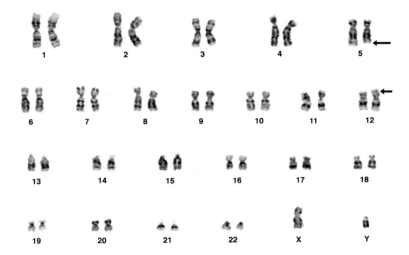

Fig. 4.19 Karyogram of a patient with chronic eosinophilic leukaemia with t(5;12)(q33;p13) (same patient as Figs 4.17 and 4.18, courtesy of Sofia Dória, Porto).

Table 4.5 Cytogenetic abnormality and fusion genes in chronic myeloproliferative/myelodysplastic disorders with t(5;12)(q33;p13) or related translocations resulting in rearrangement of *PDGFRB* gene [49, 51, 64].

Translocation	Fusion gene	Reference
t(5;7)(q33;q11.2)*	*HIP1-PDGFRB*	[66]
t(5;10)(q33;q21)†	*H4/D10S170-PDGFRB*	[67, 68]
t(5;12)(q31~33;p13)	*ETV6-PDGFRB*	[64]
t(5;17)(q33;p13)*	*RAB5-PDGFRB*	[69]

*Single cases.
†Two cases.

Table 4.6 Cytogenetic abnormality and fusion genes in chronic myeloproliferative/myelodysplastic disorders with t(5;12)(q31~33;p13) or related translocations resulting in rearrangement of the *ETV6* gene [49, 51].

Translocation	Fusion genes involving *ETV6*
t(3;12)(q26)(p13),	*ETV6-MDS/EVI1*
t(9;15;12)(p21;q15;p13)*,†	
t(5;12)(q31~33;p13)	*ETV6-PDGFRB*
t(9;15;12)(p24;q15;p13)*	*ETV6-JAK2‡*
t(9;12)(q22;p12)*	*ETV6-SYK‡*
t(12;14)(p12;q11–13) or	*ETV6-ABL‡*
cryptic or uncharacterized chromosomal rearrangement	

*Single cases.
†Second patient reported had RAEB-T (FAB classification of MDS) rather than CML.
‡*JAK2*, *SYK* and *ABL* encode tyrosine kinases so these cases may, as for *ETV6-PDGFRB*, involve dysregulation of a tyrosine kinase but in these cases it is a non-receptor rather than a receptor tyrosine kinase that is dysregulated.
CML chronic myeloid leukaemia; FAB French–American British classification; MDS, myelodysplastic syndrome; RAEB-T, refractory anaemia with excess of blasts in transformation.

to abnormal signal transduction. Variant translocations occur in which *PDGFRB* contributes to other fusion genes (Table 4.5). In each of the partner genes there are dimerization domains that are likely to contribute to the aberrant function of the fusion protein [64]. The identification of patients with rearrangement of *PDGFRB* and aberrant *PDGFRB*, function is important, in view of their reported responsiveness to imatinib mesylate [70]. There are also other patients with myeloproliferative/myelodysplastic syndromes who have involvement of *ETV6* but not *PDGFRB* (Table 4.6). In these patients there is often dysregulation of a tyrosine kinase.

Juvenile myelomonocytic leukaemia

Children suffer from a range of myelodysplastic and myelodysplastic/myeloproliferative disorders, which differ from those of adults [71–79]. If children who have been exposed to cytotoxic chemotherapy and those with genetic disorders such as Down's syndrome and neurofibromatosis are excluded, such disorders are much less common in children than in adults. Among the FAB categories of MDS seen in

Table 4.7 WHO criteria for a diagnosis of juvenile myelomonocytic leukaemias [79].

1 Monocyte count greater than 1×10^9/l
2 Blasts plus promonocytes less than 20% in peripheral blood and bone marrow
3 No Ph chromosome or *BCR-ABL* fusion gene
4 Two or more of the following:
   haemoglobin F percentage increased for age
   immature granulocytes in the peripheral blood
   white cell count greater than 10×10^9/l
   clonal chromosomal abnormality present
   myeloid progenitors hypersensitive to GM-CSF *in vitro*

GM-CSF, granulocyte-monocyte colony stimulating factor; Ph, Philadelphia chromosome.

children, refractory anaemia and refractory anaemia with ring sideroblasts (RARS) are uncommon, the latter so uncommon that an alternative diagnosis such as mitochondrial cytopathy or congenital sideroblastic anaemia should be considered. The FAB categories of MDS mainly observed are refractory anaemia with excess of blasts (RAEB), refractory anaemia with excess of blasts in transformation (RAEB-T) and CMML. However, these disorders differ clinically, haematologically and cytogenetically from the conditions given these designations in adults; generally there are both proliferative and dysplastic features. Two childhood syndromes previously considered to have distinctive features were designated juvenile chronic myeloid leukaemia and the infantile monosomy 7 syndrome. The WHO classification recommends that these two conditions and others with both dysplastic and proliferative features be categorized as juvenile myelomonocytic leukaemia (JMML) while cases lacking proliferative features are designated and classified as MDS. The criteria for the diagnosis of JMML are summarized in Table 4.7.

Clinical and haematological features

JMML is rare. Onset is usually in infancy and there is a male predominance. Ten to 15% of cases occur in children with neurofibromatosis, type 1, and in a similar percentage a mutation of the *NF1* gene is present without clinical features of the disease. Common clinical features of JMML include fever, anaemia, hepatosplenomegaly, lymphadenopathy, a rash and a bleeding tendency. Infections, including tonsillitis and bronchitis, are common.

The peripheral blood (Fig. 4.20) shows leucocytosis, neutrophilia and prominent monocytosis. Granulocyte precursors including blasts are often present. Some cases have eosinophilia or basophilia. Anaemia, thrombocytopenia and circulating nucleated red blood cells are common. Macrocytosis may be present, particularly in those with monosomy 7. Microcytosis is sometimes present but in the majority of cases, red cells are normocytic.

The bone marrow is hypercellular with granulocytic hyperplasia and usually an increase in monocytes and

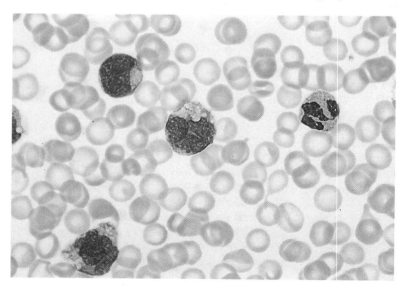

Fig. 4.20 PB film of a child with juvenile chronic myeloid leukaemia showing a blast cell and several cytologically abnormal monocytes. MGG × 870.

their precursors, eosinophils or basophils. Recognition of the monocytic component may require cytochemical stains. There may be erythroid hyperplasia. The blast percentage is often somewhat elevated. Trilineage dysplasia may be present.

There may be reversion to some characteristics of fetal erythropoiesis. The haemoglobin F level and the expression of i antigen are increased while the haemoglobin A_2 percentage, carbonic anhydrase activity, glucose-6-phosphate dehydrogenase activity and the expression of I antigen are reduced. It should be noted that haemoglobin F is elevated at birth and in normal infants may take 6 to 12 months to fall to adult levels. This should be considered when infants with an apparent myelodysplastic/myeloproliferative disorder present in early infancy. The concentration of serum immunoglobulin is increased in 50–80% of cases and some cases have a positive direct antiglobulin test or other autoantibodies. Serum lysozyme is increased.

Spontaneous colony growth from peripheral blood or bone marrow cells [76], resulting from hypersensitivity to granulocyte-macrophage colony-stimulating factor (GM-CSF), is characteristically present and is an important diagnostic criterion.

Although blast transformation occurs in only a minority of cases [75] the prognosis is poor, particularly in those with an onset after the age of 6–12 months. Unless bone marrow transplantation is carried out the median survival is less than a year [72]. Bad prognostic features include a later age of onset, a low platelet count and an elevated percentage of haemoglobin F [79].

Cytogenetic and molecular genetic features

Most cases are cytogenetically normal at diagnosis, although a variety of clonal chromosomal abnormalities have been described, either at diagnosis or during disease progression. Trisomy 8 occurs and as many as a quarter of cases have monosomy 7 at presentation or develop it during the course of the disease.

Molecular genetic abnormalities observed include a high frequency of *N-RAS* or *H-RAS* mutations [73]. Children with neurofibromatosis who develop myeloid neoplasms often show deletion of the normal *NF1* allele [74]. Other children may also have mutation of this gene. Neurofibromin, the protein encoded by *NF1*, is important in regulating the *RAS* family of oncogenes so that the two most common

molecular genetic abnormalities can be related to each other.

By definition, the Ph chromosome and the *BCR-ABL* fusion gene are absent.

References

1 Vardiman JW, Brunning RD and Harris NL (2001) Chronic myeloproliferative diseases: introduction. In Jaffe ES, Harris NL, Stein H and Vardiman JW (Eds), *World Health Organization Classification of Tumours: Pathology and Genetics of Tumours of Haematopoietic and Lymphoid Tissues*, IARC Press, Lyon, pp. 17–19.

2 Vardiman JW (2001) Myelodysplastic/myeloproliferative disease: introduction. In Jaffe ES, Harris NL, Stein H and Vardiman JW (Eds), *World Health Organization Classification of Tumours: Pathology and Genetics of Tumours of Haematopoietic and Lymphoid Tissues*, IARC Press, Lyon, pp. 47–48.

3 Lee SJ (2000) Chronic myelogenous leukaemia. *Br J Haematol*, **111**, 993–1009.

4 Spiers ASD, Bain BJ and Turner JE (1977) The peripheral blood in chronic granulocytic leukaemia. *Scand J Haematol*, **18**, 25–38.

5 Melo JV (1996) The diversity of BCR-ABL fusion proteins and their relationship to leukemia phenotype. *Blood*, **88**, 2375–2384.

6 Sokal JE, Cox EB, Baccarani M, Tura S, Gomez GA, Robertson JE *et al.* (1984) Prognostic discrimination in 'good-risk' chronic granulocytic leukemia. *Blood*, **63**, 789–799.

7 Hasford J, Pfirrmann M, Hehlmann R, Allan NC, Baccarani M, Kluin-Nelemans JC *et al.* (1998) A new prognostic score for survival of patients with chronic myeloid leukemia treated with interferon alfa. Writing Committee for the Collaborative CML Prognostic Factors Project Group. *J Natl Cancer Inst*, **90**, 850–858.

8 Thomas MJ, Irving JA, Lennard AL, Proctor SJ and Taylor PR (2001) Validation of the Hasford score in a demographic study in chronic granulocytic leukaemia. *J Clin Pathol*, **54**, 491–493.

9 Nowell PC and Hungerford DA (1960) A minute chromosome in human CML. *Science*, **132**, 1497.

10 Rowley JD (1973) A new consistent chromosomal abnormality in chronic myelogenous leukemia identified by quinacrine staining and Giemsa staining. *Nature*, **243**, 290–293.

11 Chase A, Huntly BJP and Cross NCP (2001) Cytogenetics of chronic myeloid leukaemia. *Bailliére's Clin Haematol*, **14**, 553–571.

12 Dewald GW, Juneau AL, Schad CR and Tefferi A (1997) Cytogenetic and molecular genetic methods for diagnosis and treatment response in chronic granulocytic leukemia. *Cancer Genet Cytogenet*, **97**, 59–66.

13 Sinclair RB, Nacheva EP, Leversha M, Telford N, Chang J, Reid A *et al.* (2000) Large deletions at the t(9;22)

breakpoint are common and may identify a poor-prognosis subgroup of patients with chronic myeloid leukemia. *Blood*, **95**, 738–744.

14 Herens C, Tassin F, Lemaire V, Beguin Y, Collard E, Lampertz S *et al.* (2000) deletion of the 5'-ABL region: a recurrent anomaly detected by fluorescence *in situ* hybridization in about 10% of Philadelphia-positive chronic myeloid leukaemia patients. *Br J Haematol*, **110**, 214–216.

15 Cohen N, Rozenfeld-Granot G, Hardan I, Brok-Simoni F, Amariglio N, Rechavi G and Trakhtenbrot L (2001) Subgroup of patients with Philadelphia-positive chronic myelogenous leukemia characterized by a deletion of 9q proximal to ABL gene: expression profiling, resistance to interferon therapy, and poor prognosis. *Cancer Genet Cytogenet*, **128**, 114–119.

16 Huntly BJP, Reid AG, Bench AJ, Campbell LJ, Telford N, Shepherd P *et al.* (2001) Deletions of the derivative chromosome 9 occur at the time of the Philadelphia translocation and provide a powerful and independent prognostic indicator in chronic myeloid leukaemia. *Blood*, **98**, 1732–1738.

17 Kaeda J, Chase A and Goldman JM (2002) Cytogenetic and molecular monitoring of residual disease in chronic myeloid leukaemia. *Acta Haematologica*, **107**, 64–75.

18 Marktel S, Khalid G, de Melo V, Bua M, Olavaria E, Marin D *et al.* (2002) Emergence of additional chromosomal abnormalities following treatment with STI571 (imatinib mesylate) for Philadelphia-positive chronic myeloid leukaemia in chronic phase. *Br J Haematol*, **117**, Suppl. 1, 13.

19 Byrne JL, Rogers J, Martin K, Parkin T and Russell NH (2002) Clonal evolution in patients treated with imatinib mesylate for CML in chronic phase. *Br J Haematol*, **117**, Suppl. 1, 15.

20 Savage DG, Szydlo RM, Chase A, Apperley JF and Goldman JM (1997) Bone marrow transplantation for chronic myeloid leukaemia: the effects of differing criteria for defining chronic phase on probabilities of survival and relapse. *Br J Haematol*, **99**, 30–35.

21 Vardiman JW, Pierre R, Thiele J, Imbert M, Brunning RD and Flandrin G (2001) Chronic myelogenous leukaemia. In Jaffe ES, Harris NL, Stein H and Vardiman JW (Eds), *The World Health Organization Classification of Tumours: Pathology and Genetics of Tumours of Haemopoietic and Lymphoid Tissues*, IARC Press, Lyon, pp. 20–26.

22 Cervantes F, Villamor N, Esteve J, Montoto S, Rives S, Rozman C and Montserrat E (1998) 'Lymphoid' blast crisis of chronic myeloid leukaemia is associated with distinct haematological features. *Br J Haematol*, **100**, 123–128.

23 Peterson LC, Bloomfield CD and Brunning RD (1976) Blast crisis as an initial or terminal manifestation of chronic myeloid leukaemia. *Am J Med*, **60**, 209–220.

24 Brunning RD and McKenna RW (1993) *Atlas of Tumor Pathology: Tumors of the Bone Marrow*. Third Series, fascicle 9. Armed Forces Institute of Pathology, Washington.

25 Johansson B, Fieretos T and Mitelman F (2002) Cytogenetic and molecular genetic evolution of chronic myeloid leukemia. *Acta Haematol*, **107**, 76–94.

26 Secker-Walker LM, Mehta A and Bain B on behalf of the UKCCG (1995) Abnormalities of 3q21 and 3q26 in myeloid malignancy: a United Kingdom Cancer Cytogenetic Group study. *Brit J Haematol*, **91**, 490–501.

27 Hernandez-Boluda J-C, Cervantes F, Costa D, Carrio A and Montserrat E (2000) Blast crisis of Ph-positive chronic myeloid leukemia and isochromosome 17q: report of 12 cases and review of the literature. *Leuk Lymphoma*, **38**, 83–90.

28 Ahuja HG, Jat PS, Foti A, Bar-Eli M and Cline MJ (1991) Abnormalities of the retinoblastoma gene in the pathogenesis of acute leukemia. *Blood*, **78**, 3259–3268.

29 Ishikura H, Yufu Y, Yamashita S, Abe Y, Okamura T, Motomura S *et al.* (1997) Biphenotypic blast crisis of chronic myelogenous leukemia: abnormalities of p53 and retinoblastoma genes. *Leuk Lymphoma*, **25**, 573–578.

30 Gorre ME, Mohammed M, Ellwood K, Hsu N, Paquette R, Rao PN and Sawyers CL (2001) Clinical resistance to STI-571 cancer therapy caused by BCR-ABL gene mutation or amplification. *Science*, **293**, 876–880.

31 Sill H, Goldman JM and Cross NCP (1995) Homozygous deletions of the p16 tumor-suppressor gene are associated with lymphoid transformation of chronic myeloid leukemia *Blood*, **85**, 2013–2016.

32 Reilly JT (2002) Chronic neutrophilic leukaemia: a distinct clinical entity, *Br J Haematol*, **116**, 10–18.

33 Zoumbos NC, Symeonidis A and Kourakli-Symeonidis A (1989) Chronic neutrophilic leukemia with dysplastic features: a new variant of myelodysplastic syndromes? *Acta Haematol*, **82**, 156–160.

34 Silberstein ED, Zellner DC, Shivakumar BM and Burgin LA (1974) Neutrophilic leukaemia. *Ann Intern Med*, **80**, 110–111.

35 Imbert M, Bain B, Pierre R, Vardiman JW, Brunning RD and Flandrin G (2001) Chronic neutrophilic leukaemia. In Jaffe ES, Harris NL, Stein H and Vardiman JW (Eds), *The World Health Organization Classification of Tumours: Pathology and Genetics of Tumours of Haemopoietic and Lymphoid Tissues*, IARC Press, Lyon, pp. 27–28.

36 Standen GA, Steers FJ and Jones L (1993) Clonality of chronic neutrophilic leukaemia associated with myeloma; analysis using the X-linked probe M27β. *J Clin Pathol*, **46**, 297–298.

37 Dinçol G, Nalçaci M, Dogan O, Aktan M, Küçükkaya R, Agan M and Dinçol K (2002) Coexistence of chronic neutrophilic leukemia with multiple myeloma. *Leuk Lymphoma*, **43**, 649–651.

38 Hásle H, Olesen G, Kerndrup G, Philip P and Jacobsen N (1996) Chronic neutrophilic leukaemia in adolescence and young adulthood. *Br J Haematol*, **94**, 628–630.

39 Matano S, Nakamura S, Kobayashi K, Yoshida T, Matsuda T and Sugimoto T (1997) Deletion of the long arm of chromosome 20 in a patient with chronic

neutrophilic leukemia: cytogenetic findings in chronic neutrophilic leukemia. *Am J Hematol*, **54**, 72–75.

40 Hanson CA, Dewald GW and Tefferi A (1999) Chronic neutrophilic leuemia (CNL): a long-term clinical, pathologic (sic), and cytogenetic study. *Blood*, **84**, Suppl. 1, 110a.

41 Bain BJ, Pierre R, Imbert M, Vardiman JW, Brunning RD and Flandrin G (2001) Chronic eosinophilic leukaemia and the idiopathic hypereosinophilic syndrome. In Jaffe ES, Harris NL, Stein H and Vardiman JW (Eds), *The World Health Organization Classification of Tumours: Pathology and Genetics of Tumours of Haemopoietic and Lymphoid Tissues*, IARC Press, Lyon, pp. 29–31.

42 Bain BJ (1996) Eosinophilic leukaemias and the idiopathic hypereosinophilic syndrome. *Br J Haematol*, **95**, 2–9.

43 Macdonald D, Aguiar RCT, Mason PJ Goldman JM and Cross NCP (1996) A new myeloproliferative disorder associated with chromosomal translocations involving 8p11: a review. *Leukemia*, **9**, 1628–1630.

44 Roy S, Szer J, Campbell LJ and Juneja S (2002) Sequential transformation of t(8;13)-related disease. *Acta Haematol*, **107**, 95–97.

45 Macdonald D, Reiter A and Cross NCP (2002) The 8p11 myeloproliferative syndrome: a distinct clinical entity caused by constitutive activation of FGFR1. *Acta Haematol*, **107**, 101–107.

46 Michaux L, Mecucci C, Velloso ERP, Dierlamm J, Cries A, Louwagie A *et al.* (1996) About the t(8;13)(p11;q12) clinico-pathologic entity. *Blood*, **67**, 1658–1659.

47 Still IH, Chernova O, Hurd D, Stone RM and Cowell JK (1997) Molecular characterization of the t(8;13)(p11;q12) translocation associated with an atypical myeloproliferative disorder: evidence for three discrete loci involved in myeloid leukemias on 8p11. *Blood*, **90**, 3136–3141.

48 Al-Obaidi MJ, Rymes N, White P, Pomfret M, Smith H, Starcznski J and Johnson R (2002) A fourth case of 8p11 myeloproliferative disorder transforming to B-lineage acute lymphoblastic leukaemia. A case report. *Acta Haematol*, **107**, 98–101.

49 Bain BJ (2002) An overview of translocation-related oncogenesis in the chronic myeloid leukaemias. *Acta Haematol*, **107**, 57–63.

50 Xiao S, Nalbolu SR, Aster JC, Ma J, Abruzzo L, Jaffe ES *et al.* (1998) FGFR1 is fused with a novel zinc-finger gene, ZNF198, in the t(8;13) leukaemia/lymphoma syndrome. *Nature Genet*, **18**, 84–87.

51 Gupta R, Knight CL and Bain BJ (2002) Receptor tyrosine kinase mutations in myeloid neoplasms. *Br J Haematol*, **117**, 1–20.

52 Fioretos T, Panagopoulos J, Larsen C, Swedin A, Billström R, Isaksson M *et al.* (2001) Fusion of the *BCR* and the fibroblast growth factor receptor-1 (*FGFR1*) genes as a result of t(8;22)(p11;q11) in a myeloproliferative disorder: the first fusion gene with *BCR* but not *ABL*. *Genes Chromosomes Cancer*, **32**, 302–310.

53 Demiroglu A, Steer EJ, Heath C, Taylor K, Bentley M, Allen SL *et al.* (2001) The t(8;22) in chronic myeloid leukemia fuses BCR to FGFR1: transforming activity and specific inhibition of FGFR1 fusion proteins. *Blood*, 98, 3778–3783.

54 Brody J, Basham K, Stanek A, Liu J, Koduru P, Cross NCP, Allen SL (2001) Rapid transformation to biphenotypic (B and T cell) lymphoid blast crisis in a patient with CML associated with the fusion of BCR to FGFR1. *Blood*, 98, 255b.

55 Goh K-O and Anderson FW (1979) Cytogenetic studies in basophilic chronic myelocytic leukemia. *Arch Pathol Lab Med*, **103**, 288–290.

56 Travis WD, Li C-Y, Hoagland HC, Travis LB and Banks PM (1986) Mast cell leukemia: report of a case and review of the literature. *Mayo Clin Proc*, **61**, 957–966.

57 Gupta R, Bain BJ and Knight CL (2002) Cytogenetic and molecular genetic abnormalities in systemic mastocytosis. *Acta Haematologica*, **107**, 123–128.

58 Oscier DG (1996) Atypical chronic myeloid leukaemia, a distinct clinical entity related to the myelodysplastic syndrome? *Br J Haematol*, **92**, 582–586.

59 Bennett JM, Catovsky D, Daniel MT, Flandrin G, Galton DAG, Gralnick H, Sultan C and Cox C (1994) The chronic myeloid leukaemias: guidelines for distinguishing chronic granulocytic, atypical chronic myeloid, and chronic myelomonocytic leukaemia. Proposals by the French–American–British Cooperative Leukaemia group. *Br J Haematol*, **87**, 746–754.

60 Kantarjian HM, Keating MJ, Walters RS, McCredie KB, Smith TL, Talpaz M *et al.* (1986) Clinical and prognostic features of Philadelphia chromosome-negative chronic myelogenous leukemia. *Cancer*, **58**, 2023–2030.

61 Hughes A, McVerry BA, Walker H, Bradstock KF, Hoffbrand AV and Janossy G (1981) Heterogeneous blast crises in Philadelphia negative chronic granulocytic leukaemia. *Br J Haematol*, **46**, 563–569.

62 Dreazen O, Klisak I, Rassool F, Goldman JM, Sparkes and RS Gale RP (1987) Do oncogenes determine clinical features in chronic myeloid leukaemia? *Lancet*, **i**, 1402–1405.

63 Vardiman JW, Pierre R, Bain B, Bennett JM, Imbert M, Brunning RD and Flandrin G (2001) Chronic myelomonocytic leukaemia. In Jaffe ES, Harris NL, Stein H and Vardiman JW (Eds), *The World Health Organization Classification of Tumours: Pathology and Genetics of Tumours of Haemopoietic and Lymphoid Tissues*, IARC Press, Lyon, pp. 49–52.

64 Steer EJ and Cross NCP (2002) Myeloproliferative disorders with translocations of chromosome 5q31-35: role of the platelet derived growth factor receptor beta. *Acta Haematol*, **107**, 113–122.

65 Wlodarska I, Mecucci C, Baens M, Marynen P and van den Berghe H (1996) *ETV-6* gene rearrangements in hematopoietic malignant disorders. *Leuk Lymphoma*, **23**, 287–295.

66 Ross TS, Bernard OA, Berger R and Gilliland DG (1998) Fusion of Huntingtin Interacting Protein 1 to platelet-derived growth factor β receptor (PDGFβR) in chronic

myelomonocytic leukemia with t(5;7)(q33;q11.2). *Blood*, **91**, 4419–4426.

67 Kulkarni S, Heath C, Parker S, Chase A, Iqbal S, Pocock CF *et al.* (2000) Fusion of H4/D10S170 to the platelet-derived growth factor receptor B in BCR-ABL negative myeloproliferative disorders with a t(5;10)(q33;q21). *Cancer Res*, **60**, 3592–3598.

68 Schwaller J, Anastasiadou E, Cain D, Kutok J, Wojiski S, Williams IR *et al.* (2001) *H4(D10S170)*, a gene frequently rearranged in papillary thyroid carcinoma, is fused to the platelet-derived growth factor receptor β gene in atypical chronic myeloid leukemia with t(5;10)(q33;q22). *Blood*, 97, 3910–3918.

69 Magnusson MK, Brown KE, Krueger LA, Arthur DC, Barrett J and Dunbar KE (2000) Rabaptin-5, a novel fusion partner to platelet-derived growth factor beta receptor in chronic myelomonocytic leukemia. *Blood*, **96**, 692a.

70 Apperley JF, Gardenbas M, Melo JV, Russell-Jones R, Bain BJ, Baxter EJ *et al.* (2002) Chronic myeloproliferative diseases involving rearrangements of the platelet derived growth factor receptor beta (PDGFRB) showing rapid responses to the tyrosine kinase inhibitor STI571 (imatinib mesylate). *N Engl J Med*, **347**, 481–487.

71 Passmore SJ, Hann IM, Stiller CA, Ramani P, Swansbury GJ, Gibbons B *et al.* (1995) Pediatric myelodysplasia: a study of 68 children with a new prognostic scoring system. *Blood*, **85**, 1742–1750.

72 Neimeyer CM, Aricó M, Basso G, Biondi A, Rajnoldi A, Creutzig U *et al.* and members of the European Working Group on Myelodysplastic Syndromes in Childhood (EWOG-MDS) (1997) Chronic myelomonocytic leukemia in childhood: a retrospective analysis of 110 cases. *Blood*, **89**, 3534–3543.

73 Neimeyer CM, Fenu S, Hasle H, Mann G, Stary J and van Wering E (1998) Differentiating juvenile myelomonocytic leukemia from infectious disease. *Blood*, **91**, 365–367.

74 Shannon KM, O'Connell P, Martin GA, Paderanga D, Olson K, Dinndorf P and McCormick F (1994) Loss of the normal *NF1* allele from the bone marrow of children with type 1 neurofibromatosis and malignant myeloid disorders. *N Engl J Med*, **330**, 597–601.

75 Castro-Malapina H, Schaison G, Passe S, Pasquier A, Berger R, Bayle-Weisgerber C *et al.* (1984) Subacute and chronic myelomonocytic leukemia in children (juvenile chronic myeloid leukemia), *Cancer*, **54**, 675–686.

76 Aricó M, Biondi A and Pui C-H (1997) Juvenile myelomonocytic leukemia. *Blood*, **90**, 479–488.

77 Tuncer MA, Pagliuca A, Hicsonmez FG, Ytgin S, Ozsoylu S and Mufti GJ (1992) Primary myelodysplastic syndrome in children: the clinical experience in 33 cases. *Br J Haematol*, **82**, 347–352.

78 Miyauchi J, Asada M, Sasaki M, Tsunematsu Y, Kojima S and Mizutani S (1994) Mutations of the N-ras gene in juvenile chronic myelogenous leukaemia. *Blood*, **83**, 2248–2254.

79 Vardiman JW, Pierre R, Imbert M, Bain B, Brunning RD and Flandrin G (2001) Juvenile myelomonocytic leukaemia. In Jaffe ES, Harris NL, Stein H and Vardiman JW (Eds), *The World Health Organization Classification of Tumours: Pathology and Genetics of Tumours of Haemopoietic and Lymphoid Tissues*, IARC Press, Lyon, pp. 55–57.

CHAPTER 5

CHRONIC LYMPHOID LEUKAEMIAS

In 1989 the FAB group published a proposed classification for chronic B- and T-lymphoid leukaemias [1]. The classification was based on cytology, immunophenotype and histology, which should now be supplemented by information derived from cytogenetic and molecular genetic analysis. This has been done in the World Health Organization (WHO) classifiction [2]. The chronic lymphoid leukaemias are broadly separated into those of B lineage and those of T lineage with a minority being of natural killer (NK) cell lineage. Non-Hodgkin's lymphomas (NHL) are closely related to chronic lymphoid leukaemias. Some lymphomas that may involve the bone marrow and peripheral blood are therefore included in the French–American–British (FAB) classification of chronic lymphoid leukaemias. For a more detailed classification of these and other lymphomas the WHO classification [2], which is based on the Revised European–American Lymphoma (REAL) classification [3], is recommended.

Cytological and immunophenotypic features are of major importance in the diagnosis and further categorization of lymphoid leukaemias. Neither provides a reliable diagnosis without the other. Sometimes precise diagnosis also requires trephine biopsy histology, lymph node or splenic histology or cytogenetic or molecular genetic analysis. Cytochemistry also has a role, albeit minor.

Cytology

Assessment of cytological features is usually best carried out on peripheral blood films but can also be done on films prepared from aspirates of bone marrow or other tissues or imprints from trephine biopsies or other tissue biopsies.

Immunophenotypic analysis

Immunophenotyping is essential for establishing if a leukaemia is of B or T lineage and will also help to distinguish acute lymphoblastic leukaemia (ALL) and lymphoblastic lymphoma from chronic lymphoid leukaemias. In addition, many chronic lymphoproliferative disorders have an immunophenotype that is sufficiently characteristic to be useful in diagnosis. In the case of B-lineage leukaemias, immunophenotyping will establish clonality and help to distinguish neoplastic from reactive conditions; neoplastic populations show light-chain restriction, i.e. cells express either κ or λ light chain but not both. Specific panels of monoclonal antibodies (McAb) have been recommended for the initial assessment and for the further characterization of lymphoproliferative disorders [1, 4, 5] (Tables 5.1 and 5.2). As for the acute leukaemias, immunophenotyping can be carried out by immunocytochemistry or by flow cytometry but the latter modality is the one now mainly employed.

The role of immunophenotyping in the investigation of lymphoproliferative disorders can be summarized as follows: (i) demonstration of light-chain restriction, generally indicative of clonal B-cell expansion and, for 65–75% of mature T-cell neoplasms, demonstration of clonal T-cell receptor (TCR)αβ molecule expression by means of antibodies to the variable (V) domains of TCR β chains [6]; (ii) recognition of characteristic immunophenotypic patterns that

Table 5.1 Panel of monoclonal antibodies recommended by the US-Canadian Consensus group for immunophenotyping in chronic lymphoproliferative disorders [4].

Lineage	Core panel	Supplementary panel
B	CD5, CD10, CD19, CD20, kappa, lambda	CD11c, CD22, CD23, FMC7
T/NK cell	CD3, CD4, CD5, CD7, CD8	CD2, CD16, CD56, CD57, TCR αβ, TCR γδ
Non-lineage restricted	CD45	CD25, CD38, BB4

NK, natural killer cells; TCR, T-cell receptor.

Table 5.2 Panel of monoclonal antibodies recommended by the British Committee for Standards in Haematology for immunophenotyping in chronic lymphoproliferative disorders [5].

Lineage	Core panel	Supplementary panel
B	CD19, CD23, CD22, CD79b, FMC7, Sm kappa and lambda	CD11c, CD103, HC2, cytoplasmic kappa and lambda, CD79a, CD138, cyclin D1
T/NK cell	CD2, CD5	CD3, CD7, CD4, CD8, CD11b, CD16, CD56, CD57, TIA-1
Non-lineage restricted	CD5	CD25, TdT

NK, natural killer cells; Sm, surface membrane; TdT, terminal deoxynucleotidyl transferase.

distinguish the chronic lymphoproliferative disorders from acute lymphoblastic leukaemia (ALL) and often support a specific diagnosis; (iii) recognition of different patterns of antigen expression within a specific disease category, sometimes indicative of differing prognosis, e.g. expression of p53 or, in chronic lymphocytic leukaemia, expression of CD38; (iv) confirmation of expression of a specific antigen (e.g. CD20 or CD52) when a monoclonal antibody is to be used in therapy; (v) monitoring of minimal residual disease, e.g. in CLL, monitoring of CD19-positive, CD5-positive, CD20-weak and CD79b-weak cells. Most antigens are expressed on the surface membrane but expression of cyclin D1 and p53 is nuclear so cells must be 'permeabilized' if these antigens are to be detected by flow cytometry.

Histology

In selected cases, histology of bone marrow, lymph node, spleen or skin can be useful in diagnosing chronic lymphoid leukaemias and in distinguishing them from non-Hodgkin's lymphomas. Characteristic patterns of infiltration observed in trephine biopsies and the terms conventionally used to describe them are shown in Fig. 5.1 [7]. It should be noted that the term 'interstitial' indicates that leukaemic cells are

infiltrating between the normal haemopoietic cells without disturbing the structure of the bone marrow. Conventionally the term 'diffuse' is used only to designate heavy infiltration that obliterates the normal bone marrow architecture; the term 'packed marrow' has also been used to describe this pattern of infiltration. Histology can be supplemented by immunohistochemistry. This is mainly needed in patients with only small numbers of neoplastic cells in the peripheral blood or bone marrow aspirate in whom immunophenotyping of cells in suspension is therefore not possible.

Cytogenetic and molecular genetic analysis

Cytogenetic analysis is sometimes useful in establishing clonality and in confirming the neoplastic nature of a lymphoproliferative disorder. More often it is useful in indicating a precise diagnosis since there are certain recurrent cytogenetic abnormalities that are characteristic of particular leukaemias or lymphomas. Karyotypic abnormalities may be detected by conventional cytogenetic analysis or by fluorescence *in situ* hybridization (FISH) or other *in situ* hybridization techniques.

Molecular genetic analysis is useful in establishing clonality by the detection of immunoglobulin (*IGH*)

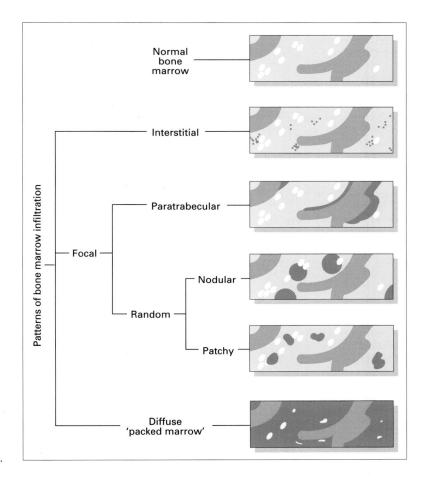

Fig. 5.1 Patterns of bone marrow (BM) infiltration observed in lymphoproliferative disorders (reproduced with permission from [7]).

or T-cell receptor *(TCR)* gene rearrangement. It is also useful in making a specific diagnosis since it is a means of identifying characteristic molecular rearrangements present in different subtypes of leukaemia or lymphoma. Molecular genetic analysis can be used for the monitoring of minimal residual disease. The most useful techniques are polymerase chain reaction (PCR), for analysis of genomic DNA, and reverse transcriptase PCR (RT-PCR), for detection of specific messenger RNA (mRNA) transcripts. Immunocytochemistry and immunohistochemistry can be regarded as extensions of molecular genetic techniques when they are used to identify the product of a specific gene. The cytogenetic and molecular genetic abnormalities most characteristic of various chronic lymphoid leukaemias are summarized in Table 5.3.

Chronic leukaemias of B-lymphocyte lineage

Chronic leukaemias of B-lymphocyte lineage express immunoglobulin on the cell surface membrane or, less often, in the cytoplasm. This may be a complete immunoglobulin or there may be expression of only heavy chain or only light chain. Since neoplastic B cells belong to a single clone, the immunoglobulin expressed is also monoclonal, i.e. it shows isotype restriction. Although monoclonal B cells express either κ or λ light chain, but not both, they may express more than one type of heavy chain (μ, δ, α, γ). Neoplastic B cells also express a variety of antigenic markers, some of which are shared with T lymphocytes or with haemopoietic cells and others of which are specific, within the haemopoietic and

Table 5.3 Cytogenetic and molecular genetic abnormalities most characteristic of chronic lymphoid leukaemias and lymphomas with a leukaemic phase.

Cytogenetic abnormality	Associated molecular genetic abnormality	Approximate frequency (where known)
Chronic lymphocytic leukaemia		
Deletion or rearrangements at 13q14	Sometimes deletion of the *RB1*, *DBM* or *BRCA2*	50%
del(11)(q22–23)	Deletion of *ATM*	20%
Trisomy 12	Unknown	20%
del(17)(p13)	Deletion or mutation of the *TP53* gene	10%
del(6)(q21)	Unknown	5%
Prolymphocytic leukaemia		
t(11;14)(q13;q32)	Dysregulation of *BCL1* by proximity to *IGH*	
Often complex, may include	As above or unknown	
trisomy 3, trisomy 12, del(6q),		
del(7q), monosomy 7,		
del(11)(q23), del(13q14)		
Splenic lymphoma with villous lymphocytes		
t(11;14)(q13;q32)	Dysregulation of *BCL1* by proximity to *IGH*	20%
Trisomy 3	Unknown	20%
Follicular lymphoma		
t(14;18)(q32;q21)	Dysregulation of *BCL2* by proximity to *IGH*	70–90%
t(2;18)(p12;q21)	Dysregulation of *BCL2* by proximity to κ	
t(18;22)(q21;q11)	Dysregulation of *BCL2* by proximity to λ	
Mantle cell lymphoma		
t(11;14)(q13;q32)	Dysregulation of *BCL1* by proximity to *IGH*, with consequent over-expression of cyclin D1 in the nucleus	90%
Lymphoplasmacytoid lymphoma		
t(9;14)(p13;q32)	Dysregulation of *PAX5* by proximity to *IGH*	
Burkitt's lymphoma		
t(8;14)(q24;q32)	Dysregulation of *MYC* by proximity to *IGH*	70–80%
t(2;8)(p12;q24)	Dysregulation of *MYC* by proximity to κ	
t(8;22)(q24;q11)	Dysregulation of *MYC* by proximity to λ	
T-cell prolymphocytic leukaemia		
inv(14)(q11q32), t(14;14)(q11;q32)	*TCL1* and *TCL1b* dysregulated by proximity to *TCRAD*	75%
t(X;14)(q28;q11)	*MTCP1* B1 dysregulated by proximity to *TCRAD*	
t(X;7)(q28;q35)	*MTCP1* B1 dysregulated by proximity to *TCRB*	

lymphoid lineages, for B lymphocytes (Table 5.4). Such antigens, expressed on the surface membrane of the cell or within the cytoplasm can be recognized by techniques employing monoclonal antibodies or, less often, polyclonal antisera (McAb, PcAb). Some of the immunophenotypic markers of leukaemic and normal lymphocytes are pan-B (characteristically positive with all B-lineage lymphocytes), some are pan-mature B, and some show selectivity for subsets of normal B lymphocytes and for cells in specific lymphoproliferative disorders. Chronic B-lineage lymphoid leukaemias do not express terminal

Table 5.4 Some monoclonal antibodies used in the characterization of chronic lymphoid leukaemias of B lineage.

Cluster designation	Specificity within haemopoietic and lymphoid lineage
CD19, CD20, CD24	B lineage; CD19 and CD24 are expressed early in B-lineage differentiation, CD20 later; CD24 is also expressed in neutrophils
CD21	CR2 (C3dR) complement receptor and also receptor for Epstein–Barr virus: subset of normal B cells, cells of majority of cases of CLL and about 50% of cases of NHL; also expressed on follicular dendritic cells
CD22	Most mature B cells and some B-cell precursors; cells of NHL, HCL and B-PLL
CD23	Low-affinity FcεR: expressed on activated B cells, cells of the majority of cases of CLL and CLL-PL and a minority of cases of PLL and NHL; also expressed on eosinophils, follicular dendritic cells and platelets
CD79a	Part of an immunoglobulin-associated heterodimeric membrane protein; expressed in cells of most B-cell lymphoproliferative disorders, both mature and immature
CD79b	Part of an immunoglobulin-associated heterodimeric membrane protein; expressed on normal B cells and in the majority of cases of most lymphoproliferative disorders; however, expressed in only a half of lymphoplasmacytoid lymphoma, a quarter of cases of HCL and only a small minority of cases of CLL
CD5*	Expressed on thymocytes and T lymphocytes and in many T-cell malignancies; expressed on a small subset of normal B cells, in a majority of cases of B-CLL and mantle cell lymphoma and in a minority of cases of B-PLL
CD10	Common ALL antigen but also expressed on some NHL, particularly follicular lymphomas and some plasma cell leukaemias and myeloma cells; more weakly expressed on some T-lineage ALL; expressed on some bone marrow stromal cells
CD25*	Interleukin 2 receptor: expressed on activated T and B cells, monocytes, hairy cells and ATLL cells
CD43	Expressed on T cells and activated B cells; expressed in CLL, small lymphocytic lymphoma and mantle cell lymphoma but not in follicular lymphoma, prolymphocytic leukaemia or hairy cell leukaemia; sometimes expressed in Burkitt's lymphoma, lymphoplasmacytic lymphoma and marginal zone lymphoma
CD38*	Early or activated T and B cells, subset of CLL haemopoietic precursors, thymic cells, plasma cells
CD103	Intra-epithelial lymphocytes, small subset of peripheral blood lymphocytes, hairy cells
FMC7	Subset of normal mature B cells (30–60%), cells of majority of cases of NHL, HCL and B-PLL but not CLL (unclustered but appears to recognize a conformational epitope of CD20 [8])
HLA-DR	Virtually all B lymphocytes and their precursors, activated T cells, haemopoietic precursors, monocytes (unclustered)
Anti-Ig,† anti-γ,† anti-α,† anti-μ,† anti-δ,† anti-κ,† anti-λ,†	Immunoglobulin and its constituent chains: SmIg is a pan-mature B marker; cytoplasmic heavy chain of IgM is detectable in pre-B cells (cμ) and in plasma cells (cIg); anti-γ, α, μ and δ, identify subsets of B cells and anti-κ and anti-λ are useful for demonstrating clonality

ALL, acute lymphoblastic leukaemia; ATLL, adult T-cell leukaemia lymphoma; CLL, chronic lymphocytic leukaemia; CLL-PL, CLL, mixed cell type; HCL, hairy cell leukaemia; NHL, non-Hodgkin's lymphoma; PLL, prolymphocytic leukaemia; SmIg, surface membrane immunoglobulin.
*Also positive in some or most T lymphocytes.
†Some polyclonal antisera are in current use.

deoxynucleotidyl transferase (TdT) or CD34 whereas lymphoblasts generally express TdT and sometimes express CD34. Conversely, lymphoma cells usually express surface membrane immunoglobulin (SmIg) and an antigen recognized by the FMC7 McAb whereas lymphoblasts do not.

DNA analysis shows that, in B-lineage chronic lymphoid leukaemias, the heavy-chain and usually the light-chain genes of immunoglobulin have undergone rearrangement; in some cases the gene for the β chain of the T-cell receptor (*TCR*) has also been rearranged.

Table 5.5 Characteristic immunophenotype of chronic B-cell leukaemias.

Marker	CLL	PLL	HCL	Follicular lymphoma	Mantle cell lymphoma	SLVL	Plasma cell leukaemia
SmIg	Weak	Strong	Strong or moderate	Strong	Moderate	Strong	Negative
CyIg	–	–/+	–/+	–	–	–/+	++
CD5	++	–/+	–	–	++	–	–
CD19, 20, 24, 79a	++*	++	++†	++	++	++	–
CD79b	–	++	–/+	++	++	++	–
CD23	++	–	–	–/+	–/+	–/+	–
FMC7, CD22	–/+	++	++	++	+	++	–
CD10	–	–/+	–	+	–/+	–	–/+
CD11c	–/+	++	++	–	–/+	+	?
CD25	–/+	–	++	–	–	–/+	–
CD38	–/+	–	–/+	–/+	–	–/+	++
HLA-DR	++	++	++	++	++	++	–

CLL, chronic lymphocytic leukaemia; CyIg, cytoplasmic immunoglobulin; HCL, hairy cell leukaemia; PLL, prolymphocytic leukaemia; SLVL, splenic lymphoma with villous lymphocytes; SmIg, surface membrane immunoglobulin.
The frequency with which a marker is positive in >30% of cells in a particular leukaemia is indicated as follows: ++, 80–100%; +, 40–80%; –/+, 10–40%; –, 0–9%.
*CLL cells express CD20 fairly weakly.
†HCL cells are negative with at least some McAb of the CD24 cluster.

The chronic leukaemias of B lineage can be further categorized as discussed below. Characteristic immunophenotypic markers of each disease entity are shown in Table 5.5.

Chronic lymphocytic leukaemia

Chronic lymphocytic leukaemia (CLL) is a chronic B-lineage lymphoproliferative disorder defined by characteristic morphology and immunophenotype. Small lymphocytic lymphoma is an equivalent lymphoma without circulating neoplastic cells [3, 9]. Mu (μ) heavy chain disease is a variant of CLL.

Clinical, haematological and cytological features

CLL is the most common leukaemia in western Europe and North America with an incidence in different surveys varying between 1 and more than 10/100 000/year. The incidence is lower in Chinese, Japanese and North American Indians and is higher in Jews. It is typically a disease of the elderly with a higher incidence in males. Some cases are familial, the pattern of inheritance suggesting a dominantly acting gene [10]. In the later stages, CLL is char-

acterized by lymphadenopathy, hepatomegaly and splenomegaly and eventually by impairment of bone marrow function. In the early stages of the disease there are no symptoms or abnormal physical findings and the diagnosis is made incidentally. Various arbitrary levels of absolute lymphocyte count have been suggested for the diagnosis of CLL (for example greater than 10×10^9/l) but the demonstration of a monoclonal population of B lymphocytes with a characteristic immunophenotype permits diagnosis at an earlier stage when the lymphocyte count is less elevated. A National Cancer Institute-sponsored working group has suggested that a lymphocyte count of greater than 5×10^9/l is sufficient for diagnosis when the immunophenotype is typical [11]. In CLL, both the lymphocyte count and its doubling time are of prognostic significance [12]. Spontaneous remission can occur in CLL but this is a rare occurrence [13]; when it occurs, the leukaemic clone may reduce to minimal levels [13].

Clinical features in μ heavy chain disease differ somewhat from those of typical CLL in that there is usually hepatosplenomegaly without peripheral lymphadenopathy [9].

The leukaemic cells are typically small with a conspicuous though usually narrow rim of cytoplasm

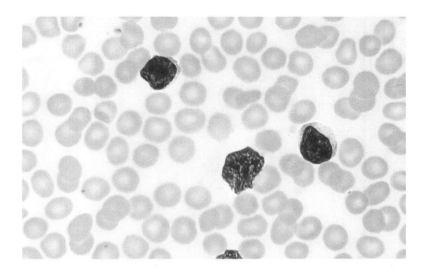

Fig. 5.2 Peripheral blood (PB) film in chronic lymphocytic leukaemia showing two mature lymphocytes and one smear cell. Nuclear chromatin is condensed and each cell contains a barely detectable nucleolus. May–Grünwald–Giemsa (MGG) × 870.

(Fig. 5.2). Cells are more uniform in their characteristics than are normal peripheral blood lymphocytes. The nuclear and cytoplasmic outlines are generally regular, although some cases have somewhat indented nuclei. Nuclear chromatin is dense and clumped with nucleoli visualized poorly if at all on light microscopy. The clumping of chromatin often gives the nucleus a mosaic pattern. Cytoplasm is weakly basophilic and sometimes contains small vacuoles and, occasionally, crystals. CLL lymphocytes are more fragile than normal lymphocytes and thus the formation of smudge cells or smear cells during the spreading of the blood film is common; this feature can be helpful in diagnosis but is not pathognomonic. The presence of up to 10% of prolymphocytes (see below for description) is compatible with the diagnosis of CLL. Some cases also show a minor population of lymphoplasmacytoid lymphocytes or cells with cleft nuclei; their presence correlates with a worse prognosis [13]. In a rare morphological variant, binucleate lymphocytes comprise a significant minority of cells [14].

In the early stages of the disease the peripheral blood abnormality is confined to the lymphocytes. Later in the disease course there is a normocytic, normochromic anaemia and thrombocytopenia. Neutropenia is uncommon unless cytotoxic therapy has been administered. Patients with CLL have a significant incidence of autoimmune disorders affecting haemopoietic lineages. Autoimmune haemolytic anaemia is particularly a feature of advanced stage disease; the blood film shows spherocytes and polychromatic macrocytes (Fig. 5.3). Autoimmune thrombocytopenia is associated more with earlier stages of the disease and may be the presenting feature [15]. The blood count and film show reduction of platelet numbers out of proportion to the degree of anaemia. Occasional patients develop Evans syndrome, i.e. autoimmune haemolytic anaemia plus autoimmune thrombocytopenia. The incidence of both autoimmune thrombocytopenia and autoimmune haemolytic anaemia has been reported to be increased by fludarabine therapy but this association has been disputed. Pure red cell aplasia is a less recognized association of CLL, which may be underreported [15]. It usually presents with anaemia of sudden onset and, if anaemia itself is excluded from the criteria for staging, it is associated mainly with early-stage disease. The blood film shows normocytic, normochromic red cells with an inappropriate lack of polychromasia and a reticulocyte count of close to zero. Severe anaemia and reticulocytopenia with preservation of a normal platelet count suggest this diagnosis. Autoimmune neutropenia occurs in about 1% of patients [16]. A case has been reported in association with fludarabine therapy [17].

Automated full blood counters produce characteristic scatterplots and histograms in patients with CLL (Figs 5.4 & 5.5).

The bone marrow aspirate is hypercellular as a consequence of infiltration by lymphocytes with similar features to those in the peripheral blood. The bone marrow lymphocyte percentage has been of

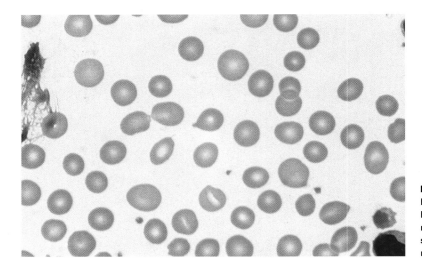

Fig. 5.3 PB film in chronic lymphocytic leukaemia complicated by autoimmune haemolytic anaemia showing one mature lymphocyte, one smear cell, spherocytes and polychromatic macrocytes. MGG × 870.

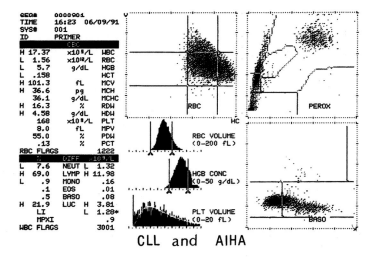

CLL and AIHA

Fig. 5.4 Histograms and scatterplots on a Bayer-Technicon H2 automated counter of peripheral blood from a patient with chronic lymphocytic leukaemia (CLL) complicated by autoimmune haemolytic anaemia. In the peroxidase channel scatterplot the neoplastic lymphocytes form a fusiform cluster extending from the 'debris' area (bottom left) through the lymphocyte box to the LUC box. (LUC = large unstained, i.e. peroxidase-negative, cells.) The presence of spherocytes has led to an increased proportion of hyperdense cells.

prognostic significance in some series of patients. In autoimmune haemolytic anaemia the bone marrow shows erythroid hyperplasia while in pure red cell aplasia there is a striking reduction in red cell precursors. In autoimmune thrombocytopenia, the bone marrow aspirate shows normal numbers of megakaryocytes. In μ heavy chain disease the bone marrow aspirate shows not only small lymphocytes but also vacuolated plasma cells [9].

Chronic lymphocytic leukaemia may undergo a prolymphocytoid transformation (see below) or a large cell transformation, referred to as Richter's syndrome. In prolymphocytoid transformation both the blood and the bone marrow show prolymphocytes whereas in Richter's syndrome the site of transformation is usually a lymph node or other tissue and the peripheral blood and bone marrow may show only the features of CLL. In other patients with Richter's syndrome, transformed cells are present in the peripheral blood and bone marrow (Fig. 5.6). It appears that Richter's syndrome represents transformation of a cell of the original clone in only two thirds of patients. When the two B-cell neoplasms are of independent clonal origin the emergence of the large cell lymphoma may be the result of immune deficiency with advanced disease. Epstein–Barr virus

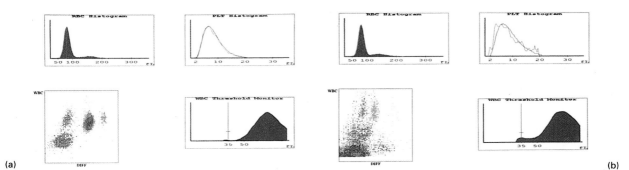

Fig. 5.5 Scatterplots on a Coulter Electronics Gen-S automated counter of PB from (a) a patient with CLL in comparison with (b) the blood of a normal volunteer. The CLL sample shows an expanded lymphocyte cluster.

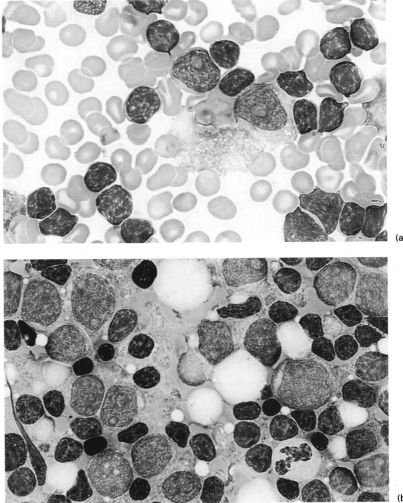

Fig. 5.6 (a) PB film in Richter's syndrome showing residual mature small lymphocytes and two large, immunoblast-like cells. (b) BM film in Richter's syndrome (same patient as Fig. 5.6a) showing a mixture of residual small mature lymphocytes and large, immunoblast-like cells. MGG × 870.

Table 5.6 The Rai staging system for chronic lymphocytic leukaemia [19].

Stage	Prognosis	Criteria
0	Favourable	Peripheral blood and bone marrow lymphocytosis only
I	Intermediate	Lymphocytosis and lymphadenopathy
II	Intermediate	Lymphocytosis plus hepatomegaly, splenomegaly or both
III	Unfavourable	Lymphocytosis and anaemia (haemoglobin concentration less than 11 g/dl)*
IV	Unfavourable	Lymphocytosis and thrombocytopenia (platelet count less than 100×10^9/l)*

*Although not specified by Rai and colleagues, anaemia or thrombocytopenia with an immune basis should not lead to categorization as stage III or IV.

Table 5.7 The Binet staging system for chronic lymphocytic leukaemia* [20].

Stage	Prognosis	Criteria
A	Favourable	Lymphocytosis with no more than two regions† having enlarged lymph nodes or other lymphoid organ; haemoglobin concentration greater than 10 g/dl and platelet count greater than 100×10^9/l
B	Intermediate	Lymphocytosis with three or more regions having enlarged lymph nodes or other lymphoid organs; haemoglobin concentration greater than 10 g/dl and platelet count greater than 100×10^9/l‡
C	Unfavourable	Haemoglobin concentration less than 10 g/dl, platelet count less than 100×10^9/l or both‡

*It is also possible to combine the Rai and Binet staging systems, giving the following stages: A(0), A(I), A(II), B(I), B(II), C(III), C(IV).
†A region being cervical, axillary, inguinal, liver or spleen.
‡Although not specified by Binet and colleagues, anaemia or thrombocytopenia with an immune basis should not lead to categorization as stage B or C.

Table 5.8 Criteria for a diagnosis of smouldering chronic lymphocytic leukaemia.

Binet stage A
Non-diffuse pattern of bone marrow infiltration
Haemoglobin concentration greater than 13 g/dl
Lymphocyte count less than 30×10^9/l
Lymphocyte doubling time greater than 12 months

(EBV) has been implicated in Richter's syndrome, both in cases showing [18] and not showing clonal identity. An uncommon transformation is to Burkitt's lymphoma.

The Rai [19] and Binet [20] staging systems for CLL incorporate clinical and haematological features (Tables 5.6 and 5.7). It is also possible to combine these two systems (see footnote to Table 5.7). In addition, it is useful to recognize a patient with 'smouldering chronic lymphocytic leukaemia' (Table 5.8) in

whom the disease is likely to run a very indolent course.

Immunophenotype

CLL cells express SmIg weakly; the heavy chain most often expressed is immunoglobulin (Ig) M, with or without IgD. Cells are positive with pan-B McAb such as CD19, CD20, CD24, CD79a and HLA-DR (see Table 5.5). In addition, leukaemic cells of the great majority of patients express CD5 (also a pan-T marker) (Fig. 5.7) and CD23 [21]. Reactivity with FMC7 and surface membrane expression of the pan-B markers CD22 and CD79b are usually absent or weak [22]; in three series of patients, CD79b was reported to be negative in 84%, 85% and 95% of cases respectively [23]. Expression of CD20 is usually weak although bone marrow and lymph node cells show stronger expression than circulating cells [24]. The complement receptor C3bR (CD35), which is

Table 5.9 A scoring system for the immunophenotypic diagnosis of chronic lymphocytic leukaemia (CLL) [21, 22].

Score 1 for each of the following:
- Weak expression of SmIg
- Expression of CD5
- Expression of CD23
- No expression of FMC7
- No expression of CD22*

A score of ≥4 points is confirmatory of CLL

---

*As an alternative, testing for CD22 can be omitted and a score of 1 can be given for negativity with CD79b [22]. This improves the discrimination between CLL and other disorders.

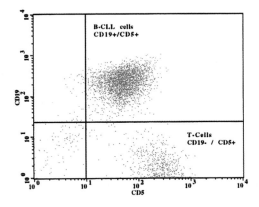

Fig. 5.7 Immunophenotyping by flow cytometry in CLL using a CD19 monoclonal antibody (McAb) labelled with phycoerythrin and a CD5 McAb labelled with fluorescein isothiocyanate; there is a major population of CD19+/CD5+ CLL cells and a minor population of CD19−/CD5+ normal T cells (courtesy of Mr R. Morilla, London).

present on normal B cells, is usually absent from CLL cells [25]. In most series of patients, CD11c and CD25 have generally been found to be expressed weakly, if at all, although in one series of patients 41% of patients were found to express CD25 in more than 30% of cells and CD11c has been reported as positive in between 13 and 70% of patients in different series [26, 27]; when positive, expression is weaker than in hairy cell leukaemia [27]. CD21, the C3d complement receptor and EBV receptor, is more weakly expressed than on normal B cells [25]. CD1c is expressed on about half of normal B cells, but is less often expressed in CLL [28]. CD45 is also often expressed more weakly than by normal B and T lymphocytes. CD45RA is expressed. CD43 is expressed

[29]; this marker may be quite useful in making a distinction from non-Hodgkin's lymphoma, although mantle cell lymphoma is also positive. CD40 is expressed and CD37 is strongly expressed. CD38 is expressed in 40–50% of cases. CLL cells show weak or moderate cytoplasmic or membrane expression of CD138, an antigen that is typically expressed by plasma cells and lymphoplasmacytoid cells [30]. Strength of expression of CD52 is similar to that of normal lymphocytes [31], a fact of relevance to the therapeutic use of this monoclonal antibody. Overexpression of *BCL2* protein, in comparison with expression on normal B lymphocytes, can be demonstrated [29]. Nuclear cyclin D1 is expressed in a significant minority of patients [32]. Nuclear expression of Ki-67 is very variable [33].

A worse prognosis in CLL has been linked to expression of both IgM and IgD rather than expression of IgD alone [34], expression of CD25 [35, 36], FMC7 [35] and CD14 [35], high levels of expression of Ki-67 [33] and expression of cyclin D1 in more than 5% of cells [32]. The most important immunophenotypic indicator of poor prognosis is CD38 expression [37–41], which correlates with expression of both IgD and IgM rather than of IgD alone [34].

CLL cells form rosettes with sheep erythrocytes whereas cells of other B-lineage lymphoproliferative disorders do not. However, with the availability of a large range of useful monoclonal antibodies this test is now redundant and will not be further discussed. The diagnosis of CLL is greatly aided by use of a scoring system that incorporates those immunophenotypic markers giving the best discrimination between CLL and NHL (Table 5.9).

In patients with early CLL, confirmation of clonality by demonstration of light-chain restriction can be facilitated by analysing κ and λ expression only on CD5-positive B cells.

Immunophenotyping of peripheral blood cells shows that absolute numbers of T cells, particularly CD8-positive T cells, are increased.

In Richter's syndrome the immunophenotype of CLL is generally retained although there may be altered expression of one or more antigen [18]. CD5 expression may, for example, be lost.

It should be noted that a small percentage of healthy adults who are apparently haematologically normal can be demonstrated to have very small numbers of B lymphocytes with the immunophenotype of CLL and with clonal rearrangement of *IGH* genes [42]; it appears that few such patients progress to overt CLL. Such clones can be demonstrated in as many as 3% of apparently haematologically normal hospital outpatients over the age of 40 years [43].

Histology

Trephine biopsy histology shows a pattern of infiltration which is either interstitial, nodular, mixed nodular and interstitial, or diffuse. The pattern of infiltration correlates with the stage of the disease, with interstitial infiltration being commonest in the earliest stages of the disease and a packed marrow pattern more characteristic of the later stages. However, the pattern of infiltration is also of prognostic significance, independent of stage. Diffuse infiltration ('packed marrow') is indicative of a worse prognosis than nodular or interstitial infiltration. The bone marrow, like lymph nodes, may show proliferation centres, a useful feature in making the distinction from non-Hodgkin's lymphoma.

Lymph node biopsy features are identical to those of small lymphocytic lymphoma; there is diffuse replacement by mature small lymphocytes with indistinct proliferation centres, containing larger nucleolated cells with the cytological features of prolymphocytes or paraimmunoblasts, which may give a pseudo-follicular pattern. The spleen shows variable infiltration of red and white pulp; white pulp infiltration usually predominates [9]. The infiltrate in the white pulp may show a pseudo-follicular pattern, attributable to the presence of proliferation centres [9].

On immunohistochemistry, CD5 expression is not always detected, even when it is detected by flow cytometry.

Cytogenetics and molecular genetics

Cytogenetic abnormalities [9, 41, 44, 45] appear to be secondary events in the development of CLL, sometimes being observed only in a subclone. The most characteristic abnormalities are deletion or rearrangements with a 13q14 breakpoint (50–60% of cases) and del(11)(q22–23) (20% of cases). Less common are trisomy 12 (10–20% of cases), del(17)(p13) (10% of cases) and del(6)(q21) (5–6% of cases). A small minority of patients (1–2%) have rearrangements of 18q21 with a heavy- or light-chain gene; in comparison with follicular lymphoma, t(14;18)

(q32;q21) is less common while t(2;18)(p12;q21) and t(18;22)(q21;q11) are more common [44]; the breakpoints on chromosome 18 differ at a molecular level from the breakpoints in follicular lymphoma [46]. A t(14;19)(q32;q13) translocation is found in less than 1% of patients, the genes involved being *IGH* and *BCL3* [47]. t(11;14)(q13;q32) and *BCL1* rearrangement have also been reported in a small proportion of cases of CLL but it is quite likely that this represents misdiagnosis of mantle cell lymphoma. Some patients have complex karyotypic abnormalities. There is a negative correlation between the presence of trisomy 12 and the presence of 13q14 abnormalities suggesting that these karyotypic abnormalities are associated with two independent leukaemogenic mechanisms. In some studies, trisomy 12 has been found to correlate with mixed cell morphology (see below) and a worse prognosis [48, 49] while isolated 13q14 abnormalities were seen in cases with typical morphology and a better prognosis. In other studies, poor prognosis appeared to be related to atypical morphology rather than to trisomy 12 in isolation [12, 50, 51]. Del(6)(q21) is associated with high white cell counts, bulky lymphadenopathy and an intermediate prognosis, similar to that of trisomy 12. Deletion of 11q23 correlates with younger age, bulky lymphadenopathy, atypical cytology, advanced disease, rapid disease progression and, in younger patients, worse survival [41, 52]. Del(17p), abnormalities of chromosome 14 and complex karyotypic abnormalities also correlate with a worse prognosis. Del(17p) may be associated with transformation. In one large series of patients, del(17p) and del(11q) were found to be independent poor prognostic features [53]. Trisomy 12, del(11q) and 13q14 rearrangements can be detected by conventional cytogenetic analysis and by FISH (Fig. 5.8). FISH is also applicable to the detection of del(6q), and del(17q). FISH techniques are more sensitive than conventional cytogenetic analysis and, in CLL, are the techniques of choice. FISH sometimes demonstrates that the cytogenetic abnormality is present only in a subclone and may show different cytogenetic abnormalities in subclones.

Some correlation between karyotype and immunophenotype has been observed. Cases with trisomy 12 are more likely to express FMC7 and show strong expression of SmIg [54]. Cases with a complex karyotype are also more likely to express FMC7 [54]. Cases with del(11q) have been found to have reduced expression of numerous adhesion molecules,

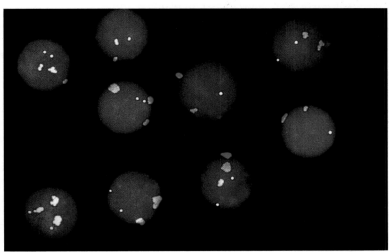

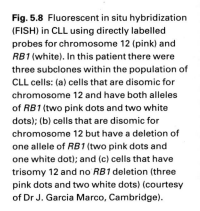

Fig. 5.8 Fluorescent in situ hybridization (FISH) in CLL using directly labelled probes for chromosome 12 (pink) and *RB1* (white). In this patient there were three subclones within the population of CLL cells: (a) cells that are disomic for chromosome 12 and have both alleles of *RB1* (two pink dots and two white dots); (b) cells that are disomic for chromosome 12 but have a deletion of one allele of *RB1* (two pink dots and one white dot); and (c) cells that have trisomy 12 and no *RB1* deletion (three pink dots and two white dots) (courtesy of Dr J. Garcia Marco, Cambridge).

including CD11a/CD18, CD11c/CD18, CD48 and CD58 [55].

Molecular genetic analysis has shown that CLL can arise either from a mutation in a naïve B cell with non-mutated V_H genes or from a post-germinal centre memory B cell with mutated V_H genes. The former has a worse prognosis [40, 56, 57]. Origin from a cell with non-mutated V_H genes was found to correlate with CD38 expression by two groups of workers [38, 58] but others observed poorer correlation [37, 40, 59]. Unmutated genes and CD38 expression have been found to be independent poor prognostic features [59]. The absence of proliferation centres in the trephine biopsy has also been found to correlate with non-mutated V_H genes [58]. Cases with trisomy 12 have predominantly unmutated V_H genes while cases

with a 13q14 abnormality more often have mutated V_H genes [9]. Median survival is about 3 years in those with non-mutated V_H genes whereas it is about 7 years in those with mutated genes [9]. The differences observed in these two subsets of CLL are summarized in Table 5.10.

At a molecular level, one study of abnormalities on chromosome 13 [60], found some patients to have deletion of the *RB1* gene at 13q14 but deletion of the *DBM* (**D**eleted in **B**-cell **M**alignancies) locus distal to *RB1* was more common and deletion at 13q12.3, encompassing the *BRCA2* (**Br**east **Ca**ncer susceptibility) gene, was the most frequent abnormality. *ATM* at 11q23 is deleted in patients with del(11q) and overall is mutated in about 20% of patients [61]; mutations are seen particularly in patients in whom the other

Table 5.10 Differences between CLL subsets with unmutated and mutated immunoglobulin variable (V_H) region genes.

	Somatic mutations of immunoglobulin variable region genes absent	Somatic mutations of immunoglobulin variable region genes present
Putative cell of origin	Pre-germinal centre naïve B cell	Post-germinal centre antigen-experienced memory B cell (CD5-positive subset)
Immunophenotype	CD38 usually expressed	CD38 not usually expressed
Cytogenetics	Increased prevalence of trisomy 12 and abnormalities of 11q and 17q	Increased prevalence of 13q14 abnormalities
Histology	Proliferation centres absent in trephine biopsy	Proliferation centres may be present in trephine biopsy
Prognosis	Worse	Better

allele is deleted [62]. The *BCL6* gene is mutated in about a quarter of patients [63]. The leukaemogenic mutation associated with trisomy 12 has not yet been elucidated but amplification of the *MDM2* gene at 12q13–15 has been suggested as a possible mechanism [45]. Mutations of the gene encoding CD79b are common and correlate with the lack of expression of the antigen that is likely to be responsible for the weak expression of SmIg in CLL [64]. Deletion or mutation of *TP53*, the tumour-suppressor gene that encodes p53, is relatively uncommon in typical CLL and correlates with progressive disease, refractoriness to therapy and poor prognosis [65]; overall, a *TP53* mutation or deletion is found in about 15% of patients. *TP53* deletion is usual in patients with deletions or translocations involving 17p13 and in these patients the other allele of *TP53* is usually deleted [62]. In other patients, dysfunction of p53 is the result of one or more *ATM* mutations [66]. The prevalence of various cytogenetic abnormalities and loss of specific cancer-suppressor genes can be related to whether or not immunoglobulin genes show hypermutation (see Table 5.10). Although *BCL2* is often overexpressed, rearrangement is demonstrable in only a small minority of patients [44].

Atypical CLL

Atypical CL is a chronic B-lineage lymphoproliferative disorder, which shares many features with CLL but shows cytological and sometimes immunophenotypic and cytogenetic differences.

Clinical, haematological and cytological features

The FAB group defined two cytologically atypical variants of CLL, designated collectively CLL, mixed cell type [1]; in some patients there was a spectrum of cells from small to large lymphocytes (but with fewer than 10% prolymphocytes) with an associated tendency to cytoplasmic basophilia while in others there was an increase of prolymphocytes so that they constituted more than 10 but fewer than 55% of lymphocytes (designated CLL/PL) (Fig. 5.9) [67, 68]. CLL/PL included patients who presented *de novo* with this morphology and others who underwent a 'prolymphocytoid transformation' of CLL. In one series of patients, those with CLL of mixed cell type tended to present with more advanced stage disease and to have a worse prognosis than classical CLL [69]. In another series the presence of more than 10% of prolymphocytes correlated with a worse prognosis [12]. Others have defined other atypical forms of CLL including cases with lobulated nuclei, correlating with trisomy 12 and worse prognosis [12], and cases with at least 10% of cells with deeply cleft or lobulated lymphocytes, a group associated with a higher white cell count, a lower platelet count and a worse prognosis [70].

Immunophenotype

About two-thirds of cases of CLL of mixed cell type have an immunophenotype typical of CLL. The other

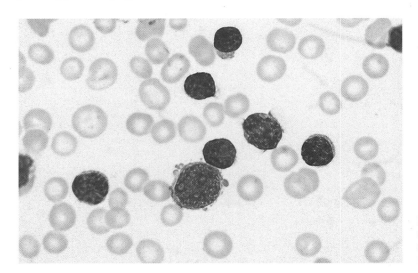

Fig. 5.9 PB film in CLL, mixed cell type, showing small mature lymphocytes and several larger cells, one with multiple nucleoli. MGG × 870.

third show atypical features such as strong expression of SmIg or CD20 or expression of CD11c or FMC7. In one study, atypical CLL with cleft or lobulated lymphocytes was associated with stronger expression of CD23 [70]. Atypical morphology is more common when there is expression of both IgD and IgM than when only IgD is expressed [34].

Cytogenetics and molecular genetics

Trisomy 12 is commoner in cases of atypical CLL than in CLL with typical cytological features whereas a normal karyotype and 13q– are less common [69]. *TP53* abnormalities are much more common than in typical CLL and are likely to be associated with progression of CLL to CLL/PL [65]. The development of trisomy 12 and of *TP53* abnormalities may represent independent pathways of transformation from CLL to CLL/PL [65].

Prolymphocytic leukaemia

Prolymphocytic leukaemia (PLL) is a chronic B-lineage lymphoproliferative disorder with prominent splenic involvement, specific cytological features and an immunophenotype resembling that of NHL rather than CLL. It was a defect of the REAL classification [3] that it did not distinguish between PLL and CLL since these are clearly quite distinct conditions. This has been remedied by the WHO classification in which B-PLL is specifically recognized [71].

Clinical, haematological and cytological features

PLL has a higher median age of onset than CLL and a higher incidence in men. It is characterized by a high white cell count and marked splenomegaly with only trivial lymphadenopathy [72].

The predominant cell is the prolymphocyte (Figs 5.10 and 5.11); a cut-off point of 55% of such cells has been found to be most useful in separating prolymphocytic leukaemia from CLL/PL [68]. The prolymphocyte is a large cell with often relatively abundant cytoplasm. The nucleus is round with relatively well condensed nuclear chromatin and with a prominent vesicular nucleolus showing perinucleolar chromatin condensation.

Immunophenotype

About two-thirds of cases of PLL have an immunophenotype that differs markedly from that of CLL. SmIg is strong, CD5 expression is low and FMC7 and CD20 expression are high. In the other third of cases, the immunophenotype is intermediate between the typical CLL phenotype and the typical PLL phenotype. In some patients cells express CD5 but show expression of FMC7 and strong expression of SmIg, thus immunophenotypically resembling cells of mantle cell lymphoma [73]. In the majority of cases of PLL there is expression of IgM with or without IgD but in a minority there is expression of IgG

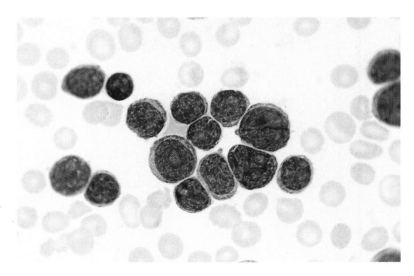

Fig. 5.10 PB film in B-prolymphocytic leukaemia showing cells that are regular in shape with round nuclei. Nuclear chromatin shows some condensation and the larger cells contain prominent vesicular nucleoli. MGG × 870.

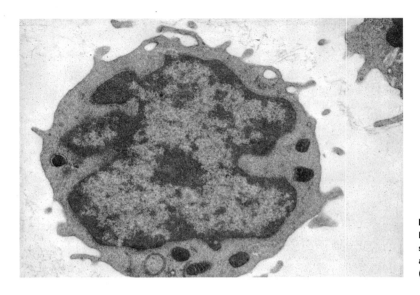

Fig. 5.11 Ultrastructural examination In B-lineage prolymphocytic leukaemia showing a prominent nucleolus and abundant cytoplasmic organelles (courtesy of Professor D. Catovsky).

or IgA. In contrast to CLL, CD79b is almost always expressed [74], as is CD22 [75]. CD11c is strongly expressed in the majority of patients [27].

Histology

The bone marrow is hypercellular with lymphoid infiltration. The trephine biopsy shows an interstitial/nodular or diffuse pattern of infiltration. Lymph node infiltration is diffuse with or without a pseudonodular pattern. Splenic infiltration is in both the red and white pulp with large proliferative nodules in the white pulp showing a characteristic bizonal appearance, dense at the centre and lighter at the periphery [76, 77].

Cytogenetics and molecular genetics

There are often complex karyotypic abnormalities. Among these have been noted trisomy 3 [75], trisomy 12 [78], del(6q), monosomy 7, del(7q), del(11)(q23), del(12)(p13), del(13)(q14) and various translocations involving chromosome 14 with a 14q32 breakpoint [75, 78–80]. Among the latter group the commonest is t(11;14)(q13;q32). However, it should be noted that some of the cases with t(11;14) and a diagnosis of PLL may actually represent mantle cell lymphoma; they express cyclin D1 and do not express CD23, which is often expressed in other cases identified as PLL; they have a worse prognosis [79]. Other trans-

locations observed have included t(6;12)(q15;p13) and t(2;3)(q35;q14) [78].

Mutations of *TP53* [81] and deletion of *RB1* occur [80].

Hairy cell leukaemia

Hairy cell leukaemia (HCL) is a chronic B-lineage lymphoproliferative disorder, usually presenting with splenomegaly and having distinctive cytological, histological and immunophenotypic features.

Clinical, haematological and cytological features

HCL occurs throughout adult life. It is considerably more common in males. The disease is characterized by splenomegaly with little lymphadenopathy. Circulating leukaemic cells are not usually numerous and many patients are pancytopenic. Severe monocytopenia is usual. Some patients have macrocytic red cells. A minority have a high white cell count with more numerous circulating hairy cells. Hairy cells are larger than normal lymphocytes or CLL lymphocytes. They have moderately abundant, weakly basophilic cytoplasm with irregular 'hairy' projections and consequently an ill-defined cell outline (Fig. 5.12). The cytoplasm may contain azurophilic granules or rod-shaped inclusions. Occasionally there are parallel linear structures in the cytoplasm

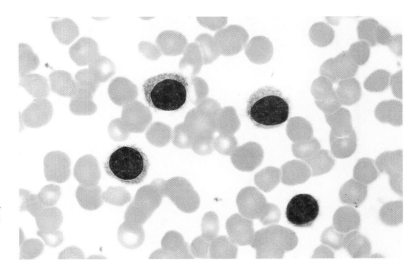

Fig. 5.12 PB film in hairy cell leukaemia. Cells have round nuclei with condensed chromatin and moderately abundant cytoplasm with ragged edges. MGG × 870.

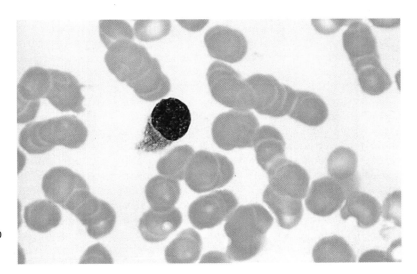

Fig. 5.13 PB film in hairy cell leukaemia showing a hairy cell containing a ribosomal lamellar complex. MGG × 100 (courtesy of Dr Laura Sainati, Padua, and Professor D. Catovsky).

(Fig. 5.13) that correspond to the ribosomal lamellar complex, which is demonstrated on ultrastructural examination. The nucleus is eccentric, and round, oval, dumbbell or kidney-shaped. The nuclear chromatin has a finely dispersed pattern and nucleoli are inconspicuous, small and usually single. In the great majority of cases of HCL the cells show tartrate-resistant acid phosphatase (TRAP) activity (Fig. 5.14). Such activity is rare, although not unknown, in other lymphoproliferative disorders. The bone marrow is usually difficult to aspirate as a consequence

of fibrosis but, when it can be aspirated, hairy cells are relatively more numerous than in the blood.

A large cell transformation may occur, most often in abdominal lymph nodes. Large cells may then be seen in the bone marrow.

Immunophenotype

Hairy cells have distinctive light-scattering characteristics on flow cytometry [73, 82]; forward light scatter is usually higher than in other chronic

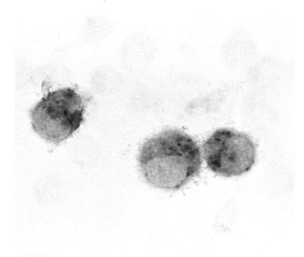

Fig. 5.14 Film prepared from a buffy coat of the PB of a patient with hairy cell leukaemia showing tartrate-resistant acid phosphatase (TRAP) activity. TRAP reaction × 870.

lymphoproliferative disorders and sideways light scatter may also be high.

Hairy cells have the immunophenotype of a relatively mature B cell. B-lineage-associated antigens CD19, CD20, CD22 and CD79a are expressed. The expression of CD22 is strong. CD79b is positive in about a quarter of patients [74]. SmIg is moderately strongly or strongly expressed with some cases also showing cytoplasmic immunoglobulin (cIg). SmIg is IgM and sometimes also IgD, IgG or IgA. CD5, CD10 and CD23 are negative. FMC7 is positive as is CD25, which represents the interleukin (IL)2 receptor and is a marker of activated T and B cells. CD11c is usually positive, and is characteristically strongly expressed. In addition to the expression of B-lineage-associated immunophenotypic markers, there are several markers that show a degree of specificity for hairy cells; they include HC2 [83], CD103 and, to a lesser extent, DBA44 [84]. CD103 is an integrin, also known as mucosal lymphocyte antigen (MLA), which is expressed on mucosa-associated T cells and some activated lymphocytes [29]. The presence of the isoenzyme of acid phosphatase identified cytochemically by TRAP activity can also be detected immunologically using a specific McAb. The use of a scoring system can help to distinguish HCL from other lymphoproliferative disorders with which it might be confused. If 1 point is scored for positivity with HC2,

CD11c, CD25 and CD103 then cases of HCL almost always score 3 or 4 while cases of hairy cell variant and splenic lymphoma with villous lymphocytes score 0, 1 or 2 [85].

Flow cytometry is a very sensitive technique for the detection of hairy cells and as few as 1% of cells may be detected. On flow cytometry, the identification of small numbers of hairy cells is aided by a comparison of side scatter of light and CD45 expression; hairy cells appear as a discrete population of cells which express CD45 more strongly than do normal lymphocytes or non-Hodgkin's lymphoma cells [86].

Histology

The trephine biopsy shows infiltration that may be interstitial in a hypocellular bone marrow, focal or diffuse. There is a highly characteristic pattern of infiltration with cells appearing to be separated from each other by a clear zone (Fig. 5.15). This pattern is more apparent on paraffin-embedded specimens than in plastic-embedded specimens, although the latter shows the cellular detail more clearly. The characteristic delicate chromatin pattern and indented or lobulated nuclei are usually readily apparent. Reticulin is increased. Spleen histology shows a distinctive pattern of red pulp infiltration with widening of the pulp cords and the formation of pseudosinuses lined by hairy cells. Immunohistochemical staining with CD20 or DBA44, assessed in relation to cytological features, can help in identification of hairy cells. Cyclin D1 is over-expressed in 50–75% of cases but this does not correlate with t(11;14) or *BCL1* rearrangement [87].

Cytogenetics and molecular genetics

A great variety of cytogenetic abnormalities have been observed including trisomy 5, trisomy 6, monosomy 10, monosomy 17, monosomy or trisomy 12, del(6q) and, most frequently, translocations with a 14q32 breakpoint (giving rise to both 14q+ and 14q–) [55, 88, 89].

Hairy cell variant

The variant form of HCL is a rare chronic B-lineage lymphoproliferative disorder, which has some clinical and cytological similarities to HCL but differs immunophenotypically, histologically and in its responsiveness to therapy.

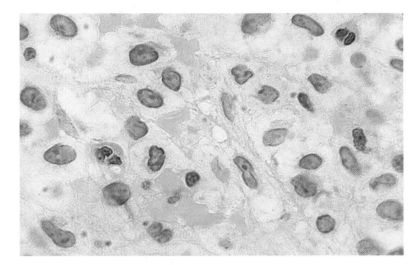

Fig. 5.15 Bone marrow trephine biopsy in hairy cell leukaemia showing cells with round, oval or irregular nuclei and scanty, ragged cytoplasm. The spacing of the nuclei is characteristic of this disorder. Two neutrophils and one erythroblast are also present. Paraffin-embedded, haematoxylin and eosin (H & E) × 870.

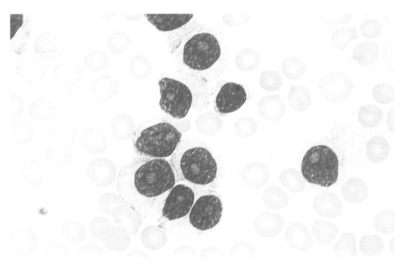

Fig. 5.16 PB film in the variant form of hairy cell leukaemia (hairy cell variant). Cells are nucleolated and it is evident that the white cell count is high. MGG × 870.

Clinical, haematological and cytological features

The variant form, like HCL, is characterized by splenomegaly with little lymphadenopathy. The white cell count, however, is usually high with peripheral blood leukaemic cells being numerous [90, 91]. In contrast to HCL, the monocyte count is usually normal. There may be mild anaemia and thrombocytopenia.

The cells of hairy cell variant leukaemia (Fig. 5.16) have a higher nucleocytoplasmic ratio than classical hairy cells, the cytoplasm is more basophilic and the nucleus has a more condensed chromatin pattern with a prominent nucleolus. The nucleus, in fact, shows more resemblance to that of a typical prolymphocyte than that of a classical hairy cell. There may be some binucleated cells and some larger cells with hyperchromatic chromatin. The TRAP reaction is almost always negative.

The distinction between HCL and hairy cell variant is clinically important since both interferon and nucleoside analogue therapy, which are, respectively, successful and highly successful in HCL, are often ineffective in hairy cell variant.

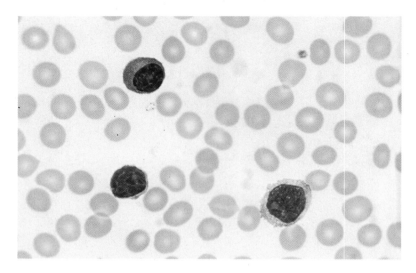

Fig. 5.17 PB film in splenic lymphoma with villous lymphocytes. The cells have small, inconspicuous nucleoli. One has villous cytoplasm and one is showing plasmacytoid differentiation. MGG × 870.

Immunophenotype

The immunophenotype is closer to that of PLL than to that of classical HCL. Negative reactions are usual with CD25 and HC2 although some cases are CD11c or, less often, CD103 positive. A scoring scheme for immunophenotypic markers has been found very useful if these four McAb are used [85]. CD79b is positive in about a quarter of patients [74].

Histology

Trephine biopsy sections most often show an interstitial infiltrate [91]. The spaced pattern of HCL may be totally absent or there may be a mixture of areas of denser infiltrate with areas in which cells are more widely spaced. Splenic infiltration is in the red pulp with a minority of cases showing blood lakes [91].

Splenic lymphoma with villous lymphocytes

Splenic lymphoma with villous lymphocytes (SLVL) is a chronic B-lineage lymphoproliferative disorder, which has in the past been confused with CLL but which differs clinically, cytologically and immunophenotypically. In the WHO classification, SLVL is regarded as a leukaemic variant of splenic marginal zone lymphoma. Transformation to a large cell lymphoma occurs in a minority of patients.

Clinical, haematological and cytological features

As suggested by the name, SLVL is predominantly a splenic lymphoma with only minor lymphadenopathy [92–94]. The incidence rises with age and is higher in men than women.

The white cell count varies from normal to moderately elevated. Up to a quarter of cases do not have an absolute lymphocytosis [94]. In patients with a high count the majority of circulating cells are abnormal lymphocytes whereas in those without lymphocytosis, villous lymphocytes may be as few as 5% of cells.

The neoplastic cells are larger than CLL cells. The nucleus is round to ovoid with clumped chromatin and, in about half the cases, a distinct small nucleolus (Fig. 5.17) [1]. The cytoplasm varies in amount, is moderately basophilic and has short villous projections, sometimes localized at one pole of the cell. The nucleocytoplasmic ratio is higher than in HCL or hairy cell variant. A minority of cells show plasmacytoid features, i.e. the nucleus is eccentric, basophilia is more pronounced and a Golgi zone is apparent. The TRAP reaction is usually negative.

Anaemia and thrombocytopenia may be present. Occasionally they are autoimmune in nature.

About a quarter of patients have a monoclonal immunoglobulin (IgG or IgM) in the serum while a smaller number have a urinary Bence Jones protein.

Immunophenotype

The SLVL cell corresponds to a relatively mature B cell with some features suggesting plasmacytoid differentiation (see Table 5.5). SmIg is strongly expressed and cytoplasmic immunoglobulin and CD38 [29] are sometimes detected. There is positivity for B-cell-associated antigens such as CD19, CD20, CD22, CD24 and CD79a and for FMC7. Expression of CD22 is strong. CD79b is positive in about three-quarters of patients [74]. Some of the markers characteristic of CLL, specifically CD23 and CD5, are usually negative (in one study 24% and 19% respectively were positive) as are CD10, CD103 and HC2 (in one study 23%, 6% and 4% respectively were positive) [93, 94]. CD11c is expressed in about 50% of patients [93, 94], CD25 in about a quarter [23, 93] and DBA44 in the majority [94]. It is important to use a panel of antibodies and to relate immunophenotype to cytology in order to distinguish SLVL from CLL, HCL and mantle cell lymphoma.

Histology

Plasmacytoid differentiation is often more prominent in histological sections than in peripheral blood cells. In contrast to CLL, the bone marrow is infiltrated in only about a half of cases. The pattern of infiltration can be either nodular or, in advanced disease, diffuse. Intrasinusoidal infiltration is characteristic and can be highlighted by immunohistochemistry. In contrast to CLL, PLL, HCL and hairy cell variant, splenic infiltration is often predominantly in the white pulp and nodular, in early cases with selective involvement of the marginal zone [1, 77, 95]. There may also be a scattering of small nodules in the red pulp.

Cytogenetics and molecular genetics

About 20% of cases have t(11;14)(q13;q32), a translocation more characteristic of mantle cell lymphoma. It has, however, been suggested on the basis of splenic histology that cases with t(11;14) and cyclin D1 expression may be more correctly categorized as mantle cell lymphoma [96]. The t(11;14)(p11;q32) translocation has been observed in a small number of patients and has been associated with an adverse prognosis [97]. Translocations with 7q22 and 2p11 breakpoints are also observed whereas trisomy 12

and 13q14 abnormalities on conventional cytogenetic analysis are uncommon [98]. Molecular mechanisms in these patients include dysregulation of the *CDK6* gene by proximity to *IGH* in t(7;14)(q21;q32) and by proximity to κ in t(2;7)(p12;q21). Del(13)(q14) is more often observed by FISH [99]. Trisomy 3 is found in approaching a fifth of patients, this abnormality also being characteristic of splenic marginal zone lymphoma.

RB1 deletion may be detected by FISH analysis [99]. A minority of cases (less than 20%) have *TP53* deletion or mutation, which is associated with a worse prognosis [100].

Other non-Hodgkin's lymphoma in leukaemic phase

Various types of non-Hodgkin's lymphoma have circulating lymphoma cells at presentation or subsequently enter a leukaemic phase [101]. The likelihood of leukaemic manifestations varies between different types of lymphoma but is relatively high in lymphomas in which the phenotype of the malignant cells corresponds to that of a relatively mature B cell such as follicular lymphoma and mantle cell lymphoma. A leukaemic phase is considerably less common in large cell lymphomas. The leukaemic phase of Burkitt's lymphoma is excluded from the FAB classification of chronic (mature) B-lymphoid leukaemias, being regarded as a form of acute lymphoblastic leukaemia (L3 category) whereas in the WHO classification it is included. The latter approach is more logical, given the immunophenotype of a mature B cell. The clinical features of lymphoma in leukaemic phase are determined largely by the nature of the underlying lymphoma. They usually include lymphadenopathy, splenomegaly or both, although occasional cases are diagnosed incidentally from a blood film before any organomegaly has occurred.

Follicular lymphoma

Follicular lymphoma [102] or follicle centre cell lymphoma [3] is a chronic B-lineage lymphoproliferative disorder with a growth pattern in lymph nodes which is, at least in part, follicular. Cells may be predominantly small, mixed small and large or predominantly large. Although this lymphoma is best defined histologically it has distinctive cytological

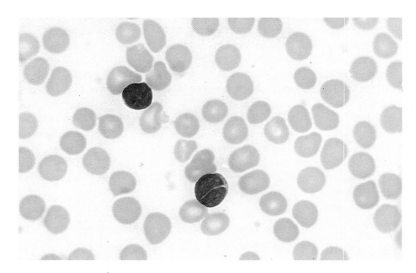

Fig. 5.18 PB film in leukaemic phase of follicular lymphoma. One cell is very small with scanty cytoplasm. The other is nucleolated and has a deep, narrow cleft. MGG × 870.

features and in the great majority of cases characteristic cytogenetic and molecular genetic features are also present.

Clinical, haematological and cytological features

Follicular lymphoma is a disease of adults, which, unusually for haematological neoplasms, shows a female predominance. Clinical features are localized or generalized lymphadenopathy with hepatomegaly and splenomegaly in those with more advanced disease. Occasionally the disease is diagnosed following an incidental blood film when there are no abnormalities on physical examination.

The circulating lymphoma cells are more pleomorphic than those of CLL. They range in size from cells that are distinctly smaller than those of CLL with small, uniformly condensed nuclei and very scanty cytoplasm, to larger cells with more abundant cytoplasm. Cells may be round or somewhat angular. Nucleoli are usually not visible. A variable but often large proportion of the cells have nuclei with deep, narrow clefts or fissures (Fig. 5.18).

Immunophenotype

The characteristic immunophenotype (Fig 5.19) is positivity for B-cell-associated antigens such as CD19, CD20, CD22 and CD24 and positivity for FMC7. CD79b is usually positive (around 80% of cases) [74]

and CD10 is often positive. The detection of CD10-positivity appears to be dependent on the specific antibody-fluorochrome used, in one study being observed to be 100% with one reagent and 0% with another [103]. CD5 is not expressed. CD23, CD43 and CD11c are usually negative. SmIg is strongly expressed. IgM is most often expressed but IgG and IgA expression are also quite common; IgD is not expressed [104]; κ expression is more common than λ expression.

Histology

Lymph node histology shows a follicular growth pattern. Bone marrow infiltration is common with paratrabecular infiltration being most characteristic. A nodular growth pattern in the bone marrow is quite uncommon. In advanced disease there is a diffuse infiltrate giving a 'packed marrow' pattern.

Cytogenetics and molecular genetics

The most characteristic cytogenetic abnormality is t(14;18)(q32;q21) (Fig. 5.20). Proximity to the immunoglobulin heavy-chain gene or associated mutation dysregulates the *BCL2* oncogene at 18q21 rendering the cells resistant to apoptosis. In the variant translocations, t(2;18)(p12;q21) and t(18;22)(q21;q11), *BCL2* is dysregulated by proximity to κ and λ genes, respectively. Classical or variant translocations are present in up to 95% of follicular lymphomas [102].

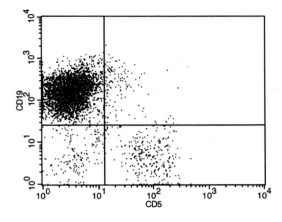

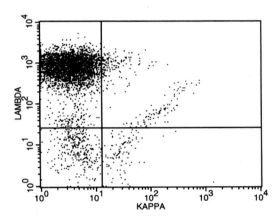

Fig. 5.19 Flow cytometric immunophenotyping in follicular lymphoma showing expression of CD19, strong expression of lambda light chain and lack of expression of CD5 (courtesy of Mr R. Morilla, London).

BCL2 rearrangement can be detected by both PCR and RT-PCR [105] and by single-colour FISH with a probe that encompasses the breakpoint on chromosome 18. t(14;18)(q32;q21) can be detected by two-colour, double-fusion FISH using probes that encompass the breakpoints on chromosome 14 and chromosome 18, respectively. *BCL2* protein expression can be detected by immunocytochemistry or immunohistochemistry with an antibody to BCL2 protein; the follicles of lymph nodes with reactive follicular hyperplasia are BCL2 negative, in contrast to the BCL2-positive neoplastic follicles of follicular lymphoma.

Secondary cytogenetic abnormalities are common and include trisomy of 5, 7, 12, 21 or X, duplica-

tion of the der(18), 6q–, 10q–, 13q– [106], der(1) t(1;17)(p36;q11-21) and der(1)t(1;11)(p36;q13) [107]. Some cases, both with and without t(14;18), show rearrangement of the *BCL6* gene at 3q27 [108]. Trisomy 7 has been related to the large cell histology and rearrangements with an 8q24 breakpoint to a blastoid variant [106]. Rearrangement of the *BCL3* gene at 17q22 correlates with transformation to more aggressive disease [109]. Disease progression can also be associated with acquisition of t(1;22)(q22;q11) in which the *FcγRIIB* gene is brought under the influence of positive regulatory elements of the λ gene [110]. Molecular genetic abnormalities that may appear with disease progression are loss of *TP53*—correlating with del(17p), and loss of p15 and p16—correlating with del(9)(p21). Follicular lymphoma is quite uncommon in children but when it occurs the proportion of patients with *BCL2* rearrangement and *BCL2* expression is higher than in adults [111]; BCL2-negative cases have more limited disease and a much better prognosis.

Mantle cell lymphoma

Mantle cell lymphoma is a chronic B-lineage lymphoproliferative disorder with variable cytological and histological features but with a characteristic cytogenetic and molecular genetic defect in the majority of patients. Although histologically low grade, its prognosis is intermediate between that of other low grade B-cell lymphomas (such as follicular lymphoma) and high grade lymphomas (such as diffuse large B-cell lymphoma).

Clinical, haematological and cytological features

Mantle cell lymphoma, previously referred to as intermediate lymphoma, lymphoma of intermediate differentiation or diffuse centrocytic lymphoma, is principally a disease of middle and old age with a marked male predominance. Presentation is usually with advanced stage disease, most often with lymphadenopathy and splenomegaly but sometimes with extranodal disease, including involvement of Waldeyer's ring and the gastrointestinal tract—multiple lymphomatous polyposis [112, 113]. There is peripheral blood involvement in about two-thirds of patients and this is indicative of a worse prognosis [114]. Cells are pleomorphic (Fig. 5.21) and most

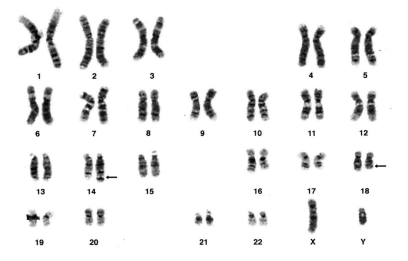

Fig. 5.20 A karyogram showing t(14;18)(q32;q21) (courtesy of Dr Fiona Ross, Salisbury).

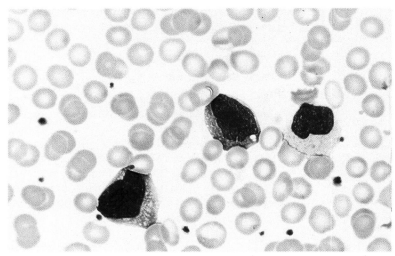

Fig. 5.21 PB film in mantle cell lymphoma. The cells are markedly pleomorphic. MGG × 870.

often mainly medium-sized with irregular nuclei [115]. Some show inconspicuous nucleoli or pronounced nuclear indentations or clefts. There may be some cells with a diffuse chromatin pattern, and in occasional patients these cells predominate [112]. When most cells have a diffuse chromatin pattern a diagnosis of blastoid variant of mantle cell lymphoma is appropriate [113]; cells in the blastoid variant may be monomorphic, resembling ALL, or pleomorphic [113]. In some patients, lymphoma cells have the cytological features of prolymphocytes [79]. One patient has been described in whom peripheral blood lymphoma cells showed platelet satellitism [116].

Immunophenotype

The characteristic immunophenotype is expression of B-cell-associated antigens such as CD19, CD20, CD22, CD24 and CD79a, expression of CD5, CD79b, FMC7 and BCL2, and lack of expression of CD10, CD11c, CD103 and BCL6. CD23 is expressed in about half of patients but expression is weak [117]. Expression of CD20 is strong. CD25 is usually not expressed. CD38 is expressed on more than 20% of cells in the majority of patients [118]. CD43 is weak or negative whereas it is strongly expressed in CLL [118]. SmIg is moderately strongly expressed. It is usually IgM with

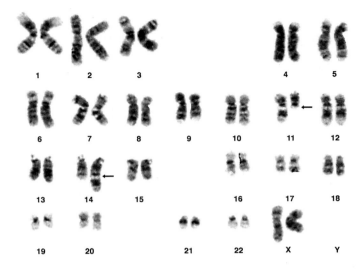

Fig. 5.22 A karyogram showing t(11;14)(q13;q32) (courtesy of Dr Fiona Ross).

or without IgD [3]. λ is more commonly expressed than κ [104]. The cells of mantle cell lymphoma express nuclear cyclin D1 (see below), which can be detected immunocytochemically and, if cells are 'permeabilized', by flow cytometry [119].

Although a typical immunophenotype can be defined, a significant minority of patients with mantle cell lymphoma have a surface membrane immunophenotype very similar to that of CLL. Demonstration of t(11;14) or of nuclear cyclin D1 expression is useful for the identification of such cases [118, 120].

Histology

Bone marrow infiltration is common, being observed in up to 80% of patients [114]. The pattern of infiltration is usually interstitial or focal with either nodules or irregularly shaped infiltrates. Paratrabecular infiltration is uncommon. Lymphoma cells in trephine biopsies may have regular round nuclei or irregular and cleaved nuclei. Chromatin is relatively dense and nucleoli are inconspicuous. Some cases have a high mitotic rate or cells with more blastic morphology; both these features are indicative of a worse prognosis. Ki-67 and p53 expression are also indicative of a worse prognosis [121]. Immunohistochemical demonstration of cyclin D1 expression is diagnostically useful [122], being detectable in almost all cases [121]. On immunohistochemistry, CD5 expression is not always detected, even when it is detected by flow cytometry.

Lymph node histology may show a diffuse infiltration, a nodular pattern or mantle zone infiltration. Splenic infiltration is mainly in the white pulp.

Cytogenetics and molecular genetics

The characteristic cytogenetic abnormality is t(11;14) (q13;q32) (Fig. 5.22) leading to rearrangement of the *BCL1* gene, which is brought into proximity to the immunoglobulin heavy-chain gene with consequent overexpression of cyclin D1 (the product of the *CCND1/PRAD/BCL1* gene). This rearrangement is not specific for mantle cell lymphoma, being detected also in a smaller proportion of patients with prolymphocytic leukaemia, splenic lymphoma with villous lymphocytes and multiple myeloma. This translocation is detected in many patients with mantle cell lymphoma by conventional cytogenetic analysis but in almost all if FISH techniques are employed [123]. FISH can be performed with commercially available probes, one centred on the *BCL1* gene and the other being a chromosome 11 centromeric probe [124]. Alternatively, specific probes for *BCL1* and *IGH* can be used, with co-localization of signals being seen; probes that encompass each gene are available, permitting dual-colour, double-fusion FISH. RT-PCR is also applicable [105] but false-negative results occur. A minority of cases of mantle cell lymphoma show a variant translocation, t(11;22)(q13;q11), which also leads to dysregulation of cyclin D1, in this case as a result of juxtaposition to the λ light-chain gene. It is unusual for t(11;14) to be present as the sole abnormality [125]. Common secondary cytogenetic abnormalities include del(1p), del(6q)(22–23), +3(q)(26–29), +3, +8q, −9, del(9p) del(10q), del(11)(q23), +12q, +12, del(13)(q14), del(13)(q31–34), del(17)(p13), −13 and −18 [121, 125–129]. Although trisomy 12 may be observed in mantle cell lymphoma, as well as in chronic lymphocytic leukaemia, trisomy 12 as a sole abnormality is not a feature of mantle cell lymphoma. Certain cytogenetic abnormalities correlate with significant numbers of circulating lymphoma cells, specifically abnormalities of 17, 21 and 22 and rearrangements with 8q24, 9p22–24 and 16q24 breakpoints [125]. Tetraploidy has been reported to be common in the blastoid variant but this was not confirmed in a second series of patients [125]. Burkitt's lymphoma-related translocations, both t(8;14)(q24;q32) and t(2;8)(p12;q24), have occurred in blastoid transformation of mantle cell lymphoma [130].

Cells of mantle cell lymphoma usually show unmutated V_H genes but in a minority there is V_H somatic mutation [113]. In addition to dysregulation of the *BCL1* gene, there is often amplification of 3q28q29 suggesting that another oncogene at that site may be relevant [131]. Amplification of part of 6p is also common [131]. Chromosomal regions that often show deletions include 1p13p32, 5p13p15.3, 6q14q27, 8p, 11q13q23 and, most frequently, 13q [131]. Inactivation of the *ATM* gene at 11q23, by point mutation or deletion, has been observed in some patients [113, 127]; in patients with loss of one allele of *ATM* as a result of del(11)(q23) the other allele is often mutated [62]. A loss of 8p21–p23 has been associated with mantle cell lymphoma with leukaemic manifestations, suggesting that there may be a tumour-suppressor gene at this locus [128]. Xq+ and 17p− have been associated with a worse prognosis [131]. Patients with the blastoid variant often have mutation of *TP53*, *CDKN2A* (encoding p16^{INK4A}) and *CDKN2C* (encoding p18^{INK4C}) [113].

Large cell lymphomas of B lineage

Large cell lymphomas of B lineage, despite being neoplasms of immunophenotypically mature cells, are clinically moderately aggressive tumours. Presentation is usually with lymphadenopathy or ex-tranodal lymphoma but in occasional cases there is peripheral blood and bone marrow involvement.

Clinical, haematological and cytological features

Most patients with large cell lymphoma present with lymphadenopathy, sometimes with associated hepatosplenomegaly. A small minority present in leukaemic phase or develop lymphoma cell leukaemia with disease progression [132]. In these patients impairment of bone marrow function may cause anaemia and cytopenia. Lymphoma cells may be present in relatively small numbers or may be very numerous. Pleomorphism is common. The cytological features are very variable from case to case. Nuclei may be round, irregular, lobulated or cleft (Fig. 5.23). Chromatin may be diffuse or show condensation. Nucleoli are common and may be conspicuous. The cell outline may be either regular or irregular. Cytoplasm is often plentiful and either weakly or strongly basophilic. A rare observation in intravascular large B-cell lymphoma is of clumps of tumour cells revealed when a film is made from the tip of the needle used for phlebotomy (Figs 5.24 & 5.25) [133].

Immunophenotype

Flow cytometry shows high forward angle light scatter [82]. The immunophenotype is that of a mature B cell but the expression of specific immunophenotypic markers varies from case to case, reflecting the heterogeneity of this condition. There is variable expression of B-cell-associated antigens, CD5 and CD10, while CD34 and TdT are not expressed. CD71 is usually expressed [82]. CD10 may be expressed and expression may correlate with follicular centre origin [103]. There may be a failure to express SmIg [82]. Immunophenotyping is important in recognizing a leukaemic presentation of large cell lymphoma since some cases have cells with cytological similarities to monoblasts.

Histology

The bone marrow is consistently involved in patients with circulating lymphoma cells but the pattern of infiltration varies. Lymph nodes usually show diffuse infiltration but occasional cases have a follicular pattern.

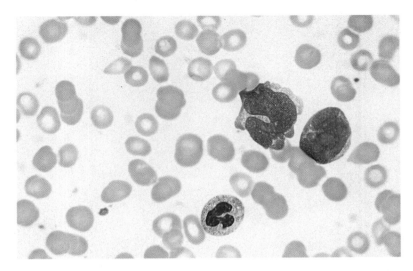

Fig. 5.23 PB film in B-lineage large cell lymphoma of centroblastic type. MGG × 870.

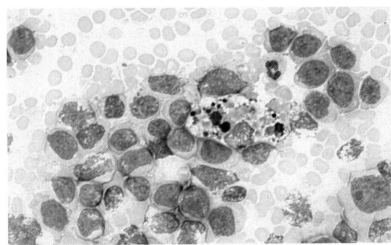

Fig. 5.24 A clump of lymphoma cells and a macrophage in a blood film of a patient with intravascular large B-cell lymphoma. The blood film was prepared from the tip of the needle following phlebotomy (courtesy of Dr R. Cobcroft, Brisbane). MGG × 870.

Cytogenetics and molecular genetics

The commonest cytogenetic abnormalities are those characteristic of follicular lymphoma. The second commonest group of abnormalities are those with rearrangement of the *BCL6/LAZ3* gene at 3q27, including t(3;14)(q27;q32). Other cases show miscellaneous cytogenetic abnormalities. Molecular genetic abnormalities include rearrangement of *BCL2* or *BCL6* and *TP53* mutations. t(3;14)(q27;q32) can be detected by two-colour FISH with probes for *BCL6* and the immunoglobulin heavy-chain gene [134]. Southern blotting and dual-colour, break-apart FISH permit detection of all *BCL6* rearrangements. Rearrangement of *MYC* and *IGH* can similarly be detected by dual-colour, break-apart FISH.

Other non-Hodgkin's lymphomas

Burkitt's lymphoma and lymphoplasmacytoid lymphoma may have a leukaemic phase. In Burkitt's lymphoma the features are identical to those of acute lymphoblastic leukaemia of FAB L3 type (see page 16). In lymphoplasmacytoid lymphoma, the circulating cells are usually small mature lymphocytes with some plasmacytoid features such as cytoplasmic

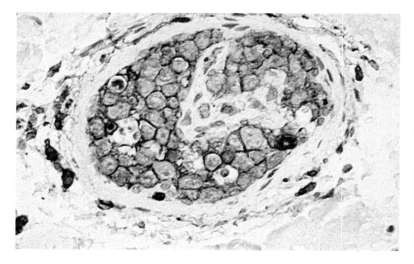

Fig. 5.25 A skin biopsy from a patient with intravascular large B-cell lymphoma showing cohesive masses of lymphoma cells within a capillary, same patient as Fig. 5.24 (with thanks to Dr R. Cobcroft and the British Journal of Haematolgy). The cells were CD45 and CD2D positive and S100 negative. Immunohistochemistry with an anti-CD20 monoclonal antibody.

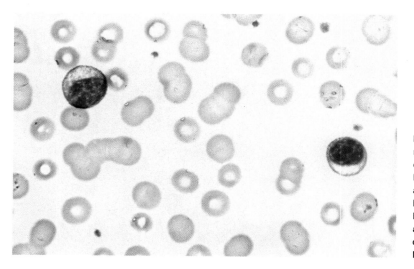

Fig. 5.26 PB film in Waldenström's macroglobulinaemia; this term describes a lymphoplasmacytoid lymphoma with production of a large amount of monoclonal IgM. The blood film shows two plasmacytoid lymphocytes together with rouleaux and abnormal staining characteristics consequent on the high level of IgM. MGG × 870.

basophilia, a small Golgi zone or an eccentric nucleus (Fig. 5.26). Occasionally these lymphoma cells have cytoplasmic crystals or large inclusions resembling Russell bodies. In addition, there may be peripheral blood features consequent on the presence of a paraprotein such as increased rouleaux formation, the presence of red cell agglutinates or, less often, a precipitated cryoprotein between or within cells. The immunophenotype is that of a late B cell with expression of cytoplasmic immunoglobulin. SmIg is expressed more strongly than in CLL cells. CD5 is not expressed. CD38 may be expressed but expression is weaker than in plasma cells [29]. The most charac-

teristic cytogenetic abnormality is t(9;14)(p13;q32) with the genes involved being the immunoglobulin heavy-chain gene and *PAX5*, a transcription factor gene [135]. Other lymphomas rarely have circulating lymphoma cells [101]. A leukaemic phase has occasionally been reported in monocytoid B-cell lymphoma [136] and MALT (mucosa-associated lymphoid tissue) lymphoma [137]. A leukaemic phase may develop in patients who initially present with nodal small lymphocytic lymphoma. When this occurs the cells have the same cytological and immunophenotypic features as CLL cells [104], this disease being regarded as the tissue equivalent of CLL.

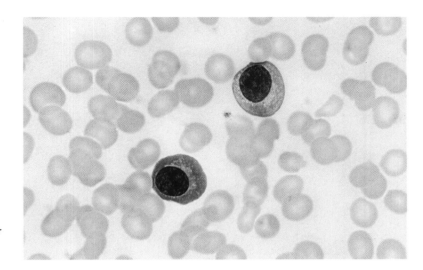

Fig. 5.27 PB film in plasma cell leukaemia. The malignant cells are identified as plasma cells by their eccentric nucleus and pale paranuclear area that represents the Golgi zone. MGG × 870.

Plasma cell leukaemia

Plasma cell leukaemia may occur *de novo* or as the terminal phase of multiple myeloma. The FAB group [1] suggested that the term plasma cell leukaemia be confined to *de novo* cases but in the WHO classification both *de novo* and secondary cases are included [138]. In *de novo* cases the patients have an acute illness, sometimes with hepatosplenomegaly and often with hypercalcaemia and renal failure. Prognosis is poor both in *de novo* and secondary cases. In one series of 18 patients with *de novo* disease the median survival was only 7 months [139].

Criteria previously suggested for a diagnosis of plasma cell leukaemia were the presence of circulating neoplastic plasma cells that both (i) constituted at least 20% of circulating cells and (ii) had an absolute count of at least 2×10^9/l. In the WHO classification, either of these criteria is accepted as sufficient for this diagnosis [138].

Clinical, haematological and cytological features

Cytological features vary considerably between cases. Some patients have mainly cells that resemble normal plasma cells with basophilic cytoplasm, a prominent Golgi zone and an eccentric nucleus (Fig. 5.27). Others have many lymphoplasmacytoid lymphocytes and only a minority of characteristic plasma cells. Yet others have more primitive cells with a higher nucleocytoplasmic ratio, a diffuse chromatin pattern, a prominent nucleolus and a less prominent Golgi zone (Fig. 5.28). In the latter group it can be difficult to recognize cells as plasma cells by light microscopy alone; in some cases there are cytological similarities with prolymphocytic leukaemia or immunoblastic lymphoma.

Immunophenotype

In addition to the markers shown in Table 5.5, positive reactions are found with McAb that show some selectivity for plasma cells such as PCA-1, BU11 [1], CD38 (when strongly expressed) and CD138 (recognizing the adhesion molecule LFA-3 or Syndecam 1) [140]. Strong expression of CD38 with weak expression of CD45 is typical of plasma cells. Of the pan-B markers CD19, CD20 and CD22 are usually negative whereas CD79a is sometimes positive [3]. Myeloma cells express CD56 strongly and do not usually express CD19 whereas normal plasma cells are usually CD19 positive and CD56 negative. Epithelial membrane antigen (EMA) may be expressed as may HLA-DR, CD43 and CD30 [3].

Histology

The appearance of histological sections of trephine biopsies or other tissues varies, depending on the degree of maturation of cells. Some cases have infiltrating cells with obvious plasma cell differentiation.

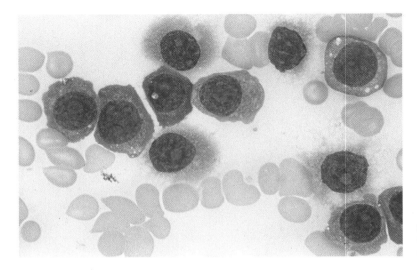

Fig. 5.28 PB film in plasma cell leukaemia with cells showing plasmablastic morphology. MGG × 870.

In other cases the histological features are similar to those of large cell (immunoblastic) lymphoma and demonstration of monotypic cytoplasmic immunoglobulin and CD138 expression is then useful in confirming the diagnosis.

Cytogenetics and molecular genetics

Plasma cell leukaemia shows cytogenetic abnormalities similar to those of multiple myeloma including t(11;14)(q13;q32) and other rearrangements with a 14q32 breakpoint and, in addition, rearrangements of chromosomes 1 and 11.

Chronic leukaemias of T-lymphocyte and NK-cell lineage

Chronic leukaemias of T-lymphocyte or NK-cell lineage are uncommon, constituting only a small proportion of chronic lymphoid leukaemias. Chronic T-lineage leukaemias express one or more T-lymphocyte markers commonly CD2, CD3, CD5 and either CD4 or CD8, and show rearrangement of one or more of the *TCR* genes (Tables 5.11 & 5.12). The cells usually form rosettes with sheep red blood cells (ERFC) but, with the ready availability of monoclonal antibodies to surface and cytoplasmic antigens of lymphocytes, this test is no longer used. TdT and CD1 are not expressed. CD38 is not usually expressed. Leukaemias of NK-cell lineage express surface antigens characteristic of cytotoxic T cells or NK cells;

they may share some antigens with T-cell leukaemias but do not express CD3 and do not show rearrangement of *TCR* genes. In neither the T nor the NK lineage is there a readily available marker of monoclonality equivalent to the light chain restriction of SmIg of the B lymphocyte. The use of antibodies to the variable (V) domains of TCRβ chains has the potential to demonstrate clonality of around 60% of mature T-cell neoplasms but this technique is not yet widely used [6]. Clonality of T-lineage or NK-lineage cells may be inferred when a cell population shows a uniform, often aberrant, immunological phenotype. However, definitive demonstration of clonality requires specialized techniques. In the case of T-lineage leukaemias, this may be either DNA analysis, to show rearrangement of one or more of the *TCR* genes, or cytogenetic analysis. For leukaemias of NK-cell lineage, usually only cytogenetic analysis is applicable but not all cases will have a clonal cytogenetic abnormality.

With advances in immunophenotyping and cytogenetic and molecular genetic analysis it is now possible to recognize many specific entities among T-cell and NK-cell neoplasms. Of the 15 entities recognized in the WHO [141] classification, four usually present with disseminated disease including leukaemia. Circulating neoplastic cells are also, by definition, present in Sézary syndrome. These conditions will be discussed in detail; conditions that do not usually have a leukaemic presentation will be dealt with more briefly.

Table 5.11 Some monoclonal antibodies used in the characterization of chronic lymphoid leukaemias of T and natural killer (NK) lineages.

Cluster designation	Specificity within haemopoietic and lymphoid lineages
CD2	Receptor for sheep red blood cell; detects E rosette-forming cells (ERFC); positive in all except the earliest of T-lineage cells and on NK cells
CD3	Part of the T-cell receptor complex; expressed on thymocytes and T cells; expressed in the cytoplasm before it is expressed on the cell surface
CD5	Expressed on thymocytes and T cells (see also Table 5.4)
CD7	Expressed on pluripotent stem cells, thymocytes and T cells; expressed in cells of some cases of acute myeloid leukaemia
CD4	Common and late thymocytes, subset (about two-thirds) of mature T cells (among which are many cells that are functionally helper/inducer) that recognize antigens in a class II context; expressed on monocytes and macrophages
CD8	Common and late thymocytes, subset (about one-third) of mature T cells (among which are many cells that are functionally cytotoxic/suppressor) that recognize antigens in a class I context
CD11b	C3bi complement receptor: expressed on monocytes, granulocytes, NK cells and hairy cells
CD16	Component of low-affinity Fc receptor, FcRIII: expressed on NK cells, neutrophils, macrophages
CD56	NK cells, activated lymphocytes, cells of some cases of acute myeloid leukaemia
CD57	NK cells, subsets of T cells, B cells and monocytes
CD25, CD38 HLA-DR	See Table 5.4
CD30	Activated B and T cells, cells of anaplastic large cell lymphoma and more weakly on cells of some cases of other types of large cell lymphoma; Hodgkin's cells and Reed–Sternberg cells

Table 5.12 12 Characteristic immunophenotype of chronic T-cell leukaemias.

Marker	LGLL–T cell	LGLL–NK	T-PLL	ATLL	Sèzary syndrome
ERFC/CD2	++	++	++	++	++
CD3	++	–	+	++	++
CD5	–/+	–/+	++	++	++
CD7	–/+	–/+	++	–/+	–/+
CD4	–	–	++	++	++
CD8	++	–/+	–/+	–	–
CD2	–	–	–/+	++	–/+

ATLL, adult T-cell leukaemia/lymphoma; ERFC, E rosette-forming cells; LGLL, large granular lymphocyte leukaemia; NK, natural killer cell; T-PLL, T-cell prolymphocytic leukaemia.
The frequency with which a marker is positive in >30% of cells in a particular leukaemia is indicated as follows: ++, 80–100%, +, 40–80%; –/+, 10–40%; –, 0–9%.

T-cell large granular lymphocyte leukaemia

Clinical, haematological and cytological features

T-cell large granular lymphocyte leukaemia occurs predominantly in the elderly [142, 143]. About a third of patients are asymptomatic at the time of diagnosis [144, 145]. Symptomatic patients usually present either with recurrent infection, resulting from neutropenia, or with signs and symptoms of anaemia. There is a strong association with Felty's syndrome (rheumatoid arthritis with neutropenia and splenomegaly) and a less strong association with other autoimmune diseases [142]. Lymphadenopathy is uncommon, but hepatomegaly and splenomegaly are

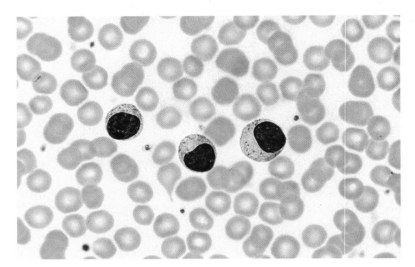

Fig. 5.29 PB film in large granular lymphocyte leukaemia. The cells have abundant weakly basophilic cytoplasm containing prominent azurophilic granules. MGG × 870.

frequent findings. Skin lesions are present in less than 20% of patients [146]. The disease typically has a prolonged survival with an actuarial median survival, in one series, of 166 months [145]. In a minority of patients, particularly those whose cells co-express CD3 and CD56, the disease has a more aggressive clinical course, similar to that of aggressive NK-cell leukaemia [147]; this variant has been referred to as natural killer-like T-cell lymphoma [148].

Most patients have an increased WBC, lymphocytosis and an increase in large granular lymphocytes (LGL) [144, 149]. Sometimes the WBC is not increased although there is an increase in the number of LGL and sometimes there is no increase in LGL although the LGL are clonal [150]. Lymphocytosis may appear only after splenectomy or with disease progression. The neoplastic cells are usually morphologically very similar to normal LGL (Fig. 5.29). Usually leukaemic cells have a round or oval nucleus with moderately condensed chromatin; the cytoplasm is voluminous and weakly basophilic and contains fine or coarse azurophilic granules. Smear cells are rare. In a minority of patients, cells are small rather than large or granules are very infrequent although the cases, in other ways, are typical of the disease. In natural killer-like T-cell lymphoma cells are larger and more pleomorphic (Fig. 5.30). Neutropenia is sometimes cyclical. Some patients have isolated neutropenia or thrombocytopenia or, less often, anaemia. These cytopenias are out of proportion to the degree of bone marrow infiltration and appear to have an immune basis. Anaemia may be due to pure red cell aplasia or to a Coombs'-positive or Coombs'-negative haemolytic anaemia [142]. Macrocytosis is sometimes present. Depending on the nature of the anaemia, the reticulocyte count may be either very low or increased. In some patients cytopenia is attributable to hypersplenism.

The bone marrow shows a variable degree of infiltration by cells with the same morphology as those in the blood. In the early stages, infiltration may be undetectable or minimal. However, in some patients without an absolute peripheral blood lymphocytosis, examination of the bone marrow is essential for diagnosis. In cases complicated by immunologically-mediated cytopenia there may be pure red cell aplasia, megaloblastic erythropoiesis or apparent arrest of granulocyte maturation. Patients with thrombocytopenia usually have normal or increased numbers of megakaryocytes but one case of amegakaryocytic thrombocytopenia has been reported (associated with pure red cell aplasia) [142].

Rheumatoid factor and antinuclear antibodies are often detectable and there is usually a polyclonal increase in immunoglobulins [142].

Immunophenotype

The immunophenotype resembles that of a normal large granular T lymphocyte [151, 152]. The most

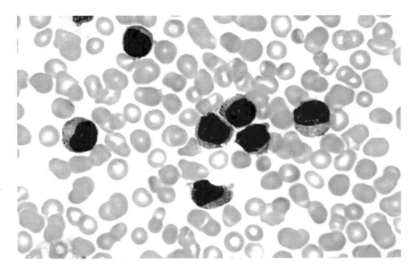

Fig. 5.30 PB film in natural killer-like large granular T-cell lymphoma. The cells are larger and more pleomorphic than in the typical form of large granular T-cell leukaemia and expressed not only CD3 but also four NK markers—CD11b, CD16, CD56 and CD57 (with thanks to Dr A. Eden and the British Journal of Haematology).

characteristic phenotype is CD2, CD3, CD8, CD57 and TCRαβ positive and TdT, CD1 and CD4 negative (see Table 5.12). The frequency of expression of CD16 has varied between different series of patients, possibly reflecting the specific antibody used for its detection. CD5, CD7, CD11b, CD56 and HLA-DR are sometimes positive. Both CD3 and CD7 are less strongly expressed than on normal T lymphocytes [153]. CD8 is also weakly expressed [29]. There is expression of cytotoxic granule contents, e.g. perforin and the antigen detectable with the monoclonal antibody, TIA-1. A minority of cases of T-cell large granular lymphocyte leukaemia have immunophenotypes rarely seen in normal peripheral blood large granular lymphocytes. These phenotypes include: CD3, CD8 and CD11b positive; CD3, CD4 and CD16 positive; CD3, CD4 and CD11b positive. One case has also been reported showing a mixed T and B immunophenotype [154].

Histology

A trephine biopsy is not usually diagnostically very useful since the specific cytological features of large granular lymphocytes cannot be discerned. Bone marrow infiltration may be undetectable or minimal. When detectable, infiltration is usually random focal or interstitial but is sometimes diffuse and occasional patients have shown nodular infiltration [155–157]. Immunohistochemistry is important in the detection of a minor degree of infiltration. Some cases have plasmacytosis [157]. Patients with red cell aplasia show few erythroid cells beyond the proerythroblast stage. In patients with neutropenia and 'maturation arrest' there are increased numbers of apoptotic cells [158]. A significant minority of patients show trilineage myelodysplasia.

Splenic infiltration is in the red pulp, sometimes with an associated plasma cell infiltrate [12].

Cytogenetics and molecular genetics

A number of clonal cytogenetic abnormalities have been described in T-cell large granular lymphocyte leukaemia but no consistent association has been recognized; T-cell receptor genes may have been involved in translocations in two patients and three reported patients have had complex chromosomal abnormalities (at least three unrelated abnormalities) [159]. Rearrangement of *TCR* genes is usually demonstrable. This is most often rearrangement of *TCRB* and *TCRG* genes, but occasionally it is the *TCRG* gene alone.

Aggressive NK-cell leukaemia

The WHO classification recognizes an aggressive leukaemia of NK lineage [160]. Because of the lack of a readily applicable clonal marker for cells of NK lineage it is difficult to determine whether a less aggressive condition with chronic NK-cell lymphocytosis also represents a neoplastic condition. Chronic NK lymphocytosis is sometimes associated with autoimmune conditions and neutropenia [142, 161].

Hepatomegaly and splenomegaly are rare and the condition shows little tendency to progress [161].

The description that follows applies to those cases with NK-cell lymphocytosis that are generally agreed to be leukaemic in nature, either because of their aggressive clinical course or because a clonal cytogenetic abnormality has been recognized. This condition is more common in the Far East (mainland China, Hong Kong, Taiwan and Japan) than in the West. In many cases the neoplastic cells show evidence of infection with EBV [162, 163].

Clinical, haematological and cytological features

The frequency of aggressive NK-cell leukaemia is about one sixth that of T-cell large granular lymphocyte leukaemia. Patients are typically younger and often have hepatosplenomegaly and B symptoms (weight loss, fever and night sweats) [142]. Gastrointestinal and central nervous system infiltration may occur. The disease shows aggressive clinical behaviour [164, 165], is highly resistant to therapy and has a poor prognosis with many patients surviving less than two months [142, 163]. Death is usually from multiorgan failure with coagulopathy [142] and sometimes a haemophagocytic syndrome. There is no association with rheumatoid arthritis [142].

The peripheral blood shows a variable increase in LGL [163]. Leukaemic cells resemble normal large granular lymphocytes but, in comparison with the cells of T-cell large granular lymphocyte leukaemia, they are often atypical—larger with more basophilic cytoplasm, hyperchromatic or diffuse chromatin, nuclear irregularity and sometimes nucleoli (Fig. 5.31a) [142, 163]. There may be circulating nucleated red blood cells and myelocytes. Anaemia and thrombocytopenia are frequent findings but severe neutropenia is less common than in T-cell large granular lymphocyte leukaemia [142].

The bone marrow aspirate shows a variable degree of infiltration by cells similar to those in the peripheral blood (Fig. 5.31b). Increased macrophages and haemophagocytosis are often prominent [163, 166].

Immunophenotype

The immunophenotype resembles that of a normal NK cell. (see Table 5.12). Leukaemic cells are CD2 positive but CD3, TCR$\alpha\beta$ and TCR $\gamma\delta$ negative; CD4 is negative and CD8 may be weakly positive or negative; there is expression of CD11b, CD16 or CD56 and sometimes CD57; CD7 and activation markers such as CD38 and HLA-DR may be expressed [3, 29, 151, 167, 168].

Histology

On trephine biopsy histology there is a variable degree of bone marrow infiltration; the pattern of infiltration may be diffuse, interstitial or angiocentric. There is a monomorphic infiltrate of medium sized cells with round nuclei and condensed chromatin [163]. The neoplastic cells express CD56 and are negative for CD3 and CD4 but the present of CD3ϵ may mean that they appear to be CD3 positive if polyclonal antisera are used. Some patients show evidence of haemophagocytosis. Bone marrow fibrosis has been reported [142].

Cytogenetics and molecular genetics

Many cases show clonal cytogenetic abnormalities. An association with duplication of 1q, rearrangements of 3q, loss of the Y chromosome, monosomy 10 and monosomy 13 has been reported [169]. *TCR* genes are not rearranged. In most cases, EBER can be detected by *in situ* hybridization [163] with a single episomal form being present [160].

Blastic natural killer-cell lymphoma/leukaemia

Blastic killer cell leukaemia/lymphoma is a rare NK, or possibly dendritic cell, neoplasm, which differs from aggressive NK-cell leukaemia in that cells are not granular and there is no EBV association [170, 171]. There is often involvement of multiple sites with a predilection for the skin, peripheral blood and bone marrow. This condition may be better defined immunologically, than morphologically, as a neoplasm of CD4-positive CD56-positive cells with no expression of B, T or myeloid immunophenotypic markers [171].

Clinical, haematological and cytological features

Patients more often present as lymphoma than as leukaemia, with the skin and lymph nodes often

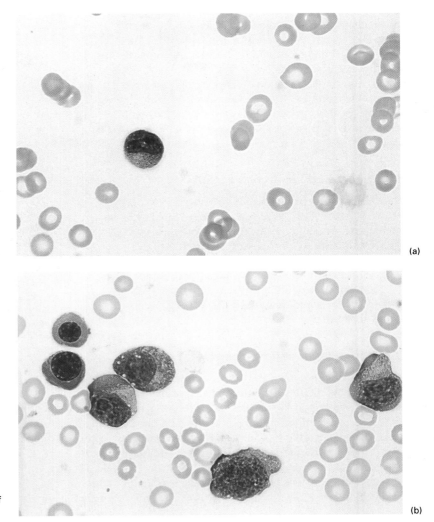

(a)

(b)

Fig. 5.31 PB and BM in aggressive natural killer-cell leukaemia; the PB (a) shows a medium sized lymphoid cell with azurophilic granules while the BM (b) shows infiltration by medium-sized, granular lymphoid cells, some of which are nucleolated. MGG × 870 (courtesy of Dr A. Martin Noya, Seville).

being infiltrated and splenomegaly sometimes being present. The peripheral blood is quite often involved at presentation and is more often involved at relapse. Anaemia, neutropenia and thrombocytopenia are common. Bone marrow infiltration is common with a diffuse pattern of infiltration. In a minority of patients, myeloid cells in the peripheral blood or bone marrow show dysplastic features such as hypogranular or pseudo-Pelger neutrophils [171].

The neoplastic cells tend to be cytologically uniform in a single patient but vary from small/medium to medium/large between patients. The nucleocytoplasmic ratio is variable. Nuclei may be regular or irregular and in some patients there are nucleoli. The cytoplasm may be granular or agranular, weakly basophilic, often vacuolated and may show pseudopodia-like extensions [171].

Immunophenotype

Cells are invariably CD3 negative. They are usually CD56 positive and often express CD4 [170, 171]. Other NK cell markers—CD11c, CD16 and CD57—are usually negative. CD7 is often expressed and occasionally there is expression of CD2 or CD5 but not CD8. CD33 expression may be quite common, unless the condition is defined as one not expressing myeloid antigens [170], possibly reflecting an origin from a myeloid-NK cell common progenitor. CD34 and terminal deoxynucleotidyl transferase are occasionally expressed [170].

On immunohistochemistry, the neoplastic cells show expression of CD4, CD43 and CD56. There is variable expression of cytoplasmic CD3ε, CD7 and cytotoxic granule-associated molecules. CD8 is not expressed.

Cytogenetics and molecular genetics

Various cytogenetic abnormalities have been described [170]. Two thirds of patients have clonal cytogenetic abnormalities [172]. These are often complex and may include del(5q), del(6q) and del(12p) [171, 172]; other chromosomes recurrently involved are 13q, 15q and 9 (monosomy 9 in a quarter of patients) [172]. Rearrangements are often unbalanced with loss of chromosomal material [172]. T-cell receptor genes are germ line.

T-cell prolymphocytic leukaemia

The FAB group proposed the term T-prolymphocytic leukaemia (T-PLL) for a group of cases that had cells showing cytological similarities to B-PLL, together with other cases that differ cytologically but can be linked to cytologically typical cases by other features (see below). This terminology is now generally accepted.

Sézary cell-like leukaemia (see below) appears to be a variant of T-PLL.

Clinical, haematological and cytological features

T-PLL is mainly a disease of the elderly and is slightly more common in males [146]. Ataxia telangiectasia predisposes to the development of this type of leukaemia. Cases of T-PLL [1, 173, 174] resemble B-PLL in presenting most commonly with marked splenomegaly and a high white cell count. They differ in that hepatomegaly, lymphadenopathy, skin infiltration and serous effusions may also be present. Fever and central nervous system infiltration sometimes occur. A small minority of patients are asymptomatic and the diagnosis is made incidentally. In most patients the clinical course is aggressive but in

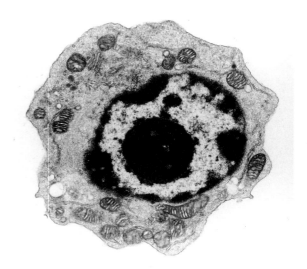

Fig. 5.32 Ultrastructural examination in T-lineage prolymphocytic leukaemia showing a regular nuclear outline, a prominent nucleolus and relatively abundant cytoplasm with a well developed Golgi zone, rough endoplasmic reticulum and numerous mitochondria (with thanks to Dr Estella Matutes, London).

about a third the disease is more indolent [175]. A single patient has been reported in whom a slow and complete spontaneous remission occurred [176].

The WBC is moderately to greatly elevated and in about a third of patients there is anaemia and thrombocytopenia [146]. In about 50% of patients, morphology of the leukaemic cells is similar to that in B-PLL although the nuclear outline may be more irregular. There may be a minor population of cells with polylobated nuclei or of Sézary-like cells. Ultrastructural examination shows the prominent nucleolus very clearly (Fig. 5.32). In other patients cells are smaller with a higher nucleocytoplasmic ratio and a less readily detectable nucleolus (Fig. 5.33). Cytoplasm is usually deeply basophilic. In about a quarter of patients the cells are small and the nucleolus is not easily detectable on light microscopy; the scanty cytoplasm is basophilic and may form blebs. Such cases have a prominent nucleolus on ultrastructural examination, have the same clinical course as other patients and show the same cytogenetic abnormality and immunophenotypic features (see below). In about 5% of patients cells have cerebriform nuclei [177].

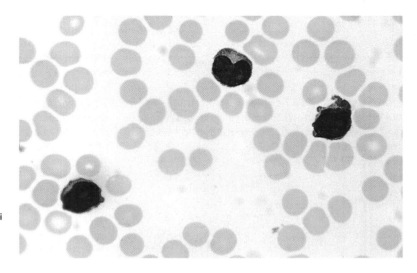

Fig. 5.33 PB film in T-prolymphocytic leukaemia (T-PLL). In this case the nuclei are more irregular and the nucleoli are less conspicuous than in B-PLL. MGG × 870.

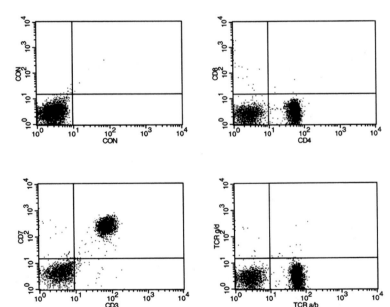

Fig. 5.34 Flow cytometry Immunophenotyping in T-lineage prolymphocytic leukaemia showing characteristic positivity for CD3, CD4 and CD7. T-cell receptor (TCR)αβ was expressed but TCR γδ was not (by courtesy of Dr Estella Matutes and Mr R. Morilla).

Immunophenotype

Most cases of T-PLL are CD2, CD3, CD5, CD7, CD4 and TCR αβ positive and CD8 negative [1] (see Table 5.12). The remainder are negative for CD4 and positive for CD8 (15% of patients) or co-express these two markers (25% of patients). Co-expression of CD4 and CD8 is otherwise uncommon in mature T-cell neoplasms. CD7 is expressed more strongly than on normal T lymphocytes and CD3 less strongly [153]; about 20% of cases fail to express surface membrane CD3 and TCR αβ [146]. A minority of cases are CD25 positive with expression being weak. CD7 positivity helps to distinguish T-PLL from other disorders of mature T cells (Fig. 5.34).

Histology

Bone marrow infiltration is usually interstitial or diffuse, although an interstitial/nodular pattern has also been reported. Lymph node infiltration is diffuse and mainly paracortical. High endothelial venules may be prominent [3]. Splenic infiltration is in the red and white pulp [177]. Cutaneous infiltration is in the dermis, particularly around vessels and skin appendages.

Cytogenetics and molecular genetics

About three-quarters of cases of T-PLL show either inv(14)(q11q32) or t(14;14)(q11;q32) [44, 178]. These chromosomal rearrangements involve the TCRAD locus at 14q11 and two oncogenes, TCL1 and TCL1b, at 14q32.1. TCL1 and TCL1b are dysregulated and, when overexpressed, inhibit apoptosis. t(X;14)(q28;q11) is a less common translocation in which the MTCP1 B1 gene at Xq28 is brought into proximity to the TCRAD locus. Dysregulation of MTCP1 B1 can also result from fusion of this gene with the TCRB gene as a result of t(X;7)(q28;q35) [179]. A further uncommon but recurring translocation is t(11;14)(q21;q32) [179]. Other common cytogenetic abnormalities include trisomy 8, 8p+, idic(8q)(p11–12) and t(8;8)(p11–12;q11–12) (all giving rise to trisomy or polysomy of 8q), deletions of the short arm of chromosome 12 [180], deletions of the long arms of chromosomes 6 and 11 and translocations with a breakpoint at 11q23, the site of the ATM (**A**taxia **T**elangiectasia **M**utated) gene. Mutations and deletions of the ATM gene are common and may coexist with the characteristic translocations involving TCL1 [181].

Adult T-cell leukaemia/lymphoma

ATLL [1, 182, 183] occurs in adults who are carriers of the retrovirus, human T cell lymphotropic virus I (HTLV-I); serology for HTLV-I is positive and proviral DNA is clonally integrated into the DNA of the neoplastic cells. Distribution of the disease relates to areas where the virus is endemic. Cases were first recognized in Japan, and subsequently in the Caribbean, in the southern United States and in West Indian immigrants to the UK. Smaller numbers of cases have been reported from the Middle East, Central and West Africa, South America (Brazil, Chile, Colombia), Taiwan and a number of other countries.

Clinical, haematological and cytological features

The disease mainly occurs in adults above the age of 40 years but cases in infants have been described in South America. Most patients present with lymphadenopathy, bone and skin lesions, hypercalcaemia and circulating lymphoma cells. Some patients have hepatomegaly or splenomegaly or infiltration of other organs. In about 10% of patients presentation is as a lymphoma with no abnormal cells in the peripheral blood. Prognosis is generally poor but some patients have a more chronic or smouldering disease. There is a significant incidence of opportunistic infections. A minority of patients suffer from other HTLV-I-related disorders such as tropical spastic paraparesis and uveitis.

The number of circulating lymphoma cells is very variable. The morphology is distinctive (Fig. 5.35). Cells vary greatly in size and form. Most cells have condensed and relatively homogeneous nuclear chromatin with nucleoli being infrequent and small. A minority of cells are blastic with basophilic cytoplasm. Some cells have convoluted nuclei, and may resemble Sézary cells, while many are polylobated, with some nuclei resembling clover leaves or flowers. Some cases have atypical cytological features—large granular lymphocytes in one case [184] and bizarre giant cells resembling Hodgkin's cells in others [185].

Some patients are anaemic and some have neutrophilia or eosinophilia. The neutrophilia may be marked, e.g. $16–55 \times 10^9$/l; and in some cases is attributable to secretion of granulocyte-colony-stimulating factor (G-CSF) by neoplastic cells [186].

The following criteria have been suggested for the diagnosis of smouldering and chronic forms of ATLL [187]. Smouldering ATLL has either at least 5% of abnormal cells in the peripheral blood or histological evidence of lung or skin infiltration but the total lymphocyte count is less than 4×10^9/l; the serum lactate dehydrogenase (LDH) is less than 1.5 times the upper limit of normal, the serum calcium is normal and there is no evidence of tissue infiltration other than in the skin or lungs. Chronic ATLL has a lymphocyte count of more than 4×10^9/l and T lymphocytes are more than 3.5×10^9/l; there are usually at least 5% of atypical cells in the circulation; the serum LDH is less than twice the upper limit of normal and the serum calcium is normal; there are no lymphomatous effusions nor infiltration of the central nervous system or

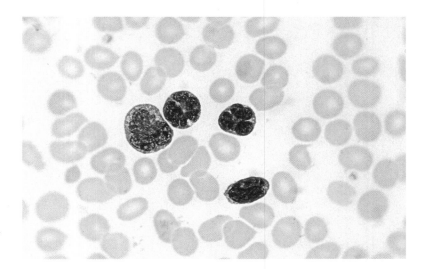

Fig. 5.35 PB film in adult T-cell leukaemia/lymphoma. Cells are pleomorphic with polylobulated nuclei, one of which resembles a clover leaf. MGG × 870.

gastrointestinal tract. Cases that do not fall into these two categories but have circulating leukaemic cells are designated ATLL; such cases are further classified as acute ATLL or the lymphomatous form of ATLL.

Immunophenotype

ATLL cells form E rosettes and usually express CD2, CD3, CD5, CD4, CD25 and HLA-DR [1, 29] (see Table 5.12). A minority of cases are positive for CD7 or CD8. Expression of CD3 is considerably weaker than on normal T lymphocytes and CD7, when expressed, is also weaker than on normal cells [153]. Positivity for CD25 helps to distinguish ATLL from other T-cell disorders, which are usually CD25 negative. Other activation markers, such as CD38 and HLA-DR, may be expressed.

Histology

The bone marrow may initially be normal or show interstitial infiltration but, with disease progression, diffuse infiltration may be seen. Increased bone destruction by osteoclasts may be apparent. In one patient the pathological features of osteitis fibrosa cystica were seen [188]. Lymph nodes show diffuse infiltration, either paracortical or effacing nodal architecture. Neoplastic cells are very pleomorphic and may include multinucleated giant cells. Infiltration in the skin is perivascular or diffuse in the middle and upper dermis; some cases show epidermotropism with formation of intraepidermal lymphoid infiltrates known as Pautrier's microabscesses, formerly thought to be confined to the Sézary syndrome.

Cytogenetics and molecular genetics

A variety of chromosomal abnormalities have been described in ATLL, most commonly trisomy 12, del(6q) and rearrangements with breakpoints at 7p14 or 15, 14q11–13 or 14q32 [189]. Rearrangements of 1p32–36 and 5q11–13 may also be preferentially associated with ATLL. Complex karyotypes and clonal evolution are common.

Mutations of tumour-suppressing genes, *CDKN2A* (p16) and *TP53* (p53), may be found in the acute and lymphomatous forms of ATLL.

HTLV-I is clonally integrated in leukaemic cells at a random site, which differs between patients. Multiple integration in different clones is associated with indolent disease whereas multiple integration into a single clone is associated with aggressive disease [190].

Mycosis fungoides–Sézary syndrome

Sézary syndrome and mycosis fungoides are related cutaneous T-cell lymphomas. Sézary syndrome is an erythrodermic variant of mycosis fungoides. Cutaneous T-cell lymphomas usually run a chronic course but transformation to an aggressive large cell lymphoma, including anaplastic large cell lymphoma, can occur.

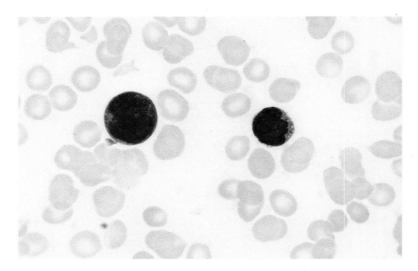

Fig. 5.36 PB film in large cell variant of Sézary syndrome. Both cells have convoluted nuclei. The smaller one has inconspicuous cytoplasmic vacuoles. MGG × 870.

Clinical, haematological and cytological features

Sézary syndrome is characterized by circulating lymphoma cells together with pruritis and a generalized exfoliative or infiltrative erythroderma, the cutaneous manifestations being consequent on infiltration. Mycosis fungoides may be restricted to the skin with the cutaneous infiltrate presenting clinically as patches, plaques or tumours; the tumours may ulcerate. When the disease becomes more generalized, lymphoma cells identical to those in Sézary syndrome may circulate in the blood. A defective retrovirus related to HTLV-I has been suspected of being an aetiological agent in this type of lymphoma [191] but this has not been confirmed; it is possible that the DNA sequence identified is not of viral origin.

Sézary cells [1] may be either large or small and one or other form usually predominates in an individual patient. Large Sézary cells are similar in size to a neutrophil or a monocyte with a high nucleocytoplasmic ratio and a round or oval nucleus with densely condensed chromatin, a grooved surface and usually no detectable nucleolus (Fig. 5.36). Small Sézary cells are similar in size to a normal small lymphocyte with a high nucleocytoplasmic ratio and a dense hyperchromatic nucleus with a grooved surface and no visible nucleolus (Fig. 5.37). Some cells show a ring of cytoplasmic vacuoles; periodic acid–Schiff (PAS) staining shows this to be due to the presence of glycogen. Small Sézary cells, in particular, may be difficult to identify on light microscopy. Electron microscopy can be very useful since it reveals the highly complex, convoluted nucleus (Fig. 5.38), which is not so readily detectable by light microscopy. Not surprisingly, an increasing number of circulating lymphoma cells correlates with worse prognosis in patients with erythrodermic cutaneous T-cell lymphoma [192]. The lymphocyte count and the percentage of Sézary cells have been found predictive of response to extracorporeal photopheresis [193].

The haemoglobin concentration and platelet count are usually normal. There may be a reactive eosinophilia.

In a rare lymphoproliferative disorder that may be more closely related to T-PLL than to Sézary syndrome there are no cutaneous lesions but there are abnormal circulating cells that cannot be distinguished from Sézary cells (see below).

Immunophenotype

The characteristic immunophenotype of Sézary cells is expression of CD2, CD3, CD4 and CD5 with no expression of CD8 or CD25 [1, 194] (see Table 5.12). CD3 and CD4 are often more weakly expressed than in normal T lymphocytes. The bimodal distribution of CD3 expression when there are both normal and neoplastic cells present can be used for the enumeration of Sézary cells [195]. A half to three quarters of cases are CD7 negative [146]. Lack of expression of CD7 and/or absent or weak expression of CD26,

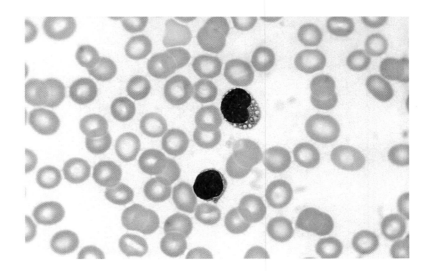

Fig. 5.37 PB film in small cell variant of Sézary syndrome. The nuclei show surface grooves and one cell has a partial circle of vacuoles around the nucleus. MGG × 870.

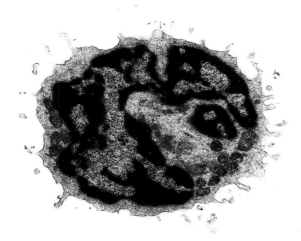

Fig. 5.38 Ultrastructural examination in Sézary syndrome showing the characteristic highly irregular nuclear outline (courtesy of Dr Estella Matutes, reproduced with permission from reference 7).

usually associated with weak expression of CD4, can be useful in identifying neoplastic cells in the blood [196]. CD25 is expressed in a minority of cases [191]. Cutaneous lymphocyte antigen (CD103) is expressed [197]. Detection of more than 11% of CD4-positive CD7-negative cells by flow cytometry has been found useful in detecting haematological involvement in mycosis fungoides and in confirming the diagnosis of Sézary syndrome in erythrodermic patients [191, 194].

Histology

Bone marrow infiltration is absent in the early stages and, even with advanced disease, is often minimal; infiltration is interstitial. Skin infiltration is in the upper dermis, particularly around the skin append-ages, and within the epidermis, forming Pautrier's microabscesses. Epidermotropism and Pautrier's micro-abscesses are characteristic of Sézary syndrome and mycosis fungoides but are not always present and are not pathognomonic since they have now also been observed in a number of cases of ATLL. In the later stages, when there is tumour formation, epidermo-tropism may be lost with tumour in both upper and lower dermis. Lymph node infiltration is paracortical.

Cytogenetics and molecular genetics

A great variety of cytogenetic abnormalities have been reported in Sézary syndrome without any con-sistent association being apparent. Random hetero-ploidy occurs. Clonal abnormalities are often highly complex and polyploid cells are not uncommon.

No specific molecular genetic abnormality has been associated with this type of lymphoma. However, demonstration of rearrangement of *TCR* genes is use-ful in confirming the diagnosis and has been found to be more sensitive in the detection of peripheral blood involvement than morphometric analysis [197].

Since it can be difficult to distinguish the small cell variant of Sézary syndrome from reactive

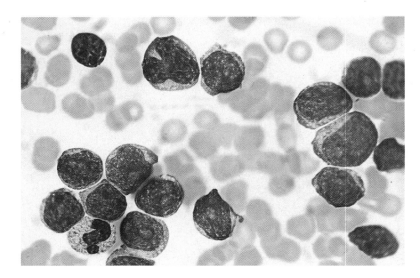

Fig. 5.39 PB film from a patient with hepatosplenic lymphoma in leukaemic phase showing large pleomorphic cells with basophilic cytoplasm. MGG × 870.

erythrodermic conditions it has been suggested that the detection of a clonal cytogenetic abnormality or demonstration of *TCR* rearrangement should be a prerequisite for the diagnosis of this form of cutaneous T-cell lymphoma [197].

Sézary cell-like leukaemia

A rare type of T-cell leukaemia has clinical and laboratory features overlapping Sézary syndrome and T-PLL [146, 198, 199]. In the WHO classification this condition is regarded as a variant of T-PLL.

Clinical, haematological and cytological features

This is a clinically aggressive disease. Of the small number of patients described, more than half have had hepatomegaly and a third lymphadenopathy. Skin lesions are not present. The white cell count is moderately to markedly elevated. Leukaemic cells have cerebriform nuclei and are more often small than large. The haemoglobin concentration and platelet count are usually normal.

Immunophenotype

The characteristic immunophenotype is positivity for CD2, CD3 and CD5. Most cases express CD7 and there is usually either expression of both CD4 and CD8 or expression of CD8 alone.

Cytogenetics and molecular genetics

The few cases studied cytogenetically have suggested a much closer relationship to T-PLL than to Sézary syndrome. All three had complex cytogenetic abnormalities including inv(14)(q11q32) and two also had iso(8q) [198].

Hepatosplenic T-cell lymphoma

This is a rare, clinically aggressive T-cell lymphoma in which the neoplastic cells typically express TCR γδ, normally expressed on a minor subset of peripheral blood T lymphocytes, but do not express TCR αβ.

Clinical, haematological and cytological features

Patients typically present with widespread disease and systemic symptoms. Hepatosplenomegaly is characteristic but there is usually no lymphadenopathy. Anaemia and thrombocytopenia are common. In one series of patients, a variable degree of peripheral blood involvement was usually detectable (Fig. 5.39) [200] but this cannot be readily distinguished from other T-cell lymphomas; however, on trephine biopsy the characteristic intravascular pattern of infiltration may suggest this diagnosis (see below). The bone marrow is hypercellular with erythroid and megakaryocytic hyperplasia. There is a scanty to moderate infiltrate of small to medium sized cells with the

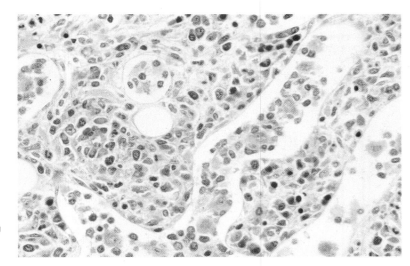

Fig. 5.40 Trephine biopsy section from a patient with hepatosplenic lymphoma in leukaemic phase showing intravascular lymphoma, same patient as Fig. 5.41. Giemsa × 348.

smaller cells having condensed chromatin while the larger cells are more blastic with a small but easily detectable nucleolus. Some cells have fine granules [200]. There may be increased plasma cells and reactive haemophagocytosis.

Immunophenotype

Characteristically there is expression of CD2, CD3, CD7, CD11b and CD56 [200, 201]. CD4, CD5 and CD8 are usually not expressed. In the majority of patients there is expression of TCR γδ but in a minority there is expression of TCR αβ expression of TCR αβ and TCR γδ. The cytotoxic granule protein, TIA-1, is expressed but not granzyme B of perforin.

Histology

Early in the disease course, bone marrow infiltration is interstitial and intrasinusoidal (Fig. 5.40). With advancing disease, there is a more extensive interstitial infiltration. There is typically hyperplasia of myeloid cells.

Cytogenetics and molecular genetics

The most characteristic cytogenetic abnormalities are trisomy 8 and an isochromosome of 7q, i(7)(q10). The majority of cases show a monoclonal rearrangement of *TCRG*, but not of *TCRB*.

Other T-cell non-Hodgkin's lymphoma

Rarely leukaemia occurs as a manifestation of T-cell lymphomas, either at presentation or during the course of the illness.

Clinical, haematological and cytological features

Clinical features may include hepatomegaly, splenomegaly and lymphadenopathy. The blood count may show anaemia or thrombocytopenia. The circulating cells may be small or medium sized with a variable degree of pleomorphism. In other patients neoplastic cells are large, usually with basophilic cytoplasm, prominent nucleoli and considerable pleomorphism (Fig. 5.41). In most cases of anaplastic large cell lymphoma, lymphoma cells are very large and pleomorphic (Fig. 5.42). Cytoplasmic granules have been reported in the small cell variant of anaplastic large cell lymphoma [202]. The neoplastic cells of T-cell lymphomas cannot be distinguished from those of B-lineage lymphomas on the basis of cytological features [132] so that immunophenotyping is essential for precise diagnosis.

Immunophenotype

Although the immunophenotype is that of a mature T cell there is no consistent pattern. Immunopheno-

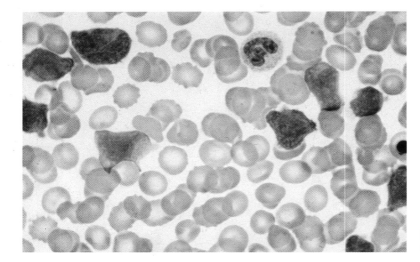

Fig. 5.41 PB film in a T-lineage lymphoma. MGG × 870.

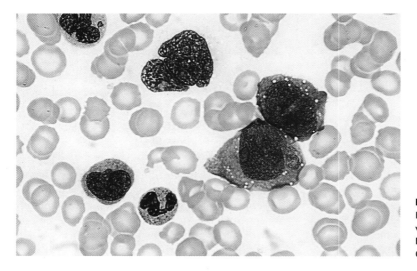

Fig. 5.42 PB in large cell anaplastic lymphoma. The lymphoma cells are very large and very pleomorphic. MGG × 870 (courtesy of Dr D. Clark, Grantham).

types rarely seen in normal peripheral blood T cells are common [132]. Abnormalities that may occur include under- or over-expression or lack of expression of CD3, under-expression or absent expression of CD7, over-expression of CD5, under- or over-expression of CD2 and failure to express either CD4 or CD8 [203]. A specific immunophenotype is recognizable when there is peripheral blood involvement by anaplastic large cell lymphoma; these cells sometimes express T-lineage markers and in addition express CD30, CD25, HLA-DR, ALK1 and often epithelial membrane antigen (EMA).

Histology

In patients with peripheral blood involvement by large cell lymphoma, lymph node biopsies usually show diffuse effacement by lymphoma cells. The bone marrow trephine biopsy usually shows extensive infiltration by large highly abnormal cells; the pattern of infiltration is random focal or diffuse. Anaplastic large cell lymphoma can be distinguished from other large cell lymphomas by the typical immunophenotype and the cytological features (very large, highly abnormal cells, often with a cohesive growth pattern).

Cytogenetics and molecular genetics

A range of cytogenetic and molecular genetic abnormalities is seen, depending on the precise type of lymphoma.

Many patients with anaplastic large cell lymphoma have a specific cytogenetic abnormality, t(2;5) (p23;q35). There is fusion of part of the *NPM* (**N**ucleo**P**hos**M**in) gene at 5q35 with part of the *ALK* (**A**naplastic **L**ymphoma **K**inase) gene from 2p23 leading to synthesis of a chimeric protein. *NPM-ALK* fusion transcripts can be detected by RT-PCR and ALK expression by immunohistochemistry (ALK is not normally expressed in lymphoid or haemopoietic cells) [105]. In a minority of patients there are other translocations and other fusion genes involving *ALK*. Rearrangements of *ALK* in typical and variant translocations can be detected by dual-colour, break-apart FISH.

References

1 Bennett JM, Catovsky D, Daniel M-T, Flandrin G, Galton DAG, Gralnick HR and Sultan C (1989) Proposals for the classification of chronic (mature) B and T lymphoid leukaemias. *J Clin Pathol*, **42**, 567–584.

2 Jaffe ES, Harris NL, Stein H and Vardiman JW (Eds) (2001) *World Health Organization Classification of Tumours: Pathology and Genetics of Tumours of Haematopoietic and Lymphoid Tissues*, IARC Press, Lyon.

3 Harris NL, Jaffe ES, Stein H, Banks PM, Chan JKC, Cleary ML *et al.* (1994) A revised European–American classification of lymphoid neoplasms: a proposal from the International Lymphoma Study group. *Blood*, **84**, 1361–1392.

4 Stewart CC, Behm FG, Carey JL, Cornbleet J, Duque RE, Hudnall SD *et al.* (1997) U.S.-Canadian consensus recommendations on the immunophenotypic analysis of hematologic neoplasia by flow cytometry: selection of antibody combinations. *Cytometry*, **30**, 231–235.

5 Bain BJ, Barnett D, Linch D, Matutes E and Reilly JT (2002) Revised guideline on immunophenotyping in acute leukaemias and lymphoproliferative disorders. *Clin Lab Haematol*, **24**, 1–13.

6 Langerak AW, van den Beemd MWM, Wolvers-Tettero ILM, Boor PP, van Lochem EG and Hooijkaas H (2001) Molecular and flow cytometric analysis of Vβ repertoire for clonality assessment in mature TCR αβ T-cell proliferations, *Blood*, **98**, 165–173.

7 Bain BJ, Clark DC, Lampert IA and Wilkins BS (2000) *Bone Marrow Pathology*. Third edition. Blackwell Science, Oxford.

8 Serke S, Schwaner I, Yordanova M, Szezepek A and Huhn D (2001) Monoclonal antibody FMC7 detects a conformational epitope on the CD20 molecule: evidence from phenotyping after rituxan therapy and transfectant cell analyses. *Cytometry*, **46**, 98–104.

9 Müller-Hermelink HK, Catovsky D, Montserrat E and Harris NL (2001) Chronic lymphocytic leukaemia/small lymphocytic lymphoma. In Jaffe ES, Harris NL, Stein H and Vardiman JW (Eds), *World Health Organization Classification of Tumours: Pathology and Genetics of Tumours of Haematopoietic and Lymphoid Tissues*, IARC Press, Lyon, pp. 127–130.

10 Yuille MR, Matutes E, Marossy A, Hilditch B, Catovsky D and Houlston RS (2000) Familial chronic lymphocytic leukaemia: a survey and a review of published cases. *Br J Haematol*, **109**, 794–799.

11 Cheson BD, Bennett JM, Grever M, Kay N, Keating MJ, O'Brien S and Rai KR (1996) National Cancer Institute-Sponsored Working Group Guidelines for chronic lymphocytic leukemia: revised guidelines for diagnosis and treatment. *Blood*, **87**, 4990–4997.

12 Oscier DG, Matutes E, Copplestone A, Pickering RM, Chapman R, Gillingham R *et al.* (1997) Atypical lymphocyte morphology: an adverse prognostic factor for disease progression in stage A CLL independent of trisomy 12. *Br J Haematol*, **98**, 934–939.

13 Thomas R, Ribeiro I, Shepherd P, Johnson P, Cook M, Lakhani A *et al.* (2002) Spontaneous clinical regression in chronic lymphocytic leukaemia. *Br J Haematol*, **116**, 341–345.

14 Amoureaux I, Mossafa H, Gentilhomme O, Girot R, Flandrin G and Troussard X (1997) Chronic lymphocytic leukaemia with binucleated lymphocytes. *Leuk Lymphoma*, **27**, 533–538.

15 Diehl LF and Ketchum LH (1998) Autoimmune disease and chronic lymphocytic leukemia: autoimmune hemolytic anemia, pure red cell aplasia, and autoimmune thrombocytopenia. *Semin Hematolol*, **25**, 80–97.

16 Rustagi P, Han T, Ziolkowski L, Currie M and Logue G (1983) Antigranulocyte antibodies in chronic lymphocytic leukemia and other chronic lymphoproliferative disorders. *Blood*, **62**, Suppl. 1, 106.

17 Stern SCM, Shah S and Costello C (1999) Probable autoimmune neutropenia induced by fludarabine treatment of chronic lymphocytic leukaemia. *Br J Haematol*, **106**, 836–837.

18 Kroft SH, Dawson B and McKenna RW (2001) Large cell lymphoma transformation of chronic lymphocytic leukemia/small lymphocytic lymphoma. *Am J Clin Pathol*, **115**, 385–395.

19 Rai KR, Sawitsky A, Cronkite EP, Chana AF, Levy RN and Pasternack BS (1975) Clinical staging of chronic lymphocytic leukemia. *Blood*, **46**, 219–234.

20 Binet JL, Auquier A, Dighiero G, Chastang C, Piguet H, Goasguen J *et al.* (1981) A new prognostic classification of chronic lymphocytic leukemia derived from multivariate survival analysis. *Cancer*, **48**, 198–206.

21 Matutes E, Owusu-Ankomah K, Morilla R, Garcia-Marco J, Houlihan A, Que TH and Catovsky D (1994)

The immunological profile of B-cell disorders and proposal of a scoring system for the diagnosis of CLL. *Leukemia*, **8**, 1640–1645.

22 Moreau EJ, Matutes E, A'Hern RP, Morilla AM, Morilla RM, Owusu-Ankomah KA *et al.* (1997) Improvement of the chronic lymphocytic leukemia scoring system with the monoclonal antibody SN8 (CD79b). *Am J Clin Pathol*, **108**, 278–382.

23 D'Arena G, Keating ML and Carotenuto M (2000) Chronic lymphoproliferative disorders: an integrated point of view for the differential diagnosis. *Leuk Lymphoma*, **36**, 225–237.

24 Huh YO, Keating MJ, Saffer HL, Jilani I, Lerner S and Albitar M (2001) Higher levels of surface CD20 expression on circulating lymphocytes compared with bone marrow and lymph nodes in B-cell chronic lymphocytic leukemia. *Am J Clin Pathol*, **116**, 437–443.

25 Freedman AS, Boyd AW, Bieber F, Daley J, Rosen K, Horowitz JC *et al.* (1987) Normal cellular counterparts of B cell chronic lymphocytic leukemia, *Blood*, **70**, 418–427.

26 Molica S, Dattilo A and Mannella A (1993) CD11c expression in B-cell chronic lymphocytic leukemia, *Blood*, **81**, 2466.

27 Marotta G, Raspadori D, Sestigiani C, Scalia G, Bigazzi C and Lauria F (2000) Expression of the CD11c antigen in B-cell chronic lymphoproliferative disorders. *Leuk Lymphoma*, **37**, 145–149.

28 Orazi A, Cattoretti G, Polli N and Rilke E (1991) Distinct morphophenotypic features of chronic B lymphocytic leukemia identified with CD1c and CD23. *Eur J Haematol*, **47**, 28–35.

29 Jennings CD and Foon KA (1997) Recent advances in flow cytometry: applications to the diagnosis of hematologic malignancy. *Blood*, **90**, 2863–2892.

30 Sebastyén A, Berczi L, Mihalik R, Paku S and Matolcsy A (1999) Syndecam-1 (CD138) expression in human non-Hodgkin's lymphomas. *Br J Haematol*, **104**, 412–419.

31 Rossmann ED, Lundin J, Lenkei R, Mellstedt H and Österborg A (2001) Variability in B-cell antigen expression: implications for the treatment of B-cell lymphomas and leukemias with monoclonal anti-bodies. *Leuk Lymphoma*, **42**, Suppl. 1, 55.

32 Molica S, Dattilo A, Giulino C and Levato D (2000) Flow cytometric expression of cyclin D1 in typical B-cell CLL allows identification of patients at high risk of disease progression. *Hematol J*, **1**, Suppl. 1, 91.

33 Zupo S, Mangiola M, Rossi E, Brugiatelli M, Ferrarini M and Morabito F (2001) Nuclear protein Ki67: a novel potential prognostic marker in B-cell chronic lymphocytic leukemia (B-CLL) *Leuk Lymphoma*, **42**, Suppl. 1, 35.

34 Shen PUF, Fuller SG, Rezuke WN, Sherburne BJ and di Guiseppe JA (2001) Laboratory, morphologic, and immunophenotypic correlates of surface immunoglobulin heavy chain isotype expression in B-cell chronic lymphocytic leukemia. *Am J Clin Pathol*, **116**, 905–912.

35 Callea V, Morabito F, Oliva BM, Stelitano C, Levato D, Dattilo A *et al.* (1999) Surface CD14 positivity correlates with worse prognosis in B-cell chronic lymphocytic leukaemia. *Br J Haematol*, **107**, 347–352.

36 Hjalmar V, Hast R and Kimby E (2002) Cell surface expession of CD25, CD54, and CD95 on B- and T-cells in chronic lymphocytic leukaemia in relation to trisomy 12, atypical morphology and clinical course. *Eur J Haematol*, **68**, 127–134.

37 Hamblin TJ, Orchard JA, Gardiner A, Oscier DG, Davis Z and Stevenson FK (2000) Immunoglobulin V genes and CD38 expression in CLL. *Blood*, **95**, 2455.

38 Damle R, Wasil T, Allen S, Schulman P, Rai KR, Chiorazzi N and Ferrarini M (2000) Updated data on V gene mutation status and CD38 expression in B-CLL. *Blood*, **95**, 2456–2457.

39 Ibrahim S, Keating M, Do K-A, O'Brien S, Huh YO, Jilani I *et al.* (2001) CD38 expression as an important prognostic factor in B-cell chronic lymphocytic leukemia. *Blood*, **98**, 181–186.

40 Jelinek DF, Tschumper RC, Geyer SM, Bone ND, Dewald GW, Hanson CA *et al.* (2001) Analysis of clonal B-cell CD38 and immunoglobulin variable region sequence status in relation to clinical outcome for B-chronic lymphocytic leukaemia. *Br J Haematol*, **115**, 854–861.

41 Chevallier P, Penther D, Avet-Loiseau H, Robillard N, Ifrah N, Mahé B *et al.* (2002) CD38 expression and secondary 17p deletion are important prognostic factors in chronic lymphocytic leukaemia. *Br J Haematol*, **116**, 142–150.

42 Green MJ, Kuzmicki A, Rawstron AC, Kennedy B, Evans PAS, Richards SJ *et al.* (2001) Clonal B cells with a CLL immunophenotype are frequently detectable in normal individuals. *Br J Haematol*, **113**, Suppl. 1, 64.

43 Rawstron AC, Green MJ, Kuzmicki A, Kennedy B, Jack AS and Hillmen P (2001) Monoclonal CLL-phenotype cells are present in 3% of otherwise normal individuals and have the characteristics of good prognosis CLL. *Leuk Lymphoma*, **42**, Suppl. 1, 29.

44 Reed JC (1998) Molecular biology of chronic lymphocytic leukemia. *Semin Oncol*, **25**, 11–18.

45 Juliusson G and Merup M (1998) Cytogenetics in chronic lymphocytic leukemia. *Semin Oncol*, **25**, 19–26.

46 Dyer MJS, Zani VJ, Lu WZ, O'Byrne A, Mould S, Chapman R *et al.* (1994) *BCL2* translocations in leukemias of mature B cells. *Blood*, **83**, 3682–3688.

47 Michaux L, Mecucci C, Stul M, Wlodarski I, Hernandez JM, Meeus P *et al.* (1996) BCL3 rearrangement and the t(14;19)(q24;q13) in lymphoproliferative disorders. *Genes Chromosomes Cancer*, **15**, 38–47.

48 Juliusson G, Oscier DG, Fitchett M, Ross FM, Stockdill G, Mackie MJ *et al.* (1990) Prognostic subgroups in B-cell chronic lymphocytic leukemia defined by specific chromsomal abnormalities. *N Engl J Med*, **323**, 720–724.

49 Finn WG, Thangavelu M, Yelavarthi KK, Goolsby C, Tallman MS, Trayner A and Peterson LC (1996) Karyotype correlates with peripheral blood morphology and immunophenotype in chronic lymphocytic leukemia. *Am J Clin Pathol*, **105**, 458–467.

50 Geisler CH, Philip P, Egelund Christensen B, Hoa-Jensen K, Tingaard-Pedersen N, Myhre Jensen O *et al.* (1996) Trisomy 12 is found in CLL with both typical and atypical immunophenotype and has no prognostic significance. *Blood*, **88**, Suppl. 1, 237a.

51 Auer RL, Bienz N, Neilson J, Cai M, Waters JJ, Milligan DW and Fegan CD (1999) The sequential analysis of trisomy 12 in chronic lymphocytic leukaemia. *Br J Haematol*, **104**, 742–744.

52 Döhner H, Stilgenbauer S, James MR, Benner A, Weilguni T, Bentz M *et al.* (1997) 11q deletions identify a new subset of B-cell chronic lymphocytic leukemia characterized by extensive nodal involvement and inferior prognosis. *Blood*, **89**, 2516–2522.

53 Döhner H, Stilgenbauer S, Benner A, Leupolt E, Kröber A, Bullinger L *et al.* (2000) Genomic aberrations and survival in chronic lymphocytic leukemia. *N Engl J Med*, **343**, 1910–1916.

54 Criel A, Michaux L and de Wolf-Peeters S (1999) The concept of typical and atypical chronic lymphocytic leukaemia. *Leuk Lymphoma*, **33**, 33–45.

55 Sembries S, Pahl H, Stilgenbauer S, Döhner H and Schriever F (1999) Reduced expression of adhesion molecules and cell signalling receptors by chronic lymphocytic leukemia cells with 11q deletion. *Blood*, **93**, 624–634.

56 Damle R, Wasil T, Fais F, Ghiotto F, Valetto A, Allen SL *et al.* (1999) Ig V gene mutation status and CD38 expression as novel prognostic indicators in chronic lymphocytic leukemia. *Blood*, **94**, 1840–1847.

57 Hamblin TJ, Davis Z, Gardiner A, Oscier DG, and Stevenson FK (1999) Unmutated Ig VH genes are associated with a more aggressive form of chronic lymphocytic leukemia. *Blood*, **94**, 1848–1854.

58 O'Connor SJM, Evans PAS, Owen RG, Morgan GJ and Jack AS (2000) Prediction of VH gene mutation status in B-CLL using immunophenotyping and trephine histology. *Blood*, **96**, 357a.

59 Hamblin TJ, Orchard JA, Ibbotson RE, Davis Z, Thomas PW, Stevenson FK and Oscier DG (2002) CD38 expression and immunoglobulin variable region mutations are independent prognostic variables in chronic lymphocytic leukemia, but CD38 expression may vary during the course of the disease. *Blood*, **99**, 1023–1029.

60 Garcia-Marco JA, Price CM and Catovsky D (1997) Interphase cytogenetics in chronic lymphocytic leukemia. *Cancer Genet Cytogenet*, **97**, 52–58.

61 Stankovic T, Weber P, Stewart G, Bedenham T, Murray J, Byrd PJ *et al.* (1999) Inactivation of ataxia telangiectasia mutated gene in B-cell chronic lymphocytic leukemia. *Lancet*, **353**, 26–29.

62 Oscier DG and Gardiner AC (2001) Lymphoid neoplasms. *Best Pract Res Clin Haematol*. **14**, 609–630.

63 Sahota SS, Davis Z, Hamblin TJ and Stevenson FK (2000) Somatic mutation of *bcl-6* genes can occur in the absence of V_H mutations in chronic lymphocytic leukemia. *Blood*, **95**, 3534–3540.

64 Thompson AA, Talley JA, Do HN, Kagan HL, Kunkel L, Berenson J *et al.* (1997) Aberrations of the B-cell receptor B29 (CD79b) gene in chronic lymphocytic leukemia. *Blood*, **90**, 1387–1394.

65 Lens D, Dyer MJ, Garcia-Marco JM, de Schouwer JJC, Hamoudi RA, Jones D *et al.* (1997) p53 abnormalities in CLL are associated with excess of prolymphocytes and poor prognosis. *Br J Haematol*, **99**, 848–857.

66 Pettitt AR, Sherrington PD, Stewart G, Cawley JC, Taylor AMRT and Stankovic T (2001) p53 dysfunction in B-cell chronic lymphocytic leukemia: inactivation of *ATM* as an alternative to *TP53* mutation. *Blood*, **89**, 814–822.

67 Enno A, Catovsky D, O'Brien M, Cherchi M, Kumaran TO and Galton DAG (1979) 'Prolymphocytoid' transformation of chronic lymphocytic leukaemia. *Br J Haematol*, **41**, 9–18.

68 Melo JV, Catovsky D and Galton DAG (1986) The relationship between chronic lymphocytic leukaemia and prolymphocytic leukaemia. I. Clinical and laboratory features of 300 patients and characterisation of an intermediate group. *Br J Haematol*, **63**, 377–387.

69 Criel A, Verhoef G, Vlietinck R, Mecucci C, Billiet J, Michaux L *et al.* (1997) Further characterization of morphologically defined typical and atypical CLL: a clinical, immunophenotypic, cytogenetic and prognostic study of 390 cases. *Br J Haematol*, **97**, 383–391.

70 Frater JL, McCarron KF, Hammel JP, Shapiro JL, Miller ML, Tubbs RR *et al.* (2001) Typical and atypical chronic lymphocytic leukemia differ clinically and immunophenotypically. *Am J Clin Pathol*, **116**, 655–664.

71 Catovsky, Montserrat E, Müller-Hermelink HK and Harris NJ (2001) B-cell prolymphocytic leukaemia. In Jaffe ES, Harris NL, Stein H and Vardiman JW (Eds), *World Health Organization Classification of Tumours: Pathology and Genetics of Tumours of Haematopoietic and Lymphoid Tissues*, IARC Press, Lyon, pp. 131–132.

72 Galton DAG, Goldmann JM, Wiltshaw E, Catovsky D, Henry K and Goldenberg GJ (1974) Prolymphocytic leukaemia, *Br J Haematol*, **27**, 7–23.

73 DiGiuseppe JA and Borowitz MJ (1998) Clinical utility of flow cytometry in the chronic lymphoid leukemias. *Semin Oncol*, **25**, 6–10.

74 Zomas AP, Matutes E, Morilla R, Owusu-Ankomah K, Seon BK and Catovsky D (1996) Expression of the immunoglobulin-associated protein B29 in B cell disorders with the monoclonal antibody SN8 (CD79b). *Leukemia*, **10**, 1966–1970.

75 Feneux D, Choquet S, de Almeida C, Davi F, Garand R, Valensi F, Léonard C and Merle-Béral H (1996)

Cytogenetic studies by FISH on B cell prolymphocytic leukemia. *Blood*, **88**, Suppl. 1, 155b.

76 Lampert I, Catovsky D, Marsh GW, Child JA and Galton DAG (1980) The histopathology of prolymphocytic leukaemia with particular reference to the spleen: a comparison with chronic lymphocytic leukaemia. *Histopathology*, **4**, 3–19.

77 Lampert I and Thompson I (1988) The spleen in chronic lymphocytic leukemia and related disorders. In Polliack A and Catovsky D (Eds), *Chronic Lymphocytic Leukemia*, pp. 193–208. Harwood Academic Publishers, Chur.

78 Brito-Babapulle V, Pittman S, Melo JV, Pomfret M and Catovsky D (1987) Cytogenetic studies on prolymphocytic leukemia 1. B-cell prolymphocytic leukemia. *Hematol Pathol*, **1**, 27–33.

79 Schlette E, Bueso-Ramos C, Giles F, Glassman A, Hayes K and Medeiros LJ (2001) Mature B-cell leukemias with more than 55% prolymphocytes: a heterogeneous group that includes an unusual variant of mantle cell lymphoma. *Am J Clin Pathol*, **115**, 571–581.

80 Lens D, Matutes E, Catovsky D and Coignet LJA (2000) Frequent deletions of 11q23 and 13q14 in B cell prolymphocytic leukemia (B-PLL) *Leukemia*, **14**, 427–430.

81 Lens D, de Schouwer JJC, Hamoudi RA, Abdul-Rauf M, Farahat N, Matutes E *et al.* (1997) p53 abnormalities in B-cell prolymphocytic leukemia. *Blood*, **89**, 2015–2023.

82 Borowitz MJ, Bray R, Gascoyne R, Melnick S, Parker JW, Picker L and Stetler-Stevenson M (1997) U.S.-Canadian consensus recommendations on the immunophenotypic analysis of hematologic neoplasia by flow cytometry: data analysis and interpretation. *Cytometry*, **30**, 236–244.

83 Posnett DN, Marboe CC, Knowles DM, Jaffe EA and Kunkel HG (1984) A membrane marker (HC1) selectively present on hairy cell leukemia cells, endothelial cells, and epidermal basal cells. *J Immunol*, **132**, 2700–2702.

84 Cordone I, Annino L, Masi S, Pescarmona E, Rahimi S, Ferrari A *et al.* (1995) Diagnostic relevance of peripheral blood immunocytochemistry in hairy cell leukaemia. *J Clin Pathol*, **48**, 955–960.

85 Matutes E and Catovsky D (1994) The value of scoring systems for the diagnosis of biphenotypic leukemia and mature B-cell disorders. *Leuk Lymphoma*, **3**, Suppl. 1, 11–14.

86 Tytherleigh L, Taparia M and Leahy MF (2001) Detection of hairy cell leukaemia in blood and bone marrow using multidimensional flow cytometry with CD45-PECy5 and SS gating. *Clin Lab Haematol*, **23**, 385–390.

87 Foucar K and Catovsky D (2001) Hairy cell leukaemia. In Jaffe ES, Harris NL, Stein H and Vardiman JW (Eds), pp. 138–141. *World Health Organization Classification of Tumours: Pathology and Genetics of Tumours of Haematopoietic and Lymphoid Tissues*, IARC Press, Lyon.

88 Juliusson G and Gahrton G (1993) Cytogenetics in CLL and related disorders. *Bailliére's Clin Haematol*, **6**, 821–848.

89 Sambani C, Trafalis DT, Mitsoulis-Mentzikoff C, Poulakidas E, Makropoulos V, Pantelias GE and Mecucci C (2001) Clonal chromosome rearrangements in hairy cell leukemia: personal experience and review of literature. *Cancer Genet Cytogenet*, **129**, 138–144.

90 Cawley JC, Burns GF and Hayhoe FGH (1980) A chronic lymphoproliferative disorder with distinctive features: a distinct variant of hairy cell leukaemia. *Leuk Res*, **4**, 547–559.

91 Sainati L, Matutes E, Mulligan S, de Oliveira MP, Rani S, Lampert IA and Catovsky D (1990) A variant form of hairy cell leukemia resistant to α interferon: clinical and phenotypic characteristics in 17 patients. *Blood*, **76**, 157–162.

92 Melo JV, Hegde U, Parreira A, Thompson I, Lampert IA and Catovsky D (1987) Splenic B lymphoma with circulating villous lymphocytes: differential diagnosis of B cell leukaemias with large spleens. *J Clin Pathol*, **40**, 329–342.

93 Matutes E, Morilla R, Owusu-Ankomah K, Houlihan A and Catovsky D (1994) The immunophenotype of splenic lymphoma with villous lymphocytes and its relevance to the differential diagnosis with other B-cell disorders. *Blood*, **83**, 1558–1562.

94 Troussard X, Valensi F, Duchayne E, Garand R, Felman P, Tulliez M, Henry-Amar M, Bryon PA, Flandrin G et le Groupe Francais d'Hématologie Cellulaire (1996) Splenic lymphoma with villous lymphocytes: clinical presentation, biology and prognostic factors in a series of 100 patients. *Br J Haematol*, **93**, 731–736.

95 Isaacson PG, Matutes E, Burke M and Catovsky D (1994) The histopathology of splenic lymphoma with villous lymphocytes. *Blood*, **84**, 3829–3834.

96 Catovsky D and Matutes E (1999) Splenic lymphoma with circulating villous lymphocytes/splenic marginal zone lymphoma. *Semin Hematol*, **36**, 148–154.

97 Cuneo A, Bardi A, Wlodarska I, Selleslag D, Roberti MG, Bigoni R *et al.* (2001) A novel recurrent translocation t(11;14)(p11;q32) in splenic marginal zone B cell lymphoma. *Leukemia*, **15**, 1262–1267.

98 Oscier DG, Matutes E, Gardiner A, Glide S, Mould S, Brito-Babapulle V, Ellis J and Catovsky D (1993) Cytogenetic studies in splenic lymphoma with villous lymphocytes. *Br J Haematol*, **85**, 487–491.

99 Garcia-Marco JA, Nouel A, Navarro B, Matutes E, Oscier D, Proice CM and Catovsky D (1998) Molecular cytogenetic analysis in splenic lymphoma with villous lymphocytes. Frequent allelic imbalance of the RB1 gene but not the D13s25 locus on chromosome 13q14. *Cancer Res*, **58**, 1736–1740.

100 Gruszka-Westwood AM, Hamoudi RA, Matutes E, Tuset E and Catovsky D (2001) p53 abnormalities in splenic lymphoma with villous lymphocytes. *Blood*, **97**, 3552–3558.

101 Bain BJ and Catovsky D (1994) The leukaemic phase of non-Hodgkin's lymphoma. *J Clin Pathol*, **48**, 189–193.

102 Nathwani BN, Harris NL, Weisenberger D, Isaacson PG, Piris MA, Berger F, Müller-Hermelink HK, and Swerdlow SH (2001) Follicular lymphoma. In Jaffe ES, Harris NL, Stein H and Vardiman JW (Eds), *World Health Organization Classification of Tumours: Pathology and Genetics of Tumours of Haematopoietic and Lymphoid Tissues*, IARC Press, Lyon, pp. 162–167.

103 Bellido M, Rubiol E, Ubeda J, López O, Estivill C, Carnicer MJ *et al.* (2001) Flow cytometry using the monoclonal antibody CD10-Pe/Cy5 is a useful tool to identify follicular lymphoma cells. *Eur J Haematol*, **66**, 100–106.

104 Jaffe ES, Raffeld M and Medeiros LJ (1993) Histologic subtypes of indolent lymphomas: caricatures of the mature B-cell system. *Semin Oncol*, **20**, Suppl. 5, 3–30.

105 Mauvieux L and Macintyre (1996) Practical role of molecular diagnostics in non-Hodgkin's lymphomas. *Bailliére's Clin Haematol*, **9**, 653–667.

106 Mohamed AN, Palutke M, Eisenberg L and Al-Katib A (2001) Chromosomal analyses of 52 cases of follicular lymphoma with t(14;18), including blastic/blastoid variant. *Cancer Genet Cytogenet*, **126**, 45–51.

107 Aamot H, Micci F, Holte H, Delabie J and Heim S (2002) M-FISH cytogenetic analysis of non-Hodgkin's lymphomas with t(14;18)(q32;q21) and add(1)(p36) as a secondary abnormality shows that the extra material often comes from chromosome arm 17q. *Leuk Lymphoma*, **43**, 1051–1056.

108 Ohno H and Fukuhara S (1997) Significance of rearrangement of BCL6 gene in B-cell lymphoid neoplasms. *Leuk Lymphoma*, **27**, 55–63.

109 Yano T, Sander CA, Andrade RE, Gauwerky CE, Croce CM, Longo DL *et al.* (1993) Molecular analysis of the BCL-3 locus at chromosome 17q22 in B cell neoplasms. *Blood*, **82**, 1813–1819.

110 Callanan M, Le Baccon P, Mossuz P, Duley S, Bastard C, Hamoudi R *et al.* (2000) Deregulation of the ITIM-bearing IgG receptor, FcγRIIBtranslocation in malignant lymphoma. *Hematol J*, **1**, Suppl. 1, 50.

111 Lorsbach RB, Shay-Seymore D, Moore J, Banks PM, Hasserjian RP, Sandlund JT and Behm FG (2002) Clinicopathologic analysis of follicular lymphoma occurring in children. *Blood*, **99**, 1959–1964.

112 Argatoff LH, Connors JM, Klasa RJ, Horsman DE and Gascoyne RD (1997) Mantle cell lymphoma: a clinicopathologic study of 80 cases. *Blood*, **89**, 2067–2078.

113 Swerdlow SH, Berger F, Isaacson PI, Müller-Hermelink HK, Nathwani BN, Piris MA and Harris NL (2001) Mantle cell lymphoma. In Jaffe ES, Harris NL, Stein H and Vardiman JW (Eds), *World Health Organization Classification of Tumours: Pathology and Genetics of Tumours of Haematopoietic and Lymphoid Tissues*, IARC Press, Lyon, pp. 168–170.

114 Samaha H, Dumontet C, Ketterer N, Moullet I, Thieblement C, Bouafia F *et al.* (1998) Mantle cell lymphoma: a retrospective study of 121 cases. *Leukemia*, **12** 1281–1287.

115 de Oliviera MSP, Jaffe ES and Catovsky D (1989) Leukaemic phase of mantle zone (intermediate) lymphoma. *J Clin Pathol*, **42**, 962–972.

116 Cesca C, Ben-Ezra J and Riley RS (2001) Platelet satellitism as presenting finding in mantle cell lymphoma. *Am J Clin Pathol*, **115**, 567–570.

117 Gong JZ, Lagoo A, Peters D, Horvatinovich J, Benz P and Buckley PJ (2001) Value of CD23 determination by flow cytometry in differentiating mantle cell lymphoma from chronic lymphocytic leukemia/small lymphocytic lymphoma. *Am J Clin Pathol*, **116**, 893–897.

118 Alexander HD, Catherwood MA, Beattie RGG, Cuthbert RJG, Kettle PJ, Markey GM and Morris TCM (2002) Immunophenotyping in the differential diagnosis of mantle cell lymphoma/leukaemia. *Br J Haematol*, **117**, Suppl. 1, 72.

119 Elnenaei MO, Jadayel DM, Matutes E, Morilla R, Owusu-Ankomah K, Atkinson S *et al.* (2001) Cyclin D1 by flow cytometry as a useful tool in the diagnosis of B-cell malignancies. *Leuk Res*, **25**, 115–123.

120 Alexander HD, Catherwood MA, Beattie RGG, Cuthbert RJG, Kettle PJ, Markey GM and Morris TCM (2001) Immunophenotyping in the differential diagnosis of mantle cell lymphoma/leukaemia. *Leuk Lymphoma*, **42**, Suppl. 1, 41–42.

121 Barista I, Romaguera JE and Cabanillas F (2001) Mantle cell lymphoma. *Lancet Oncol*, **2**, 141–148.

122 Vasef MA, Medeiros LJ, Koo C, McCourty A and Brynes RK (1997) Cyclin D1 immunohistochemical staining is useful in distinguishing mantle cell lymphoma from other low grade B-cell neoplasms in bone marrow. *Am J Clin Pathol*, **108**, 302–307.

123 Vaandrager J-W, Schuuring E, Zwikstra E, de Boer CJ, Kleiverda KK, van Krieken JHJM *et al.* (1996) Direct visualization of dispersed 11q13 chromosomal translocations in mantle cell lymphoma by multicolour DNA fiber fluorescence *in situ* hybridization. *Blood*, **88**, 1177–1182.

124 Katz RL, Caraway NP, Gu J, Jiang F, Pasco-Miller LS, Glassman AB *et al.* (2000) Detection of chromosome 11q13 breakpoints by interphase fluorescence in situ hybridization. *Am J Clin Pathol*, **114**, 248–257.

125 Onciu M, Schlette E, Medeiros LJ, Abruzzo LV, Keating M and Lai R (2001) Cytogenetic findings in mantle cell lymphoma: cases with a high level of peripheral blood involvement have a distinct pattern of abnormalities. *Am J Clin Pathol*, **116**, 886–892.

126 Bigoni R, Cuneo AS, Milani R, Roberti MG, Bardi A, Rigolin GM *et al.* (2001) Secondary chromosome changes in mantle cell lymphoma: cytogenetic and fluorescence in situ hybridization studies. *Leuk Lymphoma*, **40**, 581–590.

127 Stilgenbauer S, Winkler D, Ott G, Schaffner C, Leupolt E Bentz M *et al.* (1999) Molecular characterization of 11q deletions points to a pathogenic role of the

ATM gene in mantle cell lymphoma. *Blood*, **94**, 3262–3264.

128 Martinez-Climent JA, Vizcarra E, Sanchez D, Blesa D, Marugan I, Benet I *et al.* (2001) Loss of a novel tumor suppressor gene locus at chromosome 8p is associated with leukemic mantle cell lymphoma. *Blood*, **98**, 3479–3482.

129 Au WY, Gascoyne RD, Viswanatha DS, Connors JM, Klasa RJ and Horsman DE (2002) Cytogenetic analysis in mantle cell lymphoma: a review of 214 cases. *Leuk Lymphoma*, **43**, 783–791.

130 Vaishampayan UN, Mohamed AN, Dugan MC, Bloom RE and Palutke M (2001) Blastic mantle cell lymphoma associated with Burkitt-type translocation and hypodiploidy. *Br J Haematol*, **115**, 66–68.

131 Allen JE, Hough RE, Goepel JR, Bottomley S, Willson GA, Alcock HE *et al.* (2002) Identification of novel regions of amplification and deletion within mantle cell lymphoma DNA by comparative genomic hybridization. *Br J Haematol*, **116**, 291–298.

132 Bain BJ, Matutes E, Robinson D, Lampert IA, Brito-Babapulle V, Morilla R and Catovsky D (1991) Leukaemia as a manifestation of large cell lymphoma. *Br J Haematol*, **7**, 301–310.

133 Cobcroft R (1999) Diagnosis of angiotropic large B-cell lymphoma from a peripheral blood film, *Br J Haematol*, **104**, 429.

134 Ueda Y, Nishida K, Miki T, Horiike T, Kaneko H, Yokota S *et al.* (1997) Interphase detection of *BCL6*/IgH fusion gene in non-Hodgkin's lymphoma by fluorescence *in situ* hybridization. *Cancer Genet Cytogenet*, **99**, 102–107.

135 Iidi S, Rao PH, Nallasivam P, Hibshoosh H, Butler M, Louie DC *et al.* (1996) The t(9;14)(p13;q32) chromosomal translocation associated with lymphoplasmacytoid lymphoma involves the *PAX-5* gene. *Blood*, **88**, 4110–4117.

136 Carbone A, Gloghini A, Pinto A, Attadia V, Zagonal V and Volpe R (1989) Monocytoid B-cell lymphoma with bone marrow and peripheral blood involvement at presentation. *Am J Clin Pathol*, **92**, 228–236.

137 Griesser H, Kaiser U, Augener W, Tiemann M and Lennert K (1990) B-cell lymphoma of the mucosa-associated lymphatic tissue (MALT) presenting with bone marrow and peripheral blood involvement. *Leuk Res*, **14**, 617–622.

138 Grogan TM, van Camp B, Kyle RA, Müller-Hermelink HK and Harris NL (2001) Plasma cell neoplasms. In Jaffe ES, Harris NL, Stein H and Vardiman JW (Eds), *World Health Organization Classification of Tumours: Pathology and Genetics of Tumours of Haematopoietic and Lymphoid Tissues*, IARC Press, Lyon, pp. 142–156.

139 Costello C, Sainty D, Bouabdallah R, Fermand J-P, Delmer A, Divie M *et al.* (2001) Primary plasma cell leukaemia: a report of 18 cases. *Leuk Res*, **25**, 103–107.

140 San Miguel JF, Garcia-Sanz R, Gonzales M and Orfao A (1995) Immunophenotype and DNA content in multiple myeloma. *Bailliére's Clin Haematol*, **8**, 735–759.

141 Jaffe ES and Ralfkiaer E (2001) Mature T-cell and NK-cell neoplasms. In Jaffe ES, Harris NL, Stein H and Vardiman JW (Eds), *World Health Organization Classification of Tumours: Pathology and Genetics of Tumours of Haematopoietic and Lymphoid Tissues*, IARC Press, Lyon, pp. 191–194.

142 Lamy T and Loughran TP (1999) Current concepts: large granular lymphocyte leukaemia *Blood Rev*, **13**, 230–240.

143 Chan WC, Catovsky D, Foucar K and Montserrat E (2001) T-cell large granular lymphocyte leukaemia. In Jaffe ES, Harris NL, Stein H and Vardiman JW (Eds), *World Health Organization Classification of Tumours: Pathology and Genetics of Tumours of Haematopoietic and Lymphoid Tissues*, IARC Press, Lyon, pp. 197–198.

144 Pandolfi F, Loughran TP, Starkebaum G, Chisesi T, Barbui T, Chan WC *et al.* (1990) Clinical course and prognosis of the lymphoproliferative disease of granular lymphocytes. A multicenter study *Cancer*, **65**, 341–8.

145 Dhodapkar MV, Li CY, Lust JA, Tefferi A and Phyliky RL (1994) Clinical spectrum of clonal proliferations of T-large granular lymphocytes: a T-cell clonopathy of undetermined significance? *Blood*, **84**, 1620–1627.

146 Matutes E (1999) T-cell Lymphoproliferative Disorders: Classification, Clinical and Laboratory Aspects, *Advances in Blood Disorders*, Series Editor, Polliak A, Harwood Academic Publishers, Australia.

147 Gentile TC, Uner AH, Hutchison RE, Wright J, Ben-Ezra J, Russell EC and Loughran TP (1994) CD3+, CD56+ aggressive variant of large granular lymphocyte leukemia *Blood*, **84**, 2315–2321.

148 Gupta V, Mills MJ and Eden AG (2001) Natural killer-like T-cell leukaemia/lymphoma. *Br J Haematol*, **115**, 490.

149 Reynolds CW and Foon KA (1984) Tγ-lymphoproliferative disease and related disorders in humans and experimental animals: a review of the clinical, cellular and functional characteristics. *Blood*, **64**, 1146–1158.

150 Akashi K, Shibuya T, Taniguchi S, Hayashi S, Iwasaki H, Teshima T *et al.* (1999) Multiple autoimmune haemopoietic disorders and insidious clonal proliferation of large granular lymphocyte leukaemia. *Br J Haematol*, **107**, 670–673.

151 Loughran JP (1993) Clonal disease of large granular lymphocytes. *Blood*, **82**, 1–14.

152 Prieto J, Rios E, Parrado A, Martin A, de Blas JM and Rodriguez JM (1996) Leukaemia of natural killer cell large granular lymphocyte type with HLA-DR-CD16-CD56bright+ phenotype. *J Clin Pathol*, **49**, 1011–1013.

153 Ginaldi L, Matutes E, Farahat N, De Martinis M, Morilla R and Catovsky D (1996) Differential expression of CD3 and CD7 in T-cell malignancies: a quantitative study by flow cytometry. *Br J Haematol*, **93**, 921–927.

154 Akashi K, Shibuya T, Nakamura M, Oogami A, Harada M and Niho Y (1998) Large granular lymphocyte leukaemia with a mixed T-cell/B-cell phenotype. *Br J Haematol*, **100**, 291–294.

155 Brouet JC, Sasportes M, Flandrin G, Preud'Homme JL and Seligmann M (1975) Chronic lymphocytic leukaemia of T-cell origin. Immunological and clinical evaluation in eleven patients *Lancet*, **2**, 890–893.

156 Palutke M, Eisenberg L, Kaplan J, Hussain M, Kithier K, Tabaczka P *et al.* (1983) Natural killer and suppressor T-cell chronic lymphocytic leukemia *Blood*, **62**, 627–634.

157 Agnarsson BA, Loughran TP, Starkebaum G and Kadin ME (1989) The pathology of large granular lymphocyte leukemia *Hum Pathol*, **20**, 643–651.

158 Kouides PA and Rowe JM (1995) Large granular lymphocyte leukemia presenting with both amegakaryocytic thrombocytopenic purpura and pure red cell aplasia: clinical course and response to immunosuppressive therapy *Am J Hematol*, **49**, 232–236.

159 Wong KF, Chan JCW, Liu HSY, Man C and Kwong YL (2002) Chromosomal abnormalities in T-cell large granular lymphocyte leukaemia: report of two cases and review of the literature. *Br J Haematol*, **116**, 598–600.

160 Chan JKC, Wong KF, Jaffe ES and Ralfkiaer E (2001) Aggressive NK-cell leukaemia. In Jaffe ES, Harris NL, Stein H and Vardiman JW (Eds), *World Health Organization Classification of Tumours: Pathology and Genetics of Tumours of Haematopoietic and Lymphoid Tissues*, IARC Press, Lyon, pp. 198–199.

161 Tefferi A, Li CY, Witzig TE, Dhodapkar MV, Okuno SH and Phyliky RL (1994) Chronic natural killer cell lymphocytosis: a descriptive clinical study. *Blood*, **84**, 2721–2725.

162 Kawa-Ha K, Ishihara S, Ninomiya T, Yumura-Yagi K, Hara J, Murayama F, Tawa A and Hirai K (1989) CD3-negative lymphoproliferative disease of granular lymphocytes containing Epstein–Barr viral DNA. *J Clin Invest*, **84**, 51–55.

163 Chan JK, Sin VC, Wong KF, Ng CS, Tsang WY, Chan CH *et al.* (1997) Nonnasal lymphoma expressing the natural killer cell marker CD56: a clinicopathologic study of 49 cases of an uncommon aggressive neoplasm. *Blood*, **89**, 4501–4513.

164 Imamura N, Kusunoki Y, Kawa-Ha K, Yumura K, Hara J, Oda K *et al.* (1990) Aggressive natural killer cell leukaemia/lymphoma: report of four cases and review of the literature. Possible existence of a new clinical entity originating from the third lineage of lymphoid cells. *Br J Haematol*, **75**, 49–59.

165 Kwong YL, Chan AC and Liang RH (1997) Natural killer cell lymphoma/leukemia: pathology and treatment. *Hematol Oncol*, **15**, 71–79.

166 Noguchi M, Kawano Y, Sato N, Oshimi K (1997) T-cell lymphoma of CD3+CD4+CD56+ granular lymphocytes with hemophagocytic syndrome. *Leuk Lymphoma*, **26**, 349–358.

167 Imamura N, Kusunoki Y, Kawa-Ha K, Yumura K, Hara J, Oda K *et al.* (1990) Aggressive natural killer leukaemia/lymphoma: report of four cases and review of the literature; possible evidence of a new clinical entity originating from the third lineage of lymphoid cells. *Br J Haematol*, **75**, 49–59.

168 Tefferi A, Li C-Y, Witzig TE, Dhodapkar IMV, Okuno SH and Phyliky RL (1994) Chronic natural killer cell lymphocytosis: a descriptive clinical study. *Blood*, **84**, 2721–2735.

169 Chou W-C, Chiang I-P, Tang J-L, Su I-J, Huang S-Y, Chen Y-C *et al.* (1998) Clonal disease of natural killer large granular lymphocyte. *Br J Haematol*, **103**, 1124–1128.

170 Bayerl MG, Rakozy CK, Mohamed AN, Vo TD, Long M, Eilender D and Palutke M (2001) Blastic natural killer cell lymphoma/leukemia: a report of seven cases. *Am J Clin Pathol*, **117**, 41–51.

171 Feuillard J, Jacob M-C, Valensi F, Maynadié M, Gressin R, Chaperot L *et al.* (2002) Clinical and biological features of CD4⁺CD56⁺ malignancies. *Blood*, **99**, 1556–1563.

172 Leroux D, Mugneret F, Callanan M, Radford-Weiss I, Dastugue N, Feuillard J *et al.*, on behalf of Groupe Français de Cytogénétique Hématologique (GFCH) (2002) CD4+, CD56+ DC2 acute leukemia is characterized by recurrent clonal chromosomal changes affecting 6 major targets: a study of 21 cases by the Groupe Français de Cytogénétique Hématologique. *Blood*, **99**, 4154–4159.

173 Matutes E, Garcia Talavera J, O'Brien M and Catovsky D (1986) The morphological spectrum of T-prolymphocytic leukaemia. *Br J Haematol*, **64**, 111–124.

174 Matutes E, Brito-Babapulle V, Swansbury J, Ellis J, Morilla R, Dearden C *et al.* (1991) Clinical and laboratory features of 78 cases of T-prolymphocytic leukemia. *Blood*, **78**, 3269–3274.

175 Garand R, Goasguen J, Brizard A, Buisine J, Charpentier A, Claisse JF *et al.* (1998) Indolent course as a relatively frequent presentation of T-prolymphocytic leukaemia. Groupe Francaise d'Hematologie Cellulaire. *Br J Haematol*, **103**, 488–490.

176 Shichishima T, Kawaguchi M, Machii T, Matsuoka R, Ogawa K and Marayama Y (2000) T-prolymphocytic leukaemia with spontaneous remission. *Br J Haematol*, **108**, 397–399.

177 Catovsky D, Ralfkiaer E and Müller-Hermelink HK (2001) T-cell prolymphocytic leukaemia. In Jaffe ES, Harris NL, Stein H and Vardiman JW (Eds), *World Health Organization Classification of Tumours: Pathology and Genetics of Tumours of Haematopoietic and Lymphoid Tissues*, IARC Press, Lyon, pp. 195–196.

178 Brito-Babapulle V, Pomfret M, Matutes E and Catovsky D (1987) Cytogenetic studies on prolymphocytic leukaemia. II. T cell prolymphocytic leukaemia. *Blood*, **70**, 926–931.

179 de Schouwer PJJC, Dyer MJS, Brito-Babapulle VB, Matutes E, Catovsky D and Yuille MR (2000) T-cell prolymphocytic leukaemia: antigen receptor gene rearrangement and a novel mode of *MTCP1* B1 activation. *Br J Haematol*, **110**, 831–838.

180 Hetet G, Dastot H, Baens M, Brizard A, Sigaux F, Grandchamp B and Stern M-H (2000) Recurrent molecular deletion of the 12p13 region, centromeric to *ETV6/TEL* in T-cell prolymphocytic leukemia. *Hematol J*, **1**, 42–47.

181 Stilgenbauer S, Schnaffner C, Litterst A, Liebisch P, Gilad S, Bar-Shira A *et al.* (1997) Biallelic mutations of the *ATM* gene in T-prolymphocytic leukemia. *Nature Med*, **3**, 1155–1159.

182 Uchiyama T, Yodoi J, Sagawa K, Takatsuki K and Uchino H (1977) Adult T-cell leukemia: clinical and hematologic features of 16 cases. *Blood*, **50**, 481–492.

183 Catovsky D, Greaves MF, Rose M, Galton DAG, Goolden AWG, McCluskey DR *et al.* (1982) Adult T-cell lymphoma–leukaemia in Blacks from the West Indies. *Lancet*, **I**, 639–643.

184 Sakamoto Y, Kawachi Y, Uchida T, Abe T, Mori M, Setsu K and Indo N (1994) Adult T-cell leukaemia/lymphoma featuring a large granular lymphocyte leukaemia morphologically. *Br J Haematol*, **86**, 383–385.

185 Kamihira S, Sohda H, Atogami S, Fukushima T, Toriya K, Miyazaki Y *et al.* (1993) Unusual morphological features of adult T-cell leukemia cells with aberrant phenotype. *Leuk Lymphoma*, **12**, 123–130.

186 Matsushita K, Arima N, Yamaguchi K, Matsumoto T, Ohtsubo H, Hidaka S *et al.* (2000) Granulocyte colony-stimulating factor production by adult T-cell leukaemia cells. *Br J Haematol*, **111**, 208–215.

187 Shimoya M and members of the Lymphoma Study Group (1984–1987) (1991) Diagnostic criteria and classification of adult T-cell leukaemia–lymphoma: a report from the Lymphoma Study group (1984–87). *Br J Haematol*, **79**, 428–437.

188 Yamaguchi T, Hirano T, Kumagai K, Tsurumoto T, Shindo H, Majima R and Arima N (1999) Osteitis fibrosa cystica generalizata with adult T-cell leukaemia: a case report. *Br J Haematol*, **107**, 892–894.

189 Fifth International Workshop on Chromosomes in Leukemia–lymphoma (1988) Correlation of chromosome abnormalities with histologic and immunologic characteristics in non-Hodgkin's lymphoma and adult T-cell leukemia lymphoma. *Blood*, **70**, 1554–1564.

190 Shimamoto Y (1997) Clinical indications of multiple integrations of human T-cell lymphotropic virus. *Leuk Lymphoma*, **27**, 43–51.

191 Diamandidou E, Cohen PR and Kurzrock R (1996) Mycosis fungoides and Sézary syndrome. *Blood*, **88**, 2385–2409.

192 Scarisbrick JJ, Whittaker S, Evans AV, Fraser-Andrews EA Child FJ, Dean A and Russell-Jones R (2001) Prognostic significance of tumor burden in the blood of patients with erythrodermic primary cutaneous T-cell lymphoma. *Blood*, **97**, 624–630.

193 Evans AV, Wood BP, Scarisbrick JJ, Fraser-Andrews EA, Chinn S, Dean A *et al.* (2001) Extracorporeal photopheresis in Sézary syndrome: hematologic parameters as predictors of response. *Blood*, **98**, 1298–1301.

194 Bogen SA, Pelley D, Charif M, McCusker M, Koh H, Foss F *et al.* (1996) Immunophenotypic identification of Sézary cells in the peripheral blood. *Am J Clin Pathol*, **106**, 739–748.

195 Edelman J and Meyerson HJ (2000) Diminished CD3 expression is useful for detecting and enumerating Sézary cells. *Am J Clin Pathol*, **114**, 467–477.

196 Jones D, Dang NH, Duvic M, Washington LT and Huh YO (2001) Absence of CD26 expression is a useful marker for diagnosis of T-cell lymphoma in peripheral blood. *Am J Clin Pathol*, **115**, 885–892.

197 Russell-Jones R and Spittle MF (1996) Management of cutaneous lymphoma. *Baillière's Clin Haematol*, **9**, 743–767.

198 Brito-Babapulle V, Maljaie SH, Matutes E, Hedges M, Yuille M and Catovsky D (1997) Relationship of T cell leukaemias with cerebriform nuclei to T-prolymphocytic leukaemia: a cytogenetic analysis with *in situ* hybridization. *Br J Haematol*, **96**, 724–732.

199 Pawson R, Matutes E, Brito-Babapulle V, Maljaie H, Hedges M, Merceica J, Dyer M and Catovsky D (1997) Sézary cell leukaemia: a distinct T cell disorder or a variant form of T prolymphocytic leukaemia? *Leukemia*, **11**, 1009–1013.

200 Vega F, Medeiros LJ, Bueso-Ramos C, Jones D, Lai R, Luthra R and Abruzzo LV (2001) Hepatosplenic gamma/delta T-cell lymphoma in bone marrow: a sinusoidal neoplasm with blastic cytological features. *Am J Clin Pathol*, **116**, 410–419.

201 Khan WA, Yu L, Eisenbrey AB, Crisan D, Al Saadi A, Davis BH *et al.* (2001) Hepatosplenic gamma/delta T-cell lymphoma in immunocompromised patients. *Am J Clin Pathol*, **116**, 41–50.

202 Lesesve J-F, Buisine J, Grégoire J, Raby P, Lederlin P, Béné M-C *et al.* (2000) Leukaemic small cell variant anaplastic large cell lymphoma during pregnancy. *Clin Lab Haematol*, **22**, 297–301.

203 Jamal S, Picker LJ, Aquino DB, McKenna RW, Dawson DB and Kroft SH (2001) Immunophenotypic analysis of peripheral T-cell neoplasms. *Am J Clin Pathol*, **116**, 512–526.

INDEX